EMERGENCY AND INTENSIVE CARE MEDICINE

RECENT ADVANCES IN STROKE THERAPEUTICS

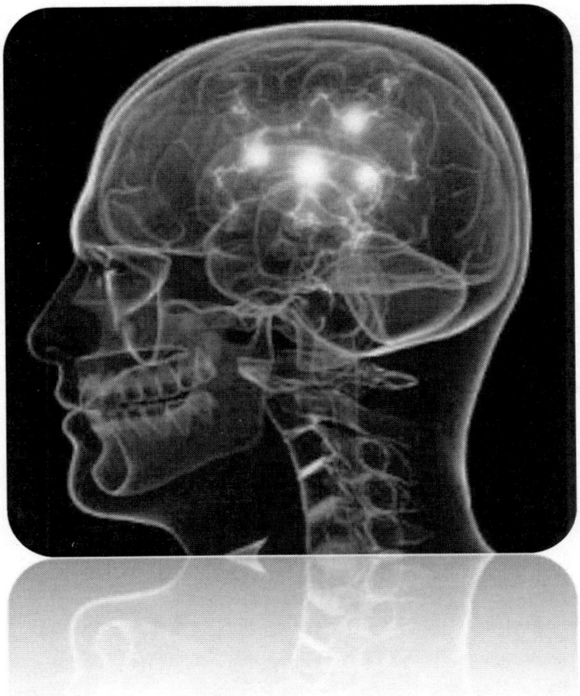

EMERGENCY AND INTENSIVE CARE MEDICINE

Additional books in this series can be found on Nova's website
under the Series tab.

Additional e-books in this series can be found on Nova's website
under the e-book tab.

EMERGENCY AND INTENSIVE CARE MEDICINE

RECENT ADVANCES IN STROKE THERAPEUTICS

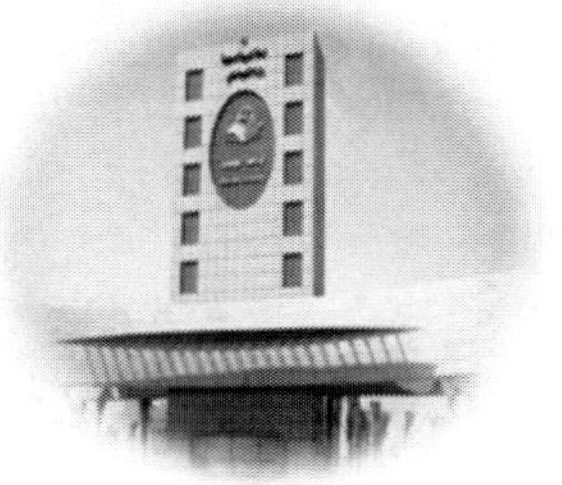

MANZOOR AHMAD MIR
RAID SALEEM ALBARADIE
AND
MALIK ALHUSSAINAWI

EDITED BY MANZOOR AHMAD MIR

Majmaah University
Almajmaa-11952
Kingdom of Saudi Arabia

New York

For permission to use material from this book please contact us:
Telephone 631-231-7269; Fax 631-231-8175
Web Site: http://www.novapublishers.com

Library of Congress Cataloging-in-Publication Data

ISBN: 978-1-63117-754-5

Published by Nova Science Publishers, Inc. † New York

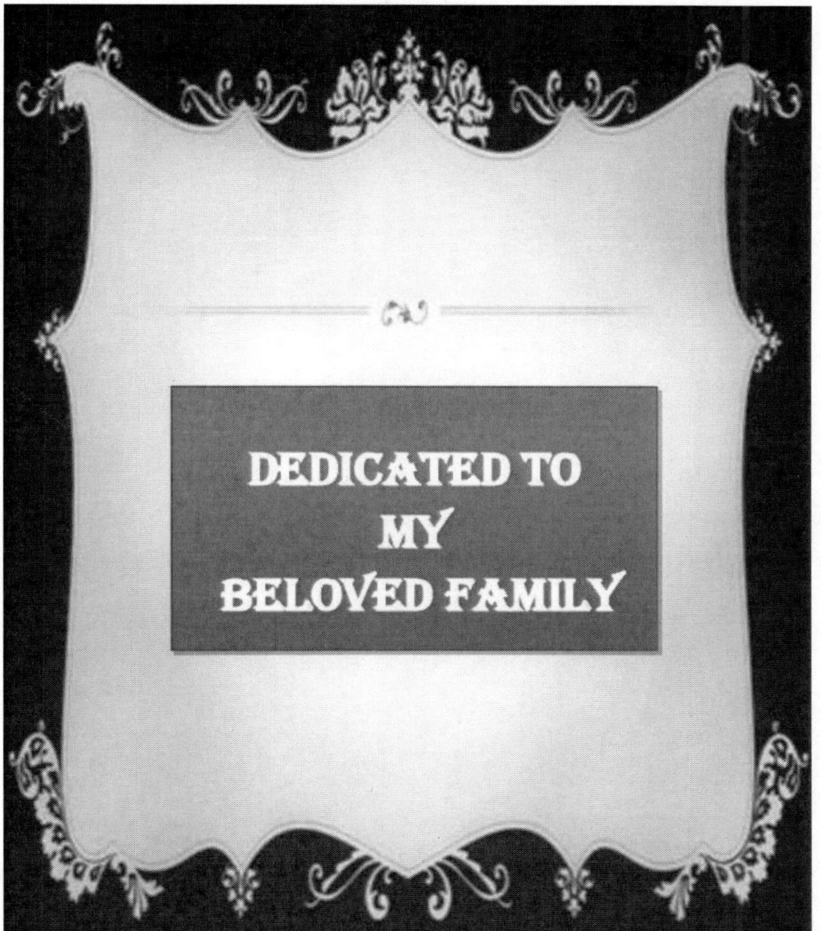

This book is dedicated to my wife, Sumaira Manzoor and son, Aariz Manzoor.

Contents

Preface

Stroke is the leading cause of disability worldwide, the second most common cause of dementia and the third leading cause of death. It has enormous clinical, social, and economic implications and demands a significant effort from both basic scientists and clinicians in the quest for understanding the underlying pathogenic mechanisms, and thereby adopting suitable preventive measures and successful therapies. Once considered exclusively a disorder of blood vessels, growing evidence has led to the realization that the biological processes underlying stroke are driven by the interaction of neurons, glia, vascular cells, and matrix components, which actively participate in mechanisms of tissue injury and repair. Stroke is a serious neurological disease, and constitutes a major cause of death and disability throughout the world. The pathophysiology of stroke is complex, and involves excitotoxicity mechanisms, inflammatory pathways, oxidative damage, ionic imbalances, apoptosis, angiogenesis and neuroprotection. The ultimate result of ischemic cascade initiated by acute stroke is neuronal death along with an irreversible loss of neuronal function. Therapeutic strategies in stroke have been developed with two main aims: restoration of cerebral flow and the minimization of the deleterious effects of ischemia on neurons. Intense research spanning over the last two decades has witnessed significant therapeutic advances in the form of carotid endarterectomy, thrombolytics, anticoagulant therapy, antiplatelet agents, neuroprotective agents, and treating associated risk factors such as hypertension and hyperlipidemia. However, the search for an effective neuroprotectant remains frustrating, and the current therapeutic protocols remain suboptimal. Till date only one FDA-approved drug is available for ischemic stroke; i.e., the serine protease tissue-type plasminogen activator (TPA), the utility of which is limited by the short therapeutic window. As new targets are identified, new opportunities emerge that build on an appreciation of acute cellular events acting in a broader context of ongoing destructive, protective, and reparative processes.

At the onset of the 21st century, it is the third-leading cause of death in most developed countries and the primary cardiovascular cause of death in Japan and China. The health burden of the disease is staggering as loss of a productive life inflicts a heavy toll on patients, families, and society. Yet this disease has no effective therapy beyond a limited group of patients (5%) who are treated with thrombolytics, which have significant adverse effects. This situation prevails despite intense research efforts and numerous clinical trials that have attempted to develop drugs to reduce morbidity and mortality from stroke. So far, drug development efforts have targeted modulators of ion channels ($Ca^{2+}$and Na^{+}), scavengers of oxygen radicals, and antagonists of excitotoxic neurotransmitters (primarily glutamate and glycine receptors).

However, current therapeutic strategies for stroke have been largely unsuccessful. One possible explanation is that research and pharmacological management have focused on very early events in brain ischemia. However, clinical trials with modulators of these targets have failed so far because of lack of efficacy, adverse effects, or other developmental difficulties. Debate on the reasons for this grim reality has sprung up in recent meetings, with finger-pointing about major possible causes of failure, including incorrect animal models, misidentified mechanisms of action, poor clinical designs, inadequate timing of treatment, and other variables. Moreover the brain ischemia and trauma elicit strong inflammatory reactions driven by both external and brain cells. The recognition of inflammation as a fundamental response to brain ischemia provides novel opportunities for new anti-inflammatory therapies. Two important pathophysiological mechanisms involved during ischemic stroke are oxidative stress and inflammation. Brain tissue is not well equipped with antioxidant defenses, so reactive oxygen species and other free radicals/oxidants, released by inflammatory cells, threaten the tissue viability in the vicinity of the ischemic core. Here in this book we will discuss the molecular aspects of oxidative stress and inflammation in ischemic stroke and potential therapeutic strategies that target neuroinflammation and the innate immune system. Further, we will present the latest findings about the cellular and humoral aspects of immune and inflammatory reactions in the brain. This will increase our understanding regarding the roles infections and immune reactions play in the brain milieu and may also have an impact on the treatment of neuroinjuries and ancillary brain diseases.

Acute ischemic stroke is treatable, and our ability to treat patients with ischemic stroke continues to improve. Perhaps the most important has been the widening of the time window for both intravenous thrombolysis as well as endovascular arterial recanalization treatments. This change in the expansion of the time window has major implications because it could dramatically increase the number of potential patients for treatment. Further expansion of the time window is possible with the likelihood that imaging will provide the necessary information for identifying suitable, individual patients. The basic imaging approaches to acute ischemic stroke patients have evolved slightly since the first edition. More importantly, there has been a deepening of our understanding of the significance of the findings observed on standard and advanced diagnostic techniques like CT and MRI. Here we will focus on the ischemic penumbra, and the other on how to use imaging to help guide endovascular therapy. All of this will reflect improved understanding of what imaging can provide the physician caring for the stroke patient to help make the wisest decision with respect to interventions that are being considered. The field continues to evolve, and better outcomes are possible and even likely. Indeed the burgeoning opportunities for treatment are so substantial that a major issue is whether there are enough trained physicians to provide optimal care to patients with acute ischemic stroke, especially those with the most severe strokes.

About the Editor

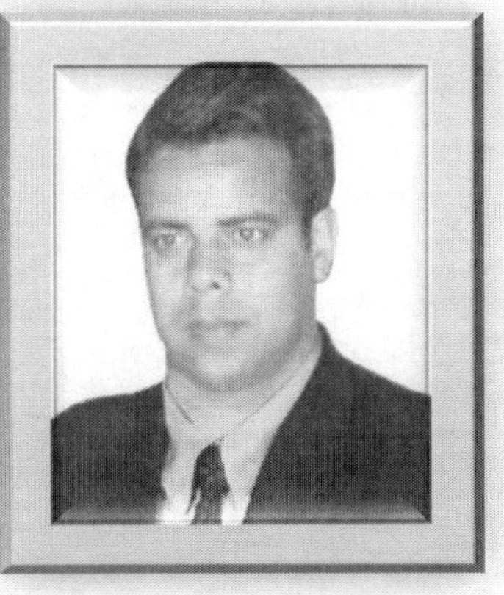

Dr Manzoor Ahmad Mir completed his masters in Life Sciences with the gold medal and then qualified the prestigious Junior Research Fellowship cum National Eligibility Test (JRF-NET) examination. He completed his Ph.D. in Immunology from Jawaharlal Nehru University New Delhi through the National Laboratory Institute of Microbial Technology (IMTECH-CSIR) in Cancer Biology and Immunology Division under the guidance of Bhatnagar Awardee Dr. Javed Naim Agrewala. His Ph. D work includes understanding the role of reverse co-stimulation in the survival of intracellular pathogens and cancer. Dr. Manzoor has many diploma courses to his credit which include Postgraduate diplomas in Higher Education (PGDHE) and Ecology and Environment (PGDEE). He has published several international papers and review articles including papers on of cancer and tuberculosis. He has also published many papers in the proceedings of international conferences and about 35 abstract papers in national and international conferences besides attending many orientation and refresher courses. He is also the author of several books on Polyphenols, Costimulation and Cancer. He is Life member of many National and International societies. He has successfully guided many students at the bachelors and masters level. Dr. Manzoor is working as an Assistant Professor at the Department of Bioresources, University of Kashmir and presently he is working as a Research Scientist with Dr. Raid Saleem Albaradie in *Sheikh Abdullah bin Abdul Mohsen Al-Tuwaijri Chair for Applied Research in Stroke* at the College of Applied Medical Sciences Majmaah University Kingdom of Saudi Arabia.

Authors

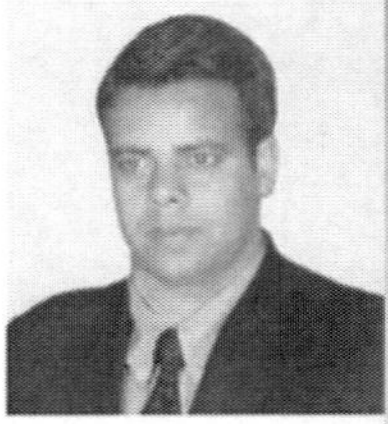

Dr. Manzoor Ahmad Mir (Ph. D)
College of Applied Medical Sciences
Majmaah University
Kingdom of Saudi Arabia and
Department of Bioresources
University of Kashmir
Srinagar India
mirmanzoor110@gmail.com

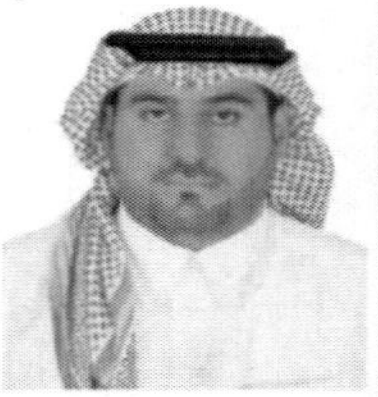

Dr. Raid Saleem Albaradie (Ph. D)
Vice Dean Research
College of Applied Medical Sciences
Majmaah University
Kingdom of Saudi Arabia
raid5555@hotmail.com

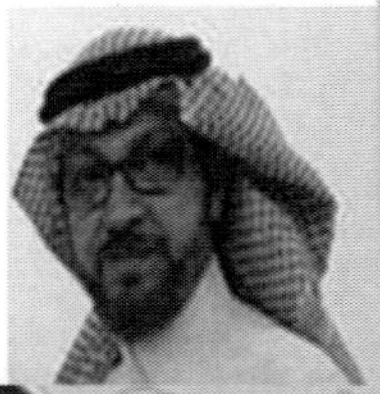

Dr. Malik D Alhussainawi, MD(KSU)
Director King Khalid Hospital
Almajmaah province
Kingdom of Saudi Arabia
drmalik7@hotmail.com

Reviewers

Professor *Mark Slevin* (Ph.D., FAHA, FIBMS, FRCPath)
Head of Genetics/Cell and Molecular Biology
Professor of Cell Pathology, SBCHS,
Manchester Metropolitan University UK
Professor of Pathology, University of Medicine and Pharmacy,
Targu Mures, Romania and Griffith University, Brisbane, Australia
Chairman of the International Research Promotions Council (Europe)

Professor *Jerks Krupinski* (Ph.D., D.Sc)
Head Clinical neuroscience, Department of Neurolgy
Hospital Universitari Mutua Terrassa
Universitat De Barcelna
Barcelona Spain

Acknowledgments

"First and foremost, I would like to thank the Prime Mover Almighty in whom I have great faith."

Although it is difficult to thank everybody and interwove in words the genuine efforts made by the people directly or indirectly to make this book possible. But I would like to take this opportunity to pen down my appreciation for a great number of people whose contribution in numerous ways immensely helped me to move towards my destination.

It gives me immense pleasure to express my sense of gratitude and respect to my mentor Dr. Raid Saleem Abroad, whose constant support, utmost patience, invaluable advice and guidance rekindled my interest in science from time to time. I will benefit for a long time to come from his sincerity, originality and truthfulness, which has nourished me intellectual maturity.

A special vote of thanks goes to Prof Mohammad Afzal Zugar and I am thankful to him for his efficient guidance to work hard with sincerity, dedication and devotion both in professional and personal life. The staff at the GDC Handwara and GDC Kupwara especially Prof Farooq Ahmad Malik , Dr. Iqbal, Dr Irshad, Mr. Mehraj, Dr. Fayaz deserves a special mention for all the help rendered at the hour of need.

The congenial company of Tajamal, Reiaz, Altaf and Riffat in the department deserves a special mention. I am short of words to justify their care, affection and untiring support showered by these very good friends. I owe my grateful attitude to Bilal Poshpori, Rahid Ashraf, Ali Sopori, Hilal Khaliq, Dr. Abid, Dr. Zahoor and Dr. Farooq Fayaz.

I owe deepest gratitude to my parents and other family members, especially my wife Sumaira and Son Aariz, Uncle Mohd Shafi Mir, my brothers Ashraf, Irshad and Tahir, my sisters Hafiza, Shafiqa and Rafiqa for continuous and unconditional support of all my undertakings, scholastic and otherwise. A seed of loyalty, hard work, dedication and sincerity sown in me by my parents played a crucial role in completion of this work. They have been a source of great strength throughout my life. Without their affection, support, best wishes, love and care this work would not have been completed.

I would also like to thank everybody who was important to the successful realization of this book, as well as expressing my apology that I could not mention personally one by one.

Finally and most importantly, I would like to thank the Almighty Allah for giving me strength, belief and good health. It is under his grace that we all live, learn and flourish.

Special Thanks

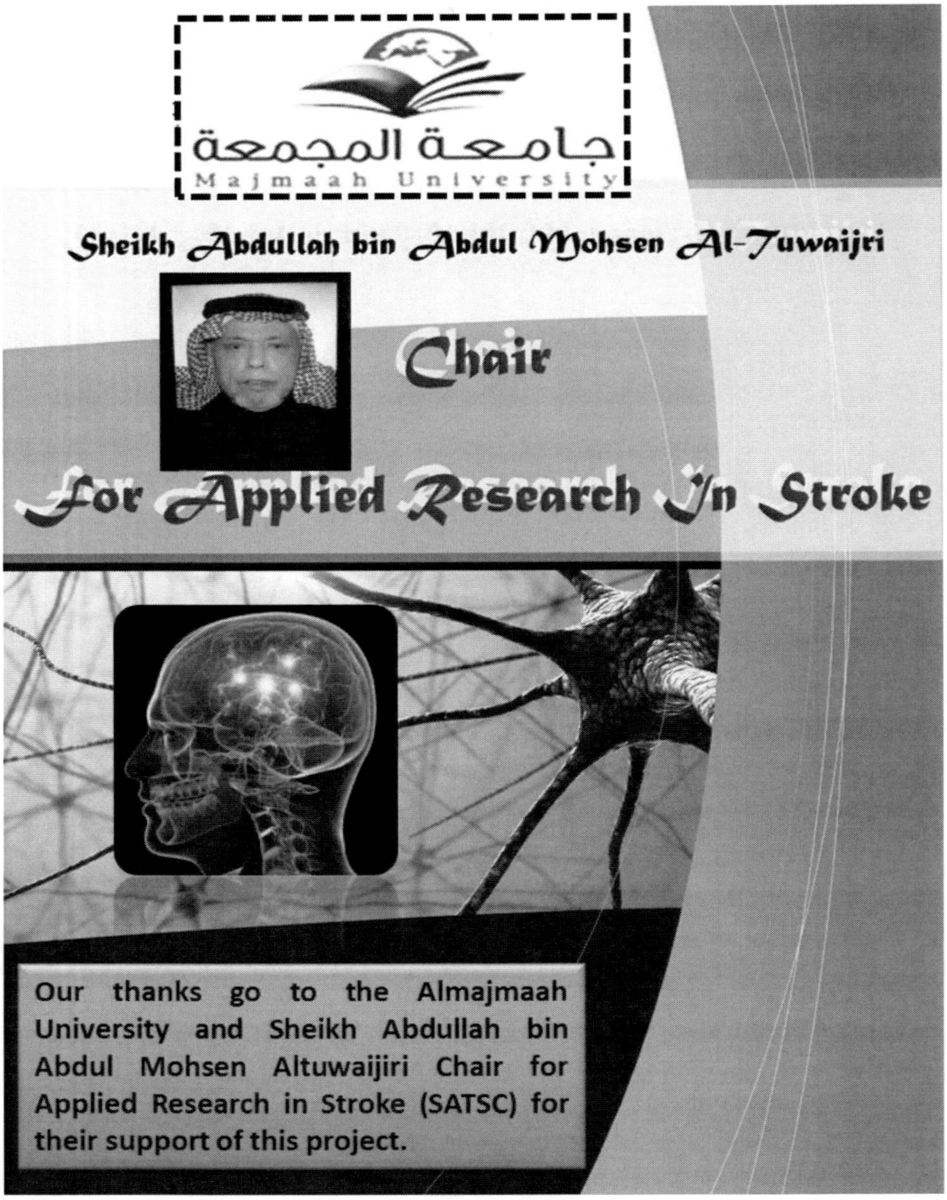

Introduction

The immune system is one of the nature's most fascinating inventions which protect us with ease against billions of bacteria, viruses and other pathogens. The immune system has evolved under a terrific selective pressure imposed by these pathogens as a result, our body has developed the ability to recognize the invading microbes and to eliminate them efficiently without causing damage to self. Our immune system is a fascinating network of cells and cell "depots." The principal task of which is to resist infection. This network protects the body from invaders, travels long distances, communicates information regarding the invaders and coordinates Special Commando Forces (effector cells) to return to the front line. It also keeps detailed records (immunological memory) about all previous intruders for many years, allowing a very rapid response in case the same "enemy" invades the body a second time.

Stroke is the second most common cause of death worldwide and a major cause of acquired disability in adults. Worldwide, around 15 million people have a stroke every year, and with about 5 million deaths, stroke is the second most common cause of death and a major cause of long-term disability. It is estimated that about 25% of people older than 85 years will develop a stroke However, current therapeutic strategies for stroke have been largely unsuccessful. One possible explanation is that research and pharmacological management have focused on very early events in brain ischemia. New research has shown that brain ischemia and trauma elicit strong inflammatory reactions driven by both external and brain cells. The recognition of inflammation as a fundamental response to brain ischemia provides novel opportunities for new anti-inflammatory therapies. Researchers are now presenting the latest findings about the cellular and humoral aspects of immune and inflammatory reactions and here in this book we will present a detailed and latest update on the current trends on the same. This will increase our understanding the roles infections and immune reactions play in the brain milieu which may have an impact on the treatment of neuroinjuries and ancillary brain diseases. Cerebral ischemia results in a number of hemodynamic, biochemical, and neurophysiology alterations. A series of complex acute, subacute and chronic events occur after the incidence of stroke and reperfusion. Ischemic injury involves energy failure, loss of cell ion homeostasis, acidosis, increased intracellular calcium excitotoxicity, free radical-mediated toxicity, and pathological permeability of the blood-brain barrier (BBB). Free radicals, specifically reactive oxygen species (ROS) that are generated soon after ischemia, as well as in later stages of ischemic reperfusion (e.g., by inflammatory cells), are the fundamental mediators of reperfusion injury.

Two important pathophysiological mechanisms involved during ischemic stroke are oxidative stress and inflammation. Brain tissue is not well equipped with antioxidant defenses, so reactive oxygen species and other free radicals/oxidants, released by inflammatory cells, threaten the tissue viability in the vicinity of the ischemic core. This book will discuss the molecular aspects of oxidative stress and inflammation in ischemic stroke and potential therapeutic strategies that target neuroinflammation and the innate immune system. Although for many years the CNS was considered an immune-privileged organ, it is now well accepted that the immune and the nervous system are engaged in bidirectional crosstalk. Moreover, mounting data suggest that in the brain, as in peripheral organs, inflammatory cells participate in tissue remodeling after injury. Microglial cells are the resident macrophages of the brain and play a critical role as resident immunocompetent and phagocytic cells in the CNS. Currently, little is known about endogenous counterregulatory immune mechanisms. However, recent studies showing that regulatory T cells are major cerebroprotective immunomodulators after stroke suggest that targeting the endogenous adaptive immune response may offer novel promising neuroprotectant therapies.

Even at the onset of 21st century, stroke has no effective therapy beyond a limited group of patients who are treated with thrombolytics, which have significant adverse effects. This situation prevails despite intense research efforts and numerous clinical trials that have attempted to develop drugs to reduce morbidity and mortality from stroke. So far, drug development efforts have targeted modulators of ion channels ($Ca^{2+}$and Na^{+}), scavengers of oxygen radicals, and antagonists of excitotoxic neurotransmitters (primarily glutamate and glycine receptors).

However, clinical trials with modulators of these targets have failed so far because of lack of efficacy, adverse effects, or other developmental difficulties. Debate on the reasons for this grim reality has sprung up in recent meetings, with finger-pointing about major possible causes of failure, including incorrect animal models, misidentified mechanisms of action, poor clinical designs, inadequate timing of treatment, and other variables. Acute ischemic stroke is treatable, and our ability to treat patients with ischemic stroke continues to improve. With the recent publications on stroke diagnostics and treatment, important changes in stroke patient management will surely occur, and most of the latest publications will be are reflected in this book. The most important advances have been the widening of the time window for both intravenous thrombolysis as well as endovascular arterial recanalization treatments. This change in the expansion of the time window has major implications because it could dramatically increase the number of potential patients for treatment. Further expansion of the time window is possible with the likelihood that imaging will provide the necessary information for identifying suitable, individual patients. The basic imaging approaches to acute ischemic stroke patients have evolved slightly in the last few years.

Despite tremendous progress in understanding the pathophysiology of stroke, translation of this knowledge into effective therapies has largely failed, with the exception of thrombolysis, which only benefits a small proportion of patients. Systemic and local immune responses have important roles in causing stroke and are implicated in the primary and secondary progression of ischemic lesions, as well as in repair, recovery, and overall outcome after a stroke. However, potential therapeutic targets in the immune system and info- amatory responses have not been well characterized. Development of novel and effective therapeutic strategies for stroke will require further investigation of these pathways in terms of their temporal profile (before, during, and after the stroke) and risk-to-benefit therapeutic ratio of modulating them.

In the past 10 years, remarkable progress in understanding stroke pathophysiology has been made, especially in ischemic stroke, which makes up 80% of all cases. These advances have led to the identification of more than 1000 molecules with brain-protective effects from experimental models and to the implementation of more than 250 clinical trials. Despite all these efforts, translation into effective therapies has failed. Reperfusion induced by alteplase (tissue plasminogen activator; TPA) is the only acute pharmacological treatment approved by the health authorities. Systemic inflammation is strongly linked to the occurrence of stroke, and inflammation might have deleterious effects during and after an event, triggering various cascades of damage. However, some recent data show that inflammatory processes might also have beneficial effects. Such inflammatory responses involve not only peripheral cells such as leukocytes, but also brain cells such as glial cells, endothelial cells, and neurons. In this Book we will also focus, assess the effects of innate and adaptive immune responses in the CNS and overall outcomes in patients with stroke, and discuss their contribution to stroke onset, ischemic brain damage, and recovery. We postulate that a better understanding of the interactions between the immune system and the CNS will foster the development of innovative therapeutic strategies for patients with stroke.

The field of Stroke research continues to evolve, and better outcomes are possible and even likely. Over the last two decades, basic science research in the field of stroke has elucidated multiple pathways of cellular injury and repair after cerebral ischemia, resulting in the identification of several promising targets for neuroprotection. A large number of neuroprotective agents have been shown to reduce stoke-related damage in animal models. To date, however, no single agent has achieved success in clinical trials. Nevertheless, analysis of the reasons behind the failure of recent drug trials, combined with the success of clot-lysing drugs in improving clinical outcome, has revealed new potential therapeutic opportunities and raised expectations that successful stroke treatment will be achieved in the near future. In this book, we will highlight the major mechanisms of neuronal injury, emphasizing those that are promising targets for stroke therapy. We will also discuss the influence of these pathways on white matter injury, and briefly touch the emerging concept of the neurovascular unit. Finally, we will discuss the emerging strategies for the treatment of acute ischemic stroke.

In: Recent Advances in Stroke Therapeutics
Editor: Manzoor Ahmad Mir
ISBN: 978-1-63117-754-5

Chapter I

The Immune System and Strokes

Abstract

The immune system is an incredible defense mechanism which protects us against a myriad of potential pathogens like viruses, bacteria, protozoa, etc. It often shows rapid, very protective and highly specific responses. When the immune system is activated, a series of complex and inter-dependent cellular responses occur. An incredible feature of the immune system is to discriminate self from non-self. This skill of the immune system is extremely essential to destroy invading pathogens and altered cancer cells. Our first line of defense against foreign organisms are barrier tissues such as the skin that stops the entry of organisms into our body. If, however, these barriers are penetrated, the body contains cells that respond rapidly to the invaders. The cells of the immune system interact with one another by a variety of signal molecules so that a coordinated response may be mounted. These signals may be secretory molecules such as lymphokines, cytokines and chemokine's or receptors and their ligands on the cell surface which stimulate cells of the immune system. Although these two arms (innate and adaptive) of the immune system have distinct functions, there is interplay between them to influence each other. Although for many years the CNS was considered an immune-privileged organ, it is now well accepted that the immune system and the nervous system are engaged in bidirectional crosstalk. Moreover, mounting data suggests that in the brain, as in peripheral organs, inflammatory cells participate in tissue remodeling after injury. Microglial cells are the resident macrophages of the brain and play a critical role as resident immunocompetent and phagocytic cells in the CNS. Stroke is the second most common cause of death worldwide and a major cause of acquired disability in adults. Despite tremendous progress in understanding the pathophysiology of stroke, the translation of this knowledge into effective therapies has largely failed, with the exception of thrombolysis, which only benefits a small proportion of patients. Systemic and local immune responses have important roles in causing a stroke. However, potential therapeutic targets in the immune system and inflammatory responses have not been well characterized. Development of novel and effective therapeutic strategies for a stroke will require further investigation of these pathways in terms of their temporal profile (before, during, and after the stroke) and risk-to-benefit therapeutic ratio of modulating them.

Introduction

Systemic and local immune responses have important roles in causing stroke and are implicated in the primary and secondary progression of ischemic lesions, as well as in repair, recovery, and overall outcome after a stroke. In this chapter, we will discuss the effects of innate and adaptive immune responses in the CNS and overall outcomes in patients with stroke, and discuss their contribution to stroke onset, ischemic brain damage, and recovery. We know that all cells of the immune system have their origin in the bone marrow and they include myeloid and lymphoid which differentiate along distinct pathways. The myeloid progenitor cell in the bone marrow gives rise to erythrocytes, platelets, neutrophils, monocytes/macrophages and dendritic cells (DCs), whereas the lymphoid progenitor cell gives rise to the natural killer (NK) cells, T cells and B cells. For T cell development, the precursor T cell must migrate to the thymus where they undergo differentiation into two distinct types, the CD4+ helper T cell and the CD8+ cytotoxic T cell. CD4+ helper T cells can be further subdivided on the basis of the cytokine profile into Th1 and Th2 cells. Th1 cells secrete mainly IL-2, IFN-γ, lymphotoxin, etc. and are responsible for cell mediated immunity. In contrast Th2 cells produce chiefly IL-4, IL-5 and IL-10 and are responsible for humoral immunity (Mossman et al. 1989). B cells originate from bone marrow in mouse, human and other mammals and from bursa of Fabricius in birds. B cells produce diverse repertoires of antibodies, synonymously called immunoglobulins (Igs).

Cells of the Immune System

The immune system consists of a wide range of distinct cells, each with a specific role to play. The myeloid lineage of cells includes macrophages, dendritic cells, monocytes, mast cells and basophils. The lymphoid lineage includes NK, B cells and T cells. Some of these cells like B cells, macrophages and dendritic cells help in antigen presentation to T cells. The cells of the immune system are found in peripheral organized tissues like spleen, lymph nodes, Payer's patches of the intestine and tonsils etc.

The immune responses occur in these sites. The cells of lymphoid origin are also found in central lymphoid organs like the thymus and bone marrow where they undergo maturation. Lymphocytes and macrophages constitute a substantial portion of recirculating pool of cells found in the blood and lymph and provide immunity at the sites where it is needed. Some specialized cells like epithelial and stromal cells provide the anatomic environment in which immunity occurs by secreting many chemical factors that regulate growth and gene activation in cells of the immune system. They also play a direct role in the induction and effector phase of the immune response.

The response to pathogens is orchestrated by the complex interactions and activities of the large number of diverse cell types involved in the immune response. The innate immune response is the first line of defense and occurs soon after pathogen exposure. It is carried out by phagocytic cells such as neutrophils and macrophages, NK cells, and granulocytes (Medzhitov et al. 2001, 1997). The subsequent adaptive immune response includes antigen-specific defense mechanisms and may take days to develop. Cell types with critical roles in adaptive immunity are T cells and B cells.

Antigen-presenting cells (APCs) are critical players in the immune response. The function of these cells is to engulf pathogens or dying cells, process them and finally present their antigenic epitopes in context with MHC molecules to T cells. However, DCs are the only cells involved in antigen presentation to the naïve T cells. For optimum activation of naïve T cells, two signals are required. The first signal is antigen specific and is delivered through binding of the T-cell receptor (TCR) to peptide/MHC complexes on the APC surface. The second signal is non-specific and is also APC driven in the form of costimulatory molecules (Lenschow et al. 1996). Among APCs only DCs constitutively express these costimulatory molecules. Several other cells, classified as non-professional APC, can be induced to express MHC-II molecules or costimulatory signals to work as an APC. Many of these cells like fibroblasts, astrocytes, epithelial cells, etc., function as an APC only for a short period during a sustained inflammatory response (Sung et al. 1997, Pechhold et al. 1997). Moreover, the main professional APCs are dendritic cells, macrophages and B cells.

Strokes are the second most common cause of death worldwide and a major cause of acquired disability in adults. Despite tremendous progress in understanding the pathophysiology of a stroke, translation of this knowledge into effective therapies has largely failed, with the exception of thrombolysis, which only benefits a small proportion of patients. Systemic and local immune responses have important roles in causing strokes and are implicated in the primary and secondary progression of ischemic lesions, as well as in repair, recovery, and overall outcome after a stroke. However, potential therapeutic targets in the immune system and inflammatory responses have not been well characterized. Development of novel and effective therapeutic strategies for strokes will require further investigation of these pathways in terms of their temporal profile (before, during, and after the stroke) and risk-to-benefit therapeutic ratio of modulating them.

Worldwide, around 15 million people have a stroke every year, and with about 5 million deaths, strokes are the second most common cause of death and a major cause of long-term disability (AHA 2010). It is estimated that about 25% of people older than 85 years will develop a stroke. In the past 10 years, remarkable progress in understanding stroke pathophysiology has been made, especially in ischemic stroke, which makes up 80% of all cases. These advances have led to the identification of more than 1000 molecules with brain-protective effects from experimental models and to the implementation of more than 250 clinical trials. Despite all these efforts, translation into effective therapies has failed. Reperfusion induced by alteplase (tissue plasminogen activator; TPA) is the only acute pharmacological treatment approved by the health authorities (Young AR 2007, NIHD 1995). Systemic inflammation is strongly linked to the occurrence of a stroke, and inflammation might have deleterious effects during and after an event, triggering various cascades of damage. However, some recent data show that inflammatory processes might also have beneficial effects (figure 1.1). Such inflammatory responses involve not only peripheral cells such as leukocytes, but also brain cells such as glial cells, endothelial cells, and neurons. In this chapter, we will focus on the effects of innate and adaptive immune responses in the CNS and overall outcomes in stroke patients, and discuss their contribution to stroke onset, ischemic brain damage, and recovery. We also discuss potential immune-based stroke therapies. We postulate that a better understanding of the interactions between the immune system and the CNS will foster the development of innovative therapeutic strategies for patients with stroke.

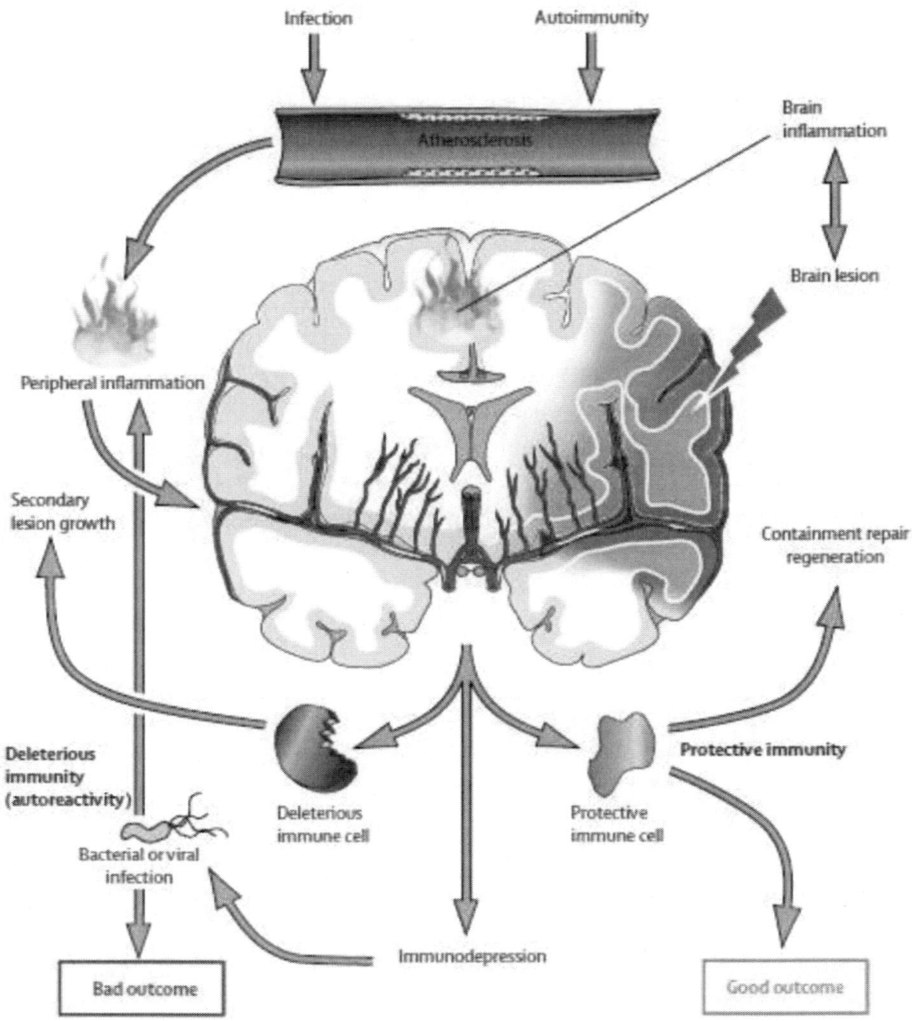

Figure 1.1. Complex interactions between peripheral inflammation (which might underlie the occurrence or atherosclerosis of a stroke), stroke-induced brain inflammation, and responses of the peripheral innate and adaptive immune systems to a stroke (inflammation, immunodepression, autoreactivity, or protective immunity).

Role of Inflammation and the Immune System in Stroke

Nearly all types of infectious agents have been suggested to increase incidence of a stroke. However, the risk of a stroke might be associated with an aggregate burden rather than with an individual pathogen. Moreover, a range of host factors, including genetic ones, probably interact with infectious or inflammatory conditions to influence the risk of vascular disease. Inflammatory processes affect stroke incidence through several mechanisms, including thrombosis through the coagulation system, vasculopathy through vasculitis or altered vascular reactivity, and, most often, by atherosclerosis (figure 1.2). The prothrombotic state reported during inflammation results from the activation of many cellular targets (e. g, monocytes, macrophages, platelets, endothelial cells, and T lymphocytes), leading to an imbalance between anticoagulant and procoagulant molecules, an increased production of chemokine's such as monocyte chemotactic protein-1), cytokines (interleukin 1β, 4, 6, and 10, tumor necrosis factor (TNF), interferon's and an altered production of adhesion molecules (P-selectin, E-selectin, L-selectin, vascular cell adhesion molecule 1 (VCAM1), intercellular adhesion molecule 1 (ICAM1), and integrin's such as CD11a-c). Circulating cells are thus recruited to the endothelial wall and promote local inflammatory events. Besides vasculitis, inflammation can also induce various processes in the cerebral microvasculature, such as blood–brain barrier leakage (partly mediated by matrix metalloproteinase (MMPs)), sequestration or adhesion of red blood cells on endothelial cells (leading to apoptosis of the latter), and platelet activation or aggregation. Among the recruited leukocytes, neutrophils, natural killer cells, dendritic cells, and macrophages produce mediators that further activate or even damage endothelial cells through activation of nitric oxide synthase (iNOS) and cyclooxygenase-2 (COX-2) pathways. Together, these events favor a T-helper-type-1 (Th1) environment for infiltrating T lymphocytes and induce their activation. Conversely, some experimental studies suggest that preinfections might have a protective role by increasing neurogenesis, promoting anti-inflammatory responses, inhibiting macrophage and T-cell accumulation within atherosclerotic lesions, and producing neuroprotective molecules and free radical scavengers, leading to a form of preconditioning. However, the consensus at present is that the cumulative effect of previous inflammation on stroke incidence is negative and suggests that inflammation is an important therapeutic target for stroke prevention. Thromboembolism is the most common mechanism of cerebrovascular occlusion, but a stroke can also manifest as a complication of systemic inflammatory disorders or autoimmune processes such as inflammatory bowel disease, primary or secondary vasculitis, rheumatoid arthritis, or antiphospholipid syndrome (Deb P 2010). Compelling evidence links inflammation (acute or chronic) and risk of a stroke to systemic infection; for example, about 30% of patients with ischemic stroke present with a recent antecedent infection and stroke incidence increases with epidemics such as influenza pandemics.

Immune System-Brain Interactions in the Acute Phase of a Stroke

An ischemic stroke results in an abrupt deprivation of nutrient supplies that quickly leads to irreversible damage in the core of the affected area. Secondary processes, such as the partly excitotoxicity, oxidative stress, and mitochondrial disturbances, spread cellular damage into preserving peri-infarct area (penumbra). Ischemic reperfusion injury also induces a robust inflammatory response that might be necessary for tissue repair and regeneration in advanced stages. Minutes to hours after onset of cerebral ischemia, a cascade of inflammatory events is initiated through the activation of resident cells (including microglia) and recruitment of circulating leukocytes. Primary signals that trigger upregulation of inflammatory mediators are endogenous molecules (damage-associated molecular patterns (DAMPs)) released from dying cells, such as high-mobility group box 1 (HMGB1), hyaluronan, or heat shock proteins (Chen GY 2010). Many DAMPs are sensed by Toll-like receptors (TLRs), a receptor family with broad cellular expression originally described as microbial sensors of the innate immune system.

Studies of TLR-2-deficient or TLR-4-deficient mice reported that these TLRs have a harmful effect through increasing stroke-induced lesions and inflammation. Recently, a study (Lahnardt S 2010) showed that TLR-2 and TLR-1 require the recruitment of CD36 as a co-receptor to promote the inflammatory responses and tissue damage evoked by cerebral ischemia in rodents. TLR-2 may also be a therapeutic target to prevent atherosclerosis, since these receptors mediated inflammation in an in-vitro model of human atherosclerosis (Monaco C 2009). However, agonists of TLR can induce protective preconditioning (Marsh BJ 2010, Leung PY 2010). Among the most studied DAMPs is HMGB1—a ligand of TLR-2, TLR-4, and advanced glycation end product (RAGE) —which is released by damaged cells and exerts a deleterious proinflammatory effect in ischemic rodents. However, HMGB1 could have a bphasic action, with an acute inflammatory noxious effect on the early stage, followed by a promotion of repair processes later on, including neurogenesis and angiogenesis; this delayed beneficial response is associated with HMGB1-positive reactive astrocytes (Hayakawa K 2010a and 2010b). Strategies that interfere with DAMP-receptor pathways might be a promising approach to restrict inflammation processes. Downstream of DAMP-receptor signaling, inflammatory mediators such as cytokines (interleukin-1β, TNF, and interleukin-6), chemokines, nitric oxide, and reactive oxygen species are released, exacerbating cell death and eventually leading to dysfunction of the blood–brain barrier. Cytokines and chemokines induce upregulation of adhesion molecules, including P-selectin, E-selectin, and ICAM1 on the vascular endothelium, attracting and homing circulating leukocytes into the cerebral parenchyma.

Immune system preserves tissue homeostasis of the host when threatened by a pathogen or sterile injury (e.g., ischemia) via two mechanisms: innate (non-specific) immunity and adaptive immunity. An immune response that begins immediately after injury or infection and relies on various cell types including polynuclear cells, macrophages, and dendritic cells, as well as resident cells from tissue lesions such as endothelial cells or microglia. These cells recognize danger signals (damage-associated molecular patterns (DAMPs)) released upon tissue injury. Engagement of broad-specificity receptors such as Toll-like receptors by DAMPs triggers an inflammatory response marked by the release of proinflammatory cytokines and chemokines and recruitment of innate immune cells. An antigen-specific immune response depends on lymphocytes that have antigen-specific receptors. Unlike innate immunity, cells of adaptive immunity develop memory against the stimulating antigen. Full activation of immune cells needs two signals the main TCR signal and the other costimulatory signal. Responses are regulated by several subsets of CD4 T-helper (Th) cells characterized by their cytokine secretion. Th1 cells produce interferon-γ, which is involved in macrophage activation and leads to cell-mediated immunity, whereas Th2 cells release interleukin-4, which stimulates the production of antibodies by B cells. Interleukin-17-producing T cells (Th17 cells) are a newly described subset implicated in the inflammatory response. The simplistic view of Th1−Th2 dichotomy is far from the true complexity in human diseases because Th polarization is relatively easy to define in murine models, whereas clear distinctions between the patterns are more difficult to establish in human beings. Innate T cells with a T-cell receptor that is distinct from that of conventional αβ T cells. γδ T cells do not recognize antigens displayed on MHC molecules, but rather recognize specific ligands expressed on stressed or infected cells but not healthy cells.

A physiological process that aims to limit tissue damage or infection, removes dead cells and debris, and promotes tissue remodeling and regeneration (irrespective of the initiating stimulus). However, inflammation might have adverse effects through collateral cellular damage, in particular in the brain parenchyma after a stroke. Some cells in the nervous system express MHC molecules and can thus act as antigen-presenting cells to regulate T cells. Notably, neurons that do not express MHC molecules can control the function of T cells.

Natural Regulatory T Cells

These cells express CD4, CD25, and the transcription factor forkhead box P3 (Foxp3) and are involved in the maintenance of peripheral tolerance. These cells act by cell-to-cell contact and by the release of immunosuppressive cytokines such as interleukin-10 or transforming growth factor-β. Other subsets of regulatory cells have also been described (e.g., CD8 T cells, B cells, or myeloid-derived suppressive cells). A peripheral tolerance mechanism induced by exposure to antigens at mucosal surfaces. The kinetics of recruitment of the different inflammatory cells are under debate, but it is accepted that neutrophils lead the migration into the brain parenchyma, followed by macrophages and lymphocytes a few days after injuring (Jin R 2010). Additionally, dendritic cells might accumulate, but the role of these key inflammatory cells in ischemic remains to be established (Gelderblom M 2009). The lymphocytes have a crucial function in inflammatory processes and are strongly associated with deleterious effects in strokes, as noted in T-cell and B-cell deficient mice, which have a strikingly reduced infarct size after transient focal ischemia (Hurn PD 2007). Administration of the immunosuppressive drug fingolimod, which, among other effects, inhibits T-cell infiltration into inflammatory tissues, also reduced infarct volumes in a mouse model of ischemia (Schichita T 2009). Progress has been made in understanding the role of different T-cell subsets in ischemic inflammation (Lo EH 2009). Shichita and colleagues (Schichita T 2009) reported that a late infiltration of γδ T cells was associated with the neurological injury. Their experiments with interleukin-17 or interleukin-23 knockout mice show that interleukin-17 produced by these γδ T cells was involved in the pathogenic mechanism and its expression was dependent on interleukin-23, which is a cytokine mainly secreted by blood-derived macrophages when they infiltrate the brain. In mice, depletion of CD4/CD25/FOXP3-positive regulatory T cells with a specific anti-CD25 monoclonal antibody increases the size of the ischemic lesion and upregulates proinflammatory cytokines such as TNF, interleukin-1β, and interferon. The neuroprotective effects of regulatory T cells were mediated by interleukin-10. Conversely, Ren and colleagues (Ren X 2010) could not confirm that regulatory T cells were involved in restricting the area of brain ischemic injury. Hence, the role of regulatory T cells in a stroke needs to be clarified. Besides infiltrating leukocytes, neurons, astrocytes, and microglia also participate in ischemic brain injury, through the release of proinflammatory mediators (McCoy 2008, Didier N 2003, Hayakawa K 2008). Under inflammatory conditions, however, activated microglia can convert to a macrophagic phenotype and thus also exert a neuroprotective info once by phagocytosis of necrotic cells and secretion of neurotrophic factors such as brain-derived neutrophic factor or insulin-like growth factor (Thored P 2009, Dennes A 2007)

Many studies suggest that inflammation has a deleterious effect (Fessbender K 1994, Hugs PM 2002) that amplifies ischemic injury and hence is a potential target for neuroprotective treatments to prevent cell death in the penumbra. However, some evidence suggests that inflammation is also involved in recovery and repair after ischemic brain damage, (Theod P 2009, Dennes A 2007) although this notion is controversial and needs further study.

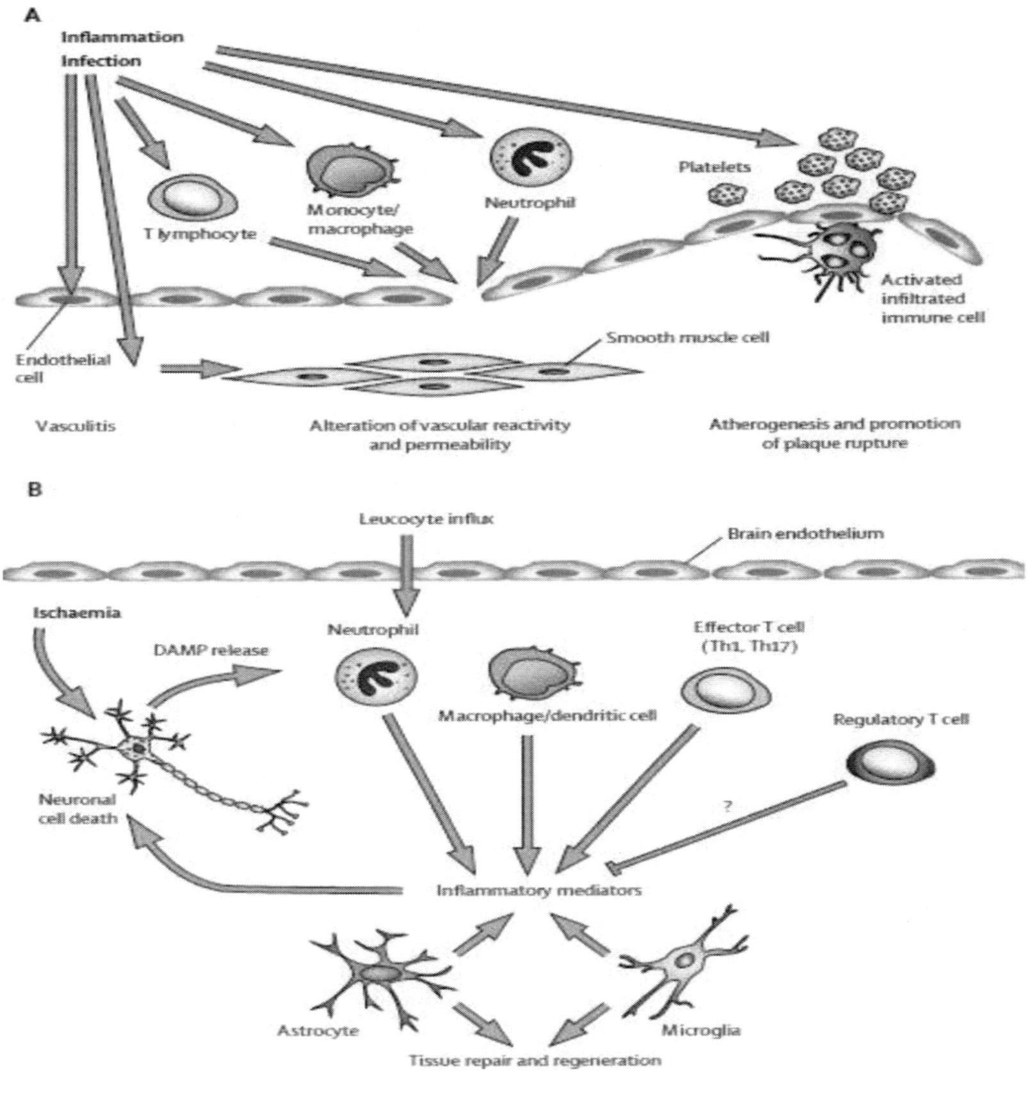

Figure 1.2. Inflammatory mechanisms before and after a stroke. (A) Inflammatory mechanisms that promote strokes: infection and inflammatory disorders can contribute to trigger cerebral ischaemia through pathophysiological processes such as vasculitis, changes of vascular reactivity, and especially atherosclerosis. (B) The acute phase of inflammation after a stroke: ischemia causes cell death in the brain parenchyma and subsequent release of endogenous molecules termed damage-associated molecular patterns (DAMPs) from dying cells. DAMPs trigger a cascade of inflammatory events that contribute to the activation of resident cells (microglia and astrocytes) and recruitment of circulating leukocytes (neutrophils, macrophages, dendritic cells, and T lymphocytes). Production of inflammatory mediators exacerbates neuronal injury. Conversely, activated resident cells might produce trophic factors that promote tissue repair and recovery. A potential role of regulatory T cells in restricting brain ischemic injury has been proposed (Liesz A et al. 2009).

Overall, a better understanding of the specific roles of inflammatory cells is needed, in particular about the kinetics of their recruitment and their relative contributions to each step of a stroke. Notably, the emerging and the intriguing role of different T-cell subsets needs to be established. Such information would help to define the therapeutic window in which the potential beneficial effects of inflammation in brain recovery in advanced stages of ischemia could be preserved (figure 1.2).

CNS and the immune system after a stroke

Nervous and immune systems engage in a bidirectional communication that aims to maintain homeostasis in the whole organism. A stroke (as any acute lesion of the CNS) can disturb this generally well balanced interaction. Briefly, ischemic brain tissue releases factors such as cytokines and neurotransmitters that can reach chemosensitive brain areas involved in immune control such as the hypothalamus, (Meisel C 2005, Chomorro A and Dirnagl U 2007, Becker KJ and Emsley HC 2010) where they can in turn activate, for instance, the sympathetic nervous system. Damage to cortical regions involved in immune regulation, such as the insula, can lead to loss of tonic inhibition and thus activation of hypothalamic areas. Furthermore, inflammatory mediators can be released from the damaged brain tissue and enter the systemic circulation where they act on cells of the immune system in the blood and secondary lymphatic organs or, through the bloodstream, activate the brain via consensus. Besides immunomodulatory signalling specific to a brain lesion, (Catania A 2009) strokes are a strong unspecific stressor (e.g., sudden loss of relevant bodily functions, fear, or sense of emergency) which activate immunomodulatory systems such as the hypothalamic–pituitary axis and the sympathetic nervous system (Elenkov IJ 2006) Within a few hours after the onset of cerebral ischemia, brain–immune system interactions can result in a downregulation of systemic immunity termed stroke-induced immunodepression (SIDS). Almost all immune cells have numerous noradrenaline receptors, which can be activated by circulating epinephrine produced by the adrenal medulla or via the dense innervation by postganglionic sympathetic fibers of lymphoid organs. Noradrenaline stimulates interleukin-10 production by blood monocytes. Overall, noradrenaline decreases the number and the activity of immune cells through its pleiotropic effects. Glucocorticoids, which are produced as a result of stress induced stimulation of the hypothalamic–pituitary-axis, are also well known immunosuppressants. After a stroke, patients often have impairments in swallowing and are therefore at high risk of aspiration. They are also exposed to the challenging microbial environment of intensive care. Infections are the most prevalent and relevant complications after a stroke: pneumonia is the main cause of death in such patients (Henon H, 1979) and has a substantial negative effect on recovery and rehabilitation. Since its description on clinical strokes, (CzlonKowska A 1979) many studies have confirmed the existence of SIDS in experimental (Prass K 2003) and clinical (Vogelgesang A 2008) strokes and shown a strong correlation between immunodepression, sympathetic nervous system activation, and outcome (Chammorro A 2007). For example, concentrations of metanephrine in the blood are as robust for prediction of clinical outcome as they are for stroke severity, (Klehmet J 2009) and markers of SIDS, such as decreased expression of HLA-DR on monocytes, predict risk of infection (Harms H 2008). Nonetheless, immunodepression after a stroke might also have an adaptive component. As the result of a stroke, the blood–brain barrier is disrupted; CNS-specific antigens are exposed to the immune system and may enter the systemic circulation. Downregulation of the immune system could help prevent aggressive responses. Although the general response to a stroke could be a decrease in the number of immune cells and subsequently of their function, further complexity ensues as some immune-cell subtypes could increase (e.g., regulatory T cells). Little is known about the consequences of these changes in circulating immune cells in the brain, but there are indications that they might be involved in brain protection and repair (Gee JM 2007). Immune responses against antigens are determined by the microenvironment of the tissue in which they occur. Co-stimulatory molecules are necessary for the priming of immune responses. Such molecules are weakly expressed in the healthy brain, but become upregulated after brain damage such as a stroke. Furthermore, systemic infection, which often occurs in patients after a stroke, leads to upregulation of co-stimulatory and MHC class I and II molecules in the periphery and the brain, thus facilitating activation of T cells and B cells against endogenous brain antigens (Becker KJ 2009). As a result of systemic inflammation, for example, during infection cytokines are produced outside and within the brain and mediate aspects of sickness behavior (Dantzer R 2008). Infection after a stroke might thus lead to an exacerbated proinflammatory phenotype. Within hours, a stroke induces systemic immune changes that last for weeks (Prass K 2003) and can affect clinical outcomes. SIDS at least partly explains the high risk of infection in patients after a stroke, and might thus be indirectly responsible for the production of inflammatory and co-stimulatory mediators that in turn negatively affect the brain lesion. Whether these deleterious effects of brain–immune interactions after a stroke are offset, at least partly, by their beneficial effect on brain repair or the restricted development of CNS integration is unclear.

Targets for Stroke Prevention: Role of Inflammation and Immunity

Numerous clinical trials have investigated the effects of anticoagulants (e.g., low-molecular-weight heparins or warfarin), anti hypertensive molecules, antiplatelet agents (e.g., aspirin, clopidogrel, Dipyridamole, ticlopidine, trifle usual, GP IIa/IIIb inhibitors, or lotrafiban), or lipid-lowering drugs (e.g., Stations) on prevention of stroke occurrence or recurrence (Stroke Trails Registry 2011). Several of these strategies are presently being used to target the immune system. The MOSES trial, (Schradar J 2005) which tested the efficacy of an angiotensin type 1-receptor antagonist (eprosartan) versus a calcium-channel blocker (nitrendipine) in 1352 patients, showed that eprosartan reduced the risk of recurrent acute strokes by about 25%. Similarly, PROGRESS88 reported a 28% relative risk reduction (95% CI 17–38%; p<00001) in the primary endpoint of cardiovascular events in 6105 patients who were randomly assigned to perindopril or control. Multiple trials have shown that anti-hypertensive drugs targeting the renin-angiotensin system can reduce stroke incidence. Beyond pharmacological strategies targeting this system, there are other interesting attempts to manipulate the immune - system targeting molecules involved in blood-pressure regulation. PMD311789 and Cyt006-AngQb90 vaccines directed against angiotensin I and angiotensin II, respectively, have been tested in phase 2 trials and were inferior in their effect on blood pressure compared with pharmacological inhibitors of the renin-angiotensin system. Nevertheless, strategies to improve the efficacy of such vaccines might confer substantial benefits for stroke prevention in the future by increasing the proportion of patients who are treated for hypertension, as these patients might more readily accept vaccination twice a year than pills every day. However, the long-term effects of such strategies remain unassessed (Brown MJ 2009)

Finally, because infectious agents seem to be risk factors for strokes, the argument for treating or preventing infection is well founded. For example, in one study (Hung IF 2007) dual pneumococcal and influenza vaccination was associated with a reduced number of cases of ischemic strokes than was reported in unvaccinated patients. Age dependent effects of vaccination, and the need to test, vaccination together with antiviral strategies such as use of neuraminidase inhibitors, are being discussed. Notably, prior infection has been suggested to increase hemorrhagic complications after thrombolysis with alteplase, but more data are needed (Urbaneck C 2010).

Immunomodulation to Restrict Brain-Tissue Damage after a Stroke

There are strong experimental evidence which supports the role of leucocyte recruitment by adhesion molecules, cytokines, and chemokines in ischemic damage. Clinical studies support the therapeutic relevance of this pathway, and show increased ICAM1 expression in the cortex and increased circulating concentrations of soluble ICAM1 after an ischemic stroke (Rallidis LS 2009) In experimental models, co-infusion of antibodies targeting ICAM1 led to a significant improvement in neurological outcome when combined with tPA-induced thrombolysis, suggesting that ICAM1 blockade might improve functional outcome and extend the therapeutic window for thrombolysis (Bowes MP 1995). Strategies have been designed to block the cytokine cascade that is induced after a stroke by use of recombinant human interleukin-1 receptor antagonist (interleukin-1Ra). Another promising strategy is the induction of mucosal tolerance with repeated low-dose intranasal administration of E-selectin, which causes a shift in immune responses from proinflammatory to anti-inflammatory and might even induce regulatory T cells. In rats, this immuno modulatory approach prevented ischemic and hemorrhagic strokes. The safety and effectiveness and maximal tolerable dose of E-selectin is under investigation in clinical trials (Emsley HC 2005, Takeda H 2002)

Other therapeutic approaches, such as the use of the antibiotic minocycline, showed promising results in animal models by reducing brain damage and promoting CNS repair (Tang XN 2007). This tetracycline might exert anti-inflammatory activities through modulation of microglial activation, immune-cell activation, and thus the subsequent release of cytokines, chemokines, lipid mediators of inflammation, and MMPs (Brundula V 2002, Stirling DP 2005). Minocycline might also reduce the harmful pro-bleeding effects of alteplase (Murata Y 2008). Experimental evidence strongly suggests that both exogenous TPA (alteplase, injected intravenously) and endogenous TPA (produced and released by injured neurons) interact with the NR1 subunit of N-methyl-Daspartate (NMDA) receptors, leading to increased glutamatergic signalling and subsequent promotion of excitotoxic or ischemic neuronal death. Strategies of active and passive immunization to prevent this interaction were shown to efficiently counteract the aggravating effect of TPA on excitotoxic or ischemic injuries (Macrez R 2010). Although the translation from bench to bedside has not been successful yet, strategies combining either anti-inflammatory drugs or neuroprotectants with thrombolytics are promising and need to be further studied.

Difficulties in Translation from Bench to Bedside and Research Priorities

With a few exceptions, positive laboratory results have not resulted in effective treatments for patients after a stroke. However, only a few trials have targeted inflammation or the immune system. What can we learn from past failures, and what are the prerequisites and prospects for future success in targeting inflammation and the immune system to prevent strokes, to minimize damage once it has occurred, and to foster regeneration and repair? First, the general question of whether the animal models of a stroke can recapitulate human pathology and predict success in clinical trials needs to be addressed. Many articles have assessed this point, (Dirnagl U 2006) which includes differences in vascular supply, kinetics of lesion evolution, confounding effects of anesthesia, difficulties in the assessment of functional outcomes, and deficiencies in the quality of preclinical trials. Accordingly, the Stroke Therapy Academic Industry Roundtable (STAIR) has provided substantial recommendations to improve the success of translation from bench to bedside. Some of these recommendations concentrate on the crucial differences between rodents and human beings and thus emphasized the need for studies into pharmacokinetics and pharmacodynamics, time to treatment, as well as inclusion of risk factors (especially ageing) and the need to use large animals (Fisher M 2005) Nonetheless, investigators need to consider specific issues about the translational roadblock when targeting immunological mechanisms. Animals used in stroke research live in conditions that are sterile or almost free of pathogens, and thus have comparatively little exposure to foreign antigens.

Moreover, rodents have a lymphatic differential blood count compared with human beings. Nevertheless, when direct comparison has been possible, it is reassuring that rodents had similar changes in adaptive and innate immunity to human beings after a stroke. However, to further improve prediction we should consider inclusion into our models of confounders related to inflammation, such as animals with atherosclerosis or pre-existing acute or chronic infections. A relevant concern relates to the potential risks involved with the use of therapeutic immunomodulation to treat strokes. Negative findings from other indications include life-threatening side-effects in a phase 1 trial of the anti-CD28 monoclonal antibody TGN1412 that was intended for the treatment of multiple sclerosis a rare but severe side-effect (progressive multifocal leucoencephalopathy) of the monoclonal antibody directed against the α4 subunit of integrins (natalizumab, an approved multiplesclerosis treatment), and meningoencephalitis as a side-effect of an amyloid-β vaccine in patients with Alzheimer's disease. Clearly, we need to be very alert to potential risks when targeting the immune system and carefully balance the risk-to-benefit ratios. Patients with chronic inflammatory diseases, such as rheumatoid arthritis, who might be at risk of infection or reactivation of viral infections, have successfully been treated with immunomodulatory therapies, such as rituximab, a chimeric anti-CD20 monoclonal antibody that depletes B cells. These findings prove that modulation of the immune system in elderly and severely ill patients, when done cautiously, can be safe. Another reason not to rush into clinical trials targeting the immune system in stroke patients lies in the fact that our current knowledge of the underlying pathophysiology is patchy at best. Importantly, although negative consequences of brain inflammation after a stroke have been documented, there is some evidence that inflammatory mechanisms contribute to lesion containment or even regeneration and repair. The good and bad sides of inflammation after a stroke need to be clarified, and the differential kinetics of deleterious and potential protective or regenerative mechanisms need to be established. For example, MMPs, such as MMP-9, was reported to show deleterious effects during the stroke, but increased concentrations of these enzymes seem to promote brain recovery after a stroke. Accordingly, pharmacological approaches targeting MMPs (or any inflammatory mediator) need to be optimized for acute inhibition at the right moment (IE, to prevent damage without compromising beneficial effects). Furthermore, weather protection of one cell type necessarily protects other cell types in the neurovascular unit is not known. In this respect, it is encouraging that Dipyridamole, a platelet inhibitor used for stroke prevention, might also have anti-inflammatory and antioxidative effects, and might indirectly protect neurons through prevention of hypoxia-induced endothelial cytotoxicity. In terms of peripheral immunity in strokes, we are only beginning to understand the effects of the adaptive immune system in the pathophysiology of a stroke. Some effects, such as SIDS, which increases the risk for infection, are negative, but in other circumstances could balance, stroke-induced autoimmunity; for example, immune cells might react against brain epitopes that are normally well shielded but get exposed after a stroke. Novel investigations are needed to disentangle destruction and protection to safely and effectively modulate the immune system in patients after a stroke.

Experimental and clinical data justify cautious optimism that inflammation and immunity might one day be targeted to prevent strokes and to minimize its effects. In view of recent failures in the development of stroke treatments, the potential risks of such therapies, and the incomplete understanding of the underlying mechanisms, we advocate a cautious approach. Indeed, because of the complexities of the interactions between the immune system and the CNS during and after a stroke, it is difficult to pinpoint a mechanism as the most promising target or approach. Although immunomodulation of peripheral immune responses might carry a risk (e.g., the phase 1 clinical trial of TGN1412, which attempted to test anti-CD28 antibodies to boost regulatory T cells), we believe that such strategies could eventually lead to a viable approach to improve the stroke outcomes. Presently, clinical translation might be near for strategies that modulate innate immunity and inflammation in the brain, first through dampening deleterious hyperinflammation (classic anti-inflammation) or chronic inflammation (e.g., pro-resolving drugs to overcome chronic inflammation and inflammation resolution deficits), and second by allowing inflammatory mechanisms to clear debris, restrict the spread of the lesion, and contribute signals that foster recovery and repair. Thus, a more comprehensive understanding of the endogenous immune responses, in particular with respect to different stages in the evolution of stroke pathology, from its prevention to recovery after a stroke, could help us to design safe immunomodulatory strategies with substantial benefits for patients.

Modulation of the Post-Ischemic Immune Response to Improve the Stroke Outcome

There are profound alterations in the systemic immune response following a stroke. The stroke induced changes include a dramatic increase in the systemic inflammation, as measured by plasma concentrations of C-reactive protein (CRP) and interleukin (IL)-6 (Beamer NB 1995). More recent data also demonstrates that a stroke leads to a sympathetically mediated dysfunction of the systemic immune response that predisposes to infection; the degree of these immunological alterations depends upon the stroke severity

(Prass K 2003, Leisz A 2009). Infection is common following a stroke, and the data demonstrate that infection in the post-stroke period, especially pneumonia (PNA), is an independent risk factor for poor outcome (Jhonston KC 1997, Aslayan S 2004, Katzan IL 2003). Why infection predisposes towards a worse outcome is unclear, but our laboratory has focused on the possibility that an infection in this vulnerable time period may lead to changes in the microenvironment of the lymphoid organs and the brain that allow for the development of a detrimental immune response towards brain antigens. The immune response is generally thought of as having an innate, or antigen non-specific, an arm and an adaptive, or antigen specific, arm. The innate immune response is also referred to as the inflammatory response and is the first line of defense against invading pathogens and the primary response to tissue injury. It is thus not surprising that there is evidence of systemic inflammation following a stroke, and that the degree of inflammation correlates to stroke severity and ultimately to the amount of tissue infected (Adebert HJ 2004, Smith CJ 2004). The amount of tissue infected is also reflected by the concentration of antigens like myelin basic protein (MBP), creatine kinase (CK)-BB, neuron specific enolase (NSE) and S100 in the peripheral circulation (Jauch EC 2006). As concerns the systemic immune system, these antigens are essentially novel, which means that lymphocyte encounter with such and antigen could lead to the development of an autoimmune response. There are many potential sites of antigen encounter in the periphery, and experimental data show that antigen is present within the cervical lymph nodes shortly after the onset of a stroke (Vanzwam M 2009). In addition, lymphocyte traffic into the infected brain tissue within days after a stroke, allowing for the possibility of novel antigen encounter within the central nervous system (CNS) itself.

For a lymphocyte to become activated to an antigen, it must generally be presented that antigen by a professional antigen presenting cell (APC) in the context of the major histocompatibility (MHC) II molecule and receive an additional costimulatory signal. The nature of the immune response is further shaped by the cytokine milieu of the environment at the site of antigen encounter. For instance, if a naïve lymphocyte recognizes its cognate antigen in the presence of interferon (IFN)-γ, a TH1 type response usually develops; if the recognition occurs in the presence of IL-4, a TH2 type response develops. Further, if antigen recognition occurs in the presence of transforming growth factor (TGF) -β1 and IL-6, a TH17 response occurs; in the absence of IL-6, a regulatory T cell response (TREG) develops. A TREG response can also be induced in the presence of IL-10. As would be expected, the type of the effector cell/response generated after antigen encounter is associated with very different immunological outcomes. For instance, TH1 cells are associated with cellular immunity and are characterized by the secretion of IFN-γ and lymphotoxin alpha (LTA) while TH2 cells are associated with humoral immunity and the secretion of IL4, IL-5, and IL-13. And while TH17 cells play a role in host defense, they also appear to be important in the genesis of autoimmunity; TH17 cells are characterized by the secretion of IL-17 (Peck A 2008). Inducible TREGS, on the other hand, are characterized by the secretion of TGF-β and IL-10 and, as the name implies, regulate immune responses.

To date, there has been little interest in exploring the possibility that autoimmune responses to brain might affect outcome from a stroke. There are, however, studies that document the fact immune responses to brain antigens do occur following a stroke. For instance, lymphocytes from stroke survivors show more activity against myelin basic protein (MBP) than the lymphocytes from patients with multiple sclerosis (Younchayud U 1974). In addition, myelin reactive T cells are found in higher numbers among patients with cerebrovascular disease (Wang WZ 1992). These data thus provide evidence that a cellular immune response to brain antigens occurs following a stroke. Further, there are increased titers of antibodies to brain antigens, including neurofilaments and portions of N-methyl-D-aspartate receptor, following a stroke, indicating that there is also the development of a humoral response to these antigens (Bornestien NM 2001, Dambinova SA 2003). The immune response to CNS antigens after stroke is likely just an epiphenomena of stroke, given that cerebral ischemic injury to the blood-brain barrier (BBB) allows for the systemic immune system to come into contact with the antigens that are normally sequestered from it. Nonetheless, it is possible that this response leads to "collateral damage"; whether these immune responses affect the outcomes of a stroke is a largely unanswered question. In an animal model of a stroke we have demonstrated that the predominant immune response to brain antigens, following a stroke is that of a TREG response characterized by secretion of TGF-β1.23 Using the paradigm of mucosal tolerance, we also found it possible to induce TREG responses prior to stroke animals that exhibit a TREG response experience both better shot (days) and long term (one month) outcome from a stroke (Gee JM 2008 and 2009, Zeerath D 2009). It is thus not surprising that a recent paper found that the absence of TREG cells is associated with worse outcome from stroke (Liesz A 2009). Induction of Treg cells characterized by the secretion of IL-10 prior to stroke also improves short term outcome and decreases infarct size. These data suggest that modulation of the post-ischemic immune response by inducting a more robust TREG response might be a viable strategy for neuroprotection. In our animal model, we also found that exposure to an inflammatory stimulus at the time of a stroke leads to a deviation of the immune response to that of a TH1 response, and the TH1 response to brain antigens is associated with worse outcome. This deviation from an endogenous TREG response to that of TH1 response induced by an inflammatory stimulus at the time of a stroke appears to be related to a change in the milieu of microenvironment at the site of antigen presentation. This observation may help to explain why persons who develop an infection in the post-stroke period have increased morbidity and mortality. It also suggests that attempts to avoid infection in the post-stroke period may be of therapeutic value. To date, however, there have only been a few trials of antibiotic prophylaxis following a stroke and these relatively small trials have conflicting results, suggesting that prophylactic antibiotic therapy may improve, worsen, or have no effect on the stroke outcome (Schwartz S 2008, Chomorro A 2005, Harms H 2008). IL-17 was recently shown to contribute to ischemic brain injury up to 7 days after the onset of a stroke (Schichita T 2009) In this study, the IL-17 was being produced by γδ T cells, which are important mediators in the antigen non-specific inflammatory response, and not by TH17 cells. Given the fact that there is robust upregulation of IL-6 following a stroke and increased expression of TGF-β1 in brain, however, the post-ischemic cytokine milieu could favor the development of TH17 cells (Krupinski J 1996, Wang X 1995) Whether or not CNS specific TH17 cells contribute to injury in cerebral ischemia has yet to be explored, but their importance in autoimmune diseases, including experimental allergic encephalomyelitis (EAE), is clear (Furuzawa-Carballeda J 2007, Hoffstetter H 2009). Recent data highlight the fact that the ratio of antigen specific TH17 cells to antigen specific TH1 cells as well as the cell type used to induce EAE (TH17 versus TH1) influence both EAE phenotype and pathology (Jager A 2009, Stromnes IM 2008). These data further suggest that the nature of the immune response to brain after a stroke has the potential to differentially affect outcome. The potential of modulating the post-ischemic immune response to improve outcome following a stroke is an intriguing neuroprotective approach as it is one of the rare interventions that could be initiated in a delayed fashion and still be expected to have an effect. There are, however, potential dangers of manipulating a response which is so complex and incompletely understood. As an example, we found that induction of MBP specific TREG cells prior to experimental strokes using the paradigm of mucosal tolerance was associated with better outcome up to one month after the ischemic injury; this benefit was not sustained to 3 months however, and there was a tendency for the animals "tolerized" to MBP exhibit a TH1 response to the antigen. Studies suggest that the phenotype of inducible TREG cells is unstable, so understanding how to prevent this "immunological drift" would be important prior to use in therapeutic trials (Zhu L 2009). And while immunosuppressive strategies might decrease the risk of developing a TH1 (and possibly TH17?) response after a stroke, such interventions might increase the risk infection, a risk which is already high in the post-stroke period. On the other hand, strategies to enhance the immune response to prevent infection in the post-stroke period might increase the risk of developing a detrimental TH1 (and possibly TH17?) immune response to brain, and as already discussed, these responses might predispose patients to worse functional outcomes following a stroke. It is also in the realm of possibility that the development of immune responses to brain antigens, be they cellular or humoral, may have more long lasting effects. For instance, it is appreciated that a stroke is a potent risk factor for dementia, and it could be that autoimmune responses to brain contribute to cognitive decline and even the progression of white matter disease (Pendlebury ST 2009) Future clinical studies will need to address the contribution of the post-ischemic immune response to these long-term outcomes. In summary, the nature of the post-ischemic immune response affects outcome from a stroke. Modulation of this response may be a viable approach to improving the outcome of a stroke, but there are potential dangers associated with immunomodulation. A more complete understanding of the endogenous immune response following a stroke is needed in order to safely manipulate this response in the post-stroke period.

References

American Heart Association. Heart Disease and Stroke Statistics—2010 update. *http://www.americanheart.org/presenter*. jhtml?identifier=3000090

Aslanyan S, Weir CJ, Diener HC, Kaste M, Lees KR. Pneumonia and urinary tract infection after acute ischemic stroke: A tertiary analysis of the gain international trial. *Eur J Neurol* 2004;11:49–53.

Audebert HJ, Rott MM, Eck T, Haberl RL. Systemic inflammatory response depends on initial stroke severity but is attenuated by successful thrombolysis. *Stroke*. 2004.

Bhuva P, Kuo SH, Claude Hemphill J, Lopez GA. Intracranial hemorrhage following thrombolytic use for stroke caused by infective endocarditis. *Neurocrit Care* 2010; 12: 79–82.

Buch MH, Smolen JS, Betteridge N, et al. Updated consensus statement on the use of rituximab in patients with rheumatoid arthritis. *Ann Rheum Dis* 2011; published online March 6.

Beamer NB, Coull BM, Clark WM, Hazel JS, Silberger JR. Interleukin-6 and interleukin-1 receptor antagonist in acute stroke. *Ann Neurol* 1995;37:800–805.

Brundula V, Rewcastle NB, Metz LM, Bernard CC, Yong VW. Targeting leukocyte MMPs and transmigration: minocycline as a potential therapy for multiple sclerosis. *Brain* 2002; 125: 1297–308.

Becker KJ. Modulation of the postischemic immune response to improve stroke outcome. *Stroke* 2010; 41 (suppl): S75–78.

Becker KJ. Sensitization and tolerization to brain antigens in stroke. *Neuroscience* 2009; 158: 1090–97.

Bowes MP, Rothlein R, Fagan SC, Zivin JA. Monoclonal antibodies preventing leukocyte activation reduce experimental neurologic injury and enhance efficacy of thrombolytic therapy. *Neurology* 1995; 45: 815–19.

Becker KJ, Kindrick DL, Lester MP, Shea C, Ye ZC. Sensitization to brain antigens after stroke is augmented by lipopolysaccharide. *J Cereb Blood Flow Metab* 2005;25:1634–1644.

Bornstein NM, Aronovich B, et al. Antibodies to brain antigens following stroke. *Neurology* 2001;56:529–530.

Becker KJ. Modulation of the postischemic immune response to improve stroke outcome. *Stroke* 2010; 41 (suppl): S75–78.

Becker KJ. Sensitization and tolerization to brain antigens in stroke. *Neuroscience* 2009; 158: 1090–97.

Brown MJ, Coltart J, et al. Randomized double-blind placebo-controlled study of an angiotensin immunotherapeutic vaccine (PMD3117) in hypertensive subjects. *Clin Sci (Lond)* 2004; 107: 167–73.

Chamorro A, Amaro S, Vargas M, et al. Catecholamines, infection, and death in acute ischemic stroke. *Neurol Sci* 2007; 252: 29–35.

Członkowska A, Cyrta B, Korlak J. Immunological observations on patients with acute cerebral vascular disease. *J Neurol Sci* 1979; 43: 455–64.

Chamorro A, Amaro S, Vargas M, et al. Catecholamines, infection, and death in acute ischemic stroke. *Neurol Sci* 2007; 252: 29–35.

Członkowska A, Cyrta B, Korlak J. Immunological observations on patients with acute cerebral vascular disease. *J Neurol Sci* 1979; 43: 455–64.

Catania A, Lonati C, Sordi A, Gatti S. Detrimental consequences of brain injury on peripheral cells. *Brain Behav Immun* 2009; 23: 877–84.

Chamorro A, Urra X, Planas AM. Infection after acute ischemic stroke: a manifestation of brain-induced immunodepression. *Stroke* 2007; 38: 1097–103.

Chen GY, Nunez G. Sterile inflammation: sensing and reacting to damage. *Nat Rev Immunol* 2010; 10: 826–37.

Catania A, Lonati C, Sordi A, Gatti S. Detrimental consequences of brain injury on peripheral cells. *Brain Behav Immun* 2009; 23: 877–84.

Chamorro A, Urra X, Planas AM. Infection after acute ischemic stroke: a manifestation of brain-induced immunodepression. *Stroke* 2007; 38: 1097–103.

Chamorro A, Horcajada JP, et al. The early systemic prophylaxis of infection after stroke study: A randomized clinical trial. *Stroke* 2005;36:1495–1500.

Chen Y, Ruetzler C, et al. Mucosal tolerance to e-selectin provides cell-mediated protection against ischemic brain injury. *Proc Natl Acad Sci U S A* 2003;100:15107–15112.

Czernichow S, Ninomiya T, Huxley R, et al. Impact of blood pressure lowering on cardiovascular outcomes in normal weight, overweight, and obese individuals: the

Perindopril Protection Against Recurrent Stroke Study trial. *Hypertension* 2010; 55: 1193–98.

Dirnagl U, Klehmet J, Braun JS, et al. Stroke-induced immunodepression: experimental evidence and clinical relevance. *Stroke* 2007; 38 (suppl): 770–73.

Denes A, Vidyasagar R, Feng J, et al. Proliferating resident microglia after focal cerebral ischaemia in mice. *J Cereb Blood Flow Metab* 2007; 27: 1941–53.

Deb P, Sharma S, Hassan KM. Pathophysiologic mechanisms of acute ischemic stroke: an overview with emphasis on therapeutic significance beyond thrombolysis. *Pathophysiology* 2010; 17: 197–218.

Dambinova SA, Khounteev GA, et al. Blood test detecting autoantibodies to n-methyl-d-aspartate neuroreceptors for evaluation of patients with transient ischemic attack and stroke. *Clin Chem* 2003;49:1752–1762.

Dirnagl U, Klehmet J, Braun JS, et al. Stroke-induced immunodepression: experimental evidence and clinical relevance. *Stroke* 2007; 38 (suppl): 770–73.

Dirnagl U. Bench to bedside: the quest for quality in experimental stroke research. *J Cereb Blood Flow Metab* 2006; 26: 1465–78.

Dayan CM, Wraith DC. Preparing for first-in-man studies: the challenges for translational immunology post-TGN1412. *Clin Exp Immunol* 2008; 151: 231–34.

Dantzer R, O'Connor JC, Freund GG, Johnson RW, Kelley KW. From inflammation to sickness and depression: when the immune system subjugates the brain. *Nat Rev Neurosci* 2008; 9: 46–56.

Didier N, Romero IA, Creminon C, Wijkhuisen A, Grassi J, Mabondzo A. Secretion of interleukin-1beta by astrocytes mediates endothelin-1 and tumor necrosis factor-alpha effects on human brain microvascular endothelial cell permeability. *J Neurochem* 2003; 86: 246–54.

Emsley HC, Smith CJ, Georgiou RF, et al; Acute Stroke Investigators. A randomised phase II study of interleukin-1 receptor antagonist in acute stroke patients. *J Neurol Neurosurg Psychiatry* 2005; 76: 1366–72.

Enlimomab Acute Stroke Trial Investigators. Use of anti-ICAM-1 therapy in ischemic stroke: results of the Enlimomab Acute Stroke Trial. *Neurology* 2001; 57: 1428–34.

Emsley HC, Hopkins SJ. Post-stroke immunodepression and infection: an emerging concept. *Infect Disord Drug Targets* 2010; 10: 91–97.

Elenkov IJ, Chrousos GP. Stress system: organization, physiology and immunoregulation. *Neuroimmunomodulation* 2006; 13: 257–67.

Emsley HC, Hopkins SJ. Post-stroke immunodepression and infection: an emerging concept. *Infect Disord Drug Targets* 2010; 10: 91–97.

Elenkov IJ, Chrousos GP. Stress system: organization, physiology and immunoregulation. *Neuroimmunomodulation* 2006; 13: 257–67.

Emsley HC, Hopkins SJ. Acute ischemic stroke and infection: recent and emerging concepts. *Lancet Neurol* 2008; 7: 341–53.

Fassbender K, Rossol S, Kammer T, et al. Proinflammatory cytokines in serum of patients with acute cerebral ischemia: kinetics of secretion and relation to the extent of brain damage and outcome of disease. *J Neurol Sci* 1994; 122: 135–39.

Fisher M, Albers GW, Donnan GA, et al; Stroke Therapy Academic Industry Roundtable IV. Enhancing the development and approval of acute stroke therapies: Stroke Therapy Academic Industry roundtable. *Stroke* 2005; 36: 1808–13.

Furuzawa-Carballeda J, Vargas-Rojas MI, Cabral AR. Autoimmune inflammation from the th17 perspective. *Autoimmun Rev* 2007;6:169–175.

Frenkel D, Huang Z, Maron R, Koldzic DN, Moskowitz MA, Weiner HL. Neuroprotection by IL-10-producing much cd4+t cells following ischemic stroke. *J Neurol Sci* 2005;233:125–132.

Gelderblom M, Leypoldt F, Steinbach K, et al. Temporal and spatial dynamics of cerebral immune cell accumulation in stroke. *Stroke* 2009; 40: 1849–57.

Gee JM, Zierath D, et al. Long term immunologic consequences of experimental stroke and mucosal tolerance. *Exp Transl Stroke Med* 2009;1:3.

Gee JM, Kalil A, Shea C, Becker KJ. Lymphocytes: potential mediators of postischemic injury and neuroprotection. *Stroke* 2007; 38 (suppl): 783–88.

Harms H, Prass K, Meisel C, et al. Preventive antibacterial therapy in acute ischemic stroke: A randomized controlled trial. *PLoS ONE* 2008;3:e2158.

Hung IF, Leung AY, Chu DW, et al. Prevention of acute myocardial infarction and stroke among elderly persons by dual pneumococcal and infl uenza vaccination: a prospective cohort study. *Clin Infect Dis* 2010; 51: 1007–16.

Hayakawa K, Nakano T, Irie K, et al. Inhibition of reactive astrocytes with fluorocitrate retards neurovascular remodeling and recovery after focal cerebral ischemia in mice. *J Cereb Blood Flow Metab* 2010; 30: 871–82.

Hayakawa K, Qiu J, Lo EH. Biphasic actions of HMGB1 signaling in inflammation and recovery after stroke. *Ann NY Acad Sci* 2010; 1207: 50–57.

Haase G, Pettmann B, Raoul C, Henderson CE. Signaling by death receptors in the nervous system. *Curr Opin Neurobiol* 2008; 18: 284–91. 52.

Hallenbeck JM. The many faces of tumor necrosis factor in stroke. *Nat Med* 2002; 8: 1363–68.

Hurn PD, Subramanian S, Parker SM, et al. T- and B-cell-deficient mice with experimental stroke have reduced lesion size and inflammation. *J Cereb Blood Flow Metab* 2007; 27: 1798–805.

Hofstetter H, Gold R, Hartung HP. Th17 cells in ms and experimental autoimmune encephalomyelitis. *Int MS J* 2009;16:12–18.

Hug A, Dalpke A, Wieczorek N, et al. Infarct volume is a major determiner of post-stroke immune cell function and susceptibility to infection. *Stroke* 2009;40:3226–3232.

Hayakawa K, Mishima K, Nozako M, et al. Delayed treatment with minocycline ameliorates neurologic impairment through activated microglia expressing a high-mobility group box1 inhibiting mechanism. *Stroke* 2008; 39: 951–58.

Hughes PM, Allegrini PR, Rudin M, Perry VH, Mir AK, Wiessner C. Monocyte chemoattractant protein-1 deficiency is protective in a murine stroke model. *J Cereb Blood Flow Metab* 2002; 22: 308–17.

Harms H, Prass K, Meisel C, et al. Preventive antibacterial therapy in acute ischemic stroke: a randomized controlled trial. *PLoS One* 2008; 3: e2158.

Henon H, Godefroy O, Leys D, et al. Early predictors of death and disability after acute cerebral ischemic event. *Stroke* 1995; 26: 392–98.

Jin R, Yang G, Li G. Inflammatorymechanisms in ischemic stroke: role of inflammatorycells. *J Leukoc Biol* 2010; 87: 779–89.

Jager A, Dardalhon V, et al. Th1, th17, and th9 effector cells induce experimental autoimmune encephalomyelitis with different pathological phenotypes. J Immunol 2009;183:7169–7177.

Johnston KC, Li JY, et al. Medical and neurological complications of ischemic stroke: Experience from the ranttas trial. Ranttas investigators. *Stroke* 1998;29:447–453.

Jauch EC, Lindsell C, et al. Association of serial biochemical markers with acute ischemic stroke: The national institute of neurological disorders and stroke recombinant tissue plasminogen activator stroke study. *Stroke* 2006;37:2508–2513.

Klehmet J, Harms H, Richter M, et al. Stroke-induced immunodepression and post-stroke infections: lessons from the preventive antibacterial therapy in stroke trial. *Neuroscience* 2009; 158: 1184–93.

Krupinski J, Kumar P, Kumar S, Kaluza J. Increased expression of tgf-beta 1 in brain tissue after ischemic stroke in humans. *Stroke* 1996;27:852–857.

Kallen B, Nilsson O, Thelin C. Effect of encephalitogenic protein on migration in agarose of leukocytes from patients with multiple sclerosis. A longitudinal study of patients with relapsing multiple sclerosis or with cerebral infarction. *Acta Neurol Scand* 1977;55:47–56.

Katzan IL, Cebul RD, Husak SH, Dawson NV, Baker DW. The effect of pneumonia on mortality among patients hospitalized for acute stroke. *Neurology* 2003;60:620–625.

Liesz A, Suri-Payer E, et al. Regulatory t cells are key cerebroprotective immunomodulators in acute experimental stroke. *Nat Med* 2009;15:192–199.

Leung PY, Packard AE, Stenzel-Poore MP. It's all in the family: multiple Toll-like receptors off er promise as novel therapeutic targets for stroke neuroprotection. *Future Neurol* 2009; 4: 201–08.

Lavallee P, Perchaud V, Gautier-Bertrand M, Grabli D, Amarenco P. Association between infl uenza vaccination and reduced risk of brain infarction. *Stroke* 2002; 33: 513–18.

Liesz A, Suri-Payer E, Veltkamp C, et al. Regulatory T cells are key cerebroprotective immunomodulators in acute experimental stroke. *Nat Med* 2009; 15: 192–99.

Lehnardt S, Lehmann S, Kaul D, et al. Toll-like receptor 2 mediates CNS injury in focal cerebral ischemia. *J Neuroimmunol* 2007; 190: 28–33.

Lee SR, Kim HY, Rogowska J, et al. Involvement of matrix metalloproteinase in neuroblast cell migration from the subventricular zone after stroke. *J Neurosci* 2006; 26: 3491–95.

Lo EH. T time in brain. *Nat Med* 2009; 15: 844–46.

Murata Y, Rosell A, Scannevin RH, Rhodes KJ, Wang X, Lo EH. Extension of the thrombolytic time window with minocycline in experimental stroke. *Stroke* 2008; 39: 3372–77.

Macrez R, Bezin L, Le Mauff B, Ali C, Vivien D. Functional occurrence of the interaction of tissue plasminogen activator with the NR1 subunit of N-methyl-D-aspartate receptors during stroke. *Stroke* 2010; 41: 2950–55.

Macrez R, Obiang P, Gauberti M, et al. Antibodies preventing the interaction of tPA with NMDA receptors reduce stroke damages and extend the therapeutic window of thrombolysis. *Stroke* (in Press).

Monaco C, Gregan SM, Navin TJ, Foxwell BM, Davies AH, Feldmann M. Toll-like receptor-2 mediates inflammation and matrix degradation in human atherosclerosis. *Circulation* 2009; 120: 2462–69.

Marsh BJ, Williams-Karnesky RL, Stenzel-Poore MP. Toll-like receptor signalling in endogenous neuroprotection and stroke. *Neuroscience* 2009; 158: 1007–20.

McCoy MK, Tansey MG. TNF signaling inhibition in the CNS: implications for normal brain function and neurodegenerative disease. *J Neuroinflammation* 2008; 5: 45.

Madinier A, Bertrand N, Mossiat C, et al. Microglial involvement in neuroplastic changes following focal brain ischemia in rats. *PLoS One* 2009; 4: e8101.

Meisel C, Schwab JM, Prass K, Meisel A, Dirnagl U. Central nervous system injury-induced immune deficiency syndrome. *Nat Rev Neurosci* 2005; 6: 775–86.

Off ner H, Vandenbark AA, Hurn PD. Effectof experimental stroke on peripheral immunity: CNS ischemia induces profound immunosuppression. *Neuroscience* 2009; 158: 1098–111.

Pendlebury ST, Rothwell PM. Prevalence, incidence, and factors associated with pre-stroke and poststroke dementia: A systematic review and meta-analysis. *Lancet Neurol* 2009;8:1006–1018.

Peck A, Mellins ED. Precarious balance: Th17 cells in host defense. *Infect Immun* 78:32–38.

Pinol-Ripoll G, de la Puerta I, Santos S, Purroy F, Mostacero E. Chronic bronchitis and acute infections as new risk factors for ischemic stroke and the lack of protection off ered by the infl uenza vaccination. *Cerebrovasc Dis* 2008; 26: 339–47.

Prass K, Meisel C, Hofl ich C, et al. Stroke-induced immunodeficiency promotes spontaneous bacterial infections and is mediated by sympathetic activation reversal by poststroke T helper cell type 1-like immunostimulation. *J Exp Med* 2003; 198: 725–36.

Rallidis LS, Zolindaki MG, Vikelis M, Kaliva K, Papadopoulos C, Kremastinos DT. Elevated soluble intercellular adhesion molecule-1 levels are associated with poor short-term prognosis in middle-aged patients with acute ischemic stroke. *Int J Cardiol* 2009; 132: 216–20.

Ren X, Akiyoshi K, Vandenbark AA, Hurn PD, Off ner H. CD4(+) FoxP3(+) regulatory T-cells in cerebral ischemic stroke. *Metab Brain Dis* 2010; published online Nov 17.

Stirling DP, Koochesfahani KM, Steeves JD, Tetzlaff W. Minocycline as a neuroprotective agent. *Neuroscientist* 2005; 11: 308–22.

Smith CJ, Emsley HC, et al. Peak plasma interleukin-6 and other peripheral markers of inflammation in the first week of ischemic stroke correlate with brain infarct volume, stroke severity and long-term outcome. *BMC Neurol* 2004;4:2.

Schwarz S, Al-Shajlawi F, et al. Effects of prophylactic antibiotic therapy with mezlocillin plus sulbactam on the incidence and height of fever after severe acute ischemic stroke: The Mannheim infection in stroke study (miss). *Stroke* 2008;39:1220–1227.

Stromnes IM, Cerretti LM, et al. Differential regulation of central nervous system autoimmunity by t(h)1 and t(h)17 cells. *Nat Med* 2008;14:337–342.

Stroke Trials Registry. *http://www.strokecenter.org/trials/* (accessed Aug 12, 2013).

Schrader J, Luders S, Kulschewski A, et al; MOSES study group. Morbidity and mortality after stroke, eprosartan compared with nitrendipine for secondary prevention: principal results of a prospective randomized controlled study (MOSES). *Stroke* 2005; 36: 1218–26.

Shichita T, Sugiyama Y, Ooboshi H, et al. Pivotal role of cerebral interleukin-17-producing gamma delta T cells in the delayed phase of ischemic brain injury. *Nat Med 2009*; 15: 946–50.

Tissot AC, Maurer P, Nussberger J, et al. Effectof immunization against angiotensin II with CYT006-AngQb on ambulatory blood pressure: a double-blind, randomised, placebo controlled phase IIa study. *Lancet* 2008; 371: 821–27.

Tang XN, Wang Q, Koike MA, et al. Monitoring the protective effects of minocycline treatment with radiolabeled annexin V in an experimental model of focal cerebral ischemia. *J Nucl Med* 2007; 48: 1822–28.

Takeda H, Spatz M, et al. Induction of mucosal tolerance to E-selectin prevents ischemic and hemorrhagic stroke in spontaneously hypertensive genetically stroke-prone rats. *Stroke* 2002; 33: 2156–63.

Thored P, Heldmann U, Gomes-Leal W, et al. Long-term accumulation of microglia with proneurogenic phenotype concomitant with persistent neurogenesis in adult subventricular zone after stroke. *Glia* 2009; 57: 835–49.

The National Institute of Neurological Disorders and Stroke rt-PA Stroke Study Group. Tissue plasminogen activator for acute ischemic stroke. *N Engl J Med* 1995; 333: 1581–87.

Uro-Coste E, Russano de Paiva G, et al. Cerebral amyloid angiopathy and microhemorrhages after amyloid beta vaccination: case report and brief review. *Clin Neuropathol* 2010; 29: 209–16.

Urra X, Cervera A, Villamor N, Planas AM, Chamorro A. Harms and benefits of lymphocyte subpopulations in patients with acute stroke. *Neuroscience* 2009; 158: 1174–83.

Urra X, Obach V, Chamorro A. Stroke induced immunodepression syndrome: from bench to bedside. *Curr Mol Med* 2009; 9: 195–202.

Urbanek C, Palm F, Grau AJ. Infl uenza and stroke risk: a key target not to be missed? *Infect Disord Drug Targets* 2010; 10: 122–31.

Vogelgesang A, Grunwald U, Langner S, et al. Analysis of lymphocyte subsets in patients with stroke and their infl uence on infection after stroke. *Stroke* 2008; 39: 237–41.

van Zwam M, Huizinga R, et al. Brain antigens in functionally distinct antigen-presenting cell populations in cervical lymph nodes in ms and eae. *J Mol Med* 2009;87:273–286.

Warnke C, Menge T, Hartung HP, et al. Natalizumab and progressive multifocal leukoencephalopathy: what are the causal factors and can it be avoided? *Arch Neurol* 2010; 67: 923–30.

Wang WZ, Olsson T, et al. Myelin antigen reactive t cells in cerebrovascular diseases. *Clin Exp Immunol* 1992;88:157–162.

Wang X, Yue TL, et al. Transforming growth factor-beta 1 exhibits delayed gene expression following focal cerebral ischemia. *Brain Res Bull* 1995;36:607–609.

Youngchaiyud U, Coates AS, Whittingham S, Mackay IR. Cellular-immune response to myelin protein: Absence in multiple sclerosis and presence in cerebrovascular accidents. *Aust N Z J Med* 1974;4:535–538.

Young AR, Ali C, Duretete A, Vivien D. Neuroprotection and stroke: time for a compromise. *J Neurochem* 2007; 103: 1302–09.

Yrjanheikki J, Tikka T, et al. A tetracycline derivative, minocycline, reduces inflammation and protects against focal cerebral ischemia with a wide therapeutic window. *Proc Natl Acad Sci USA* 1999; 96: 13496–500.

Zierath D, Thullbery M, et al. Cns immune responses following experimental stroke. *Neurocrit Care*. 2009.

Zhou L, Chong MM, Littman DR. Plasticity of cd4+ t cell lineage differentiation. *Immunity* 2009;30:646–655.

In: Recent Advances in Stroke Therapeutics
Editor: Manzoor Ahmad Mir
ISBN: 978-1-63117-754-5

Chapter II

Pathophysiology of Strokes

Abstract

Once considered exclusively a disorder of blood vessels, growing evidence has led to the realization that the biological processes underlying stroke are driven by the interaction of neurons, glia, vascular cells, and matrix components, which actively participate in mechanisms of tissue injury and repair. A stroke is a serious neurological disease, and constitutes a major cause of death and disability throughout the world. The pathophysiology of stroke is complex, and involves excitotoxicity mechanisms, inflammatory pathways, oxidative damage, ionic imbalances, apoptosis, angiogenesis and neuroprotection. The ultimate result of ischemic cascade initiated by acute stroke is neuronal death along with an irreversible loss of neuronal function. Therapeutic strategies for stroke have been developed with two main aims: restoration of cerebral flow and the minimization of the deleterious effects of ischemia on neurons. Intense research spanning over the last two decades has witnessed significant therapeutic advances in the form of carotid endarterectomy, thrombolytics, anticoagulant therapy, antiplatelet agents, neuroprotective agents, and treating associated risk factors such as hypertension and hyperlipidemia. However, the search for an effective neuroprotectant remains frustrating, and the current therapeutic protocols remain suboptimal. To date, only one FDA-approved drug is available for ischemic stroke; i.e., the serine protease tissue-type plasminogen activator (tPA), utility of which is limited by short therapeutic window. As new targets are identified, new opportunities emerge that build on an appreciation of acute cellular events acting in a broader context of ongoing destructive, protective, and reparative processes. The burden of disease is great, and its magnitude widens as a role for blood vessels and stroke in vascular and nonvascular dementias becomes more clearly established. The primary objectives of this chapter are: (1) to summarize the pathophysiology of a stroke, (2) to outline the relation of Atherosclerosis with stroke and also that of inflammatory and infective conditions associated with clinical stroke, along with role of various inflammatory mediators; (3) current status and understanding the role of genetics in stroke; (4) unifying the proposed mechanisms linking various pathogenetic processes; and (5) to discuss the emerging opportunities for novel therapeutic strategies. In this chapter we will critically evaluate the major mechanisms underlying stroke pathophysiology, with emphasis on potential novel targets for designing newer therapeutic modalities.

Keywords: Ischemic stroke; Pathophysiology; Excitotoxicity; Apoptosis; Inflammation; Therapeutic targets

Introduction

Strokes are the leading cause of disability worldwide, the second most common cause of dementia and the third leading cause of death. They have enormous clinical, social, and economic implications and demand a significant effort from both basic scientists and clinicians in the quest for understanding the underlying pathogenic mechanisms, and thereby adopting suitable preventive measures and successful therapies. A stroke is a sudden loss of brain function resulting from an interference with the blood supply to the central nervous system (CNS). Normal cerebral blood flow (CBF) is approximately 50– 60 ml/100g/min. The reduction in CBF below 20 ml/100g/min results in an electrical silence and less than 10 ml/100g/min causes irreversible neuronal injury (Hakim M 1998, Jones TH 1981). Lack of blood circulation to the brain deprives neurons of necessary glucose and oxygen. Neurons are the impulse transmitters; hence they require a constant supply of energy. Up to 85% of all strokes are of ischemic origin, with most attributable to blockage of one or more cerebral artery by blood clots, with resulting reduction in cerebral perfusion. The remaining stroke cases are hemorrhagic, involving either intracerebral or subarachnoid hemorrhage. Ischemic stroke may manifest in the form of thrombotic stroke (large vessel and small vessel types); embolic stroke (with/without knowing cardiac and/or arterial factor); systemic hypoperfusion (Watershed or Border Zone stroke); or venous thrombosis. Irrespective of the cause, compromised vascular supply to the brain is the primary event in majority (85–90%) of acute strokes. A lower respiratory reserve and complete dependence on aerobic metabolism make brain tissue particularly vulnerable to the effects of ischemia. A spectrum of severity is generally observed in the affected region of the brain, owing to the presence of collateral circulation. Thus, part of the brain parenchyma (core) undergoes immediate death, while others may only be partially injured with potential to recover (penumbra). Following the onset of ischemic stroke, cerebral blood flow is disrupted throughout the affected region of the brain. Blood flow disruption to the tissue is not uniform due to the presence of collateral circulation resulting in a flow gradient. Consequently, a "core" region of infarct develops in which flow is severely reduced, often approximating upwards of a 90% decrement, and tissue undergoes necrosis within minutes as insufficient adenosine triphosphate (ATP) is present to maintain homeostatic ionic gradients and metabolic functions (Astrup J 1977). Surrounding this core region in which blood flow is severely reduced is the "penumbra", a tissue distribution in which flow is less severely reduced and remains typically around 35% of baseline flow (Astrup J 1977). Characterized by normal cellular membrane potential but a disruption in the ability for normal action potential firing, tissue initially residing within the penumbral region progresses to cellular death, ultimately resulting in an expanded core lesion without restoration of cerebral blood flow (Lo EH 2008). As such, therapeutic development has focused on achieving reperfusion via tissue plasminogen activator (tPA) and/or restoring homeostasis via administration of 'neuroprotective' pharmacologic agents intended to disrupt the ischemic injury cascade.

Few neurological conditions are as complex and devastating as stroke, the second leading cause of death worldwide. Also called a brain attack, victims may suddenly experience paralysis impaired speech, or loss of vision due to interruption of blood flow (ischemia) caused by thrombosis or embolism. Less frequently (<15%), strokes are caused by hemorrhage or cardiac arrest. On average, strokes in the USA strike once every 40 seconds and cause death every 4 minutes, with an estimated 41.6% death rate in 2007 (Lloyd-Jones,2009). With an aging population, the absolute numbers are likely to rise. Among survivors, work capacity is compromised in 70% of victims, and 30% need assistance with self-care. Hence, the disease burden is great. The estimated stroke cost was 73.7 billion dollars in 2010 (USA) and projected to be 1.52 trillion dollars in 2050 (Lloyd-Jones, 2009). No racial or ethnic groups are spared, and the problem is global. For example, in the Russian Federation and China, the estimated death rates per 100,000 populations are five to ten times higher than in the USA (Lloyd-Jones, 2009). Hence, stroke is an affliction of mankind.

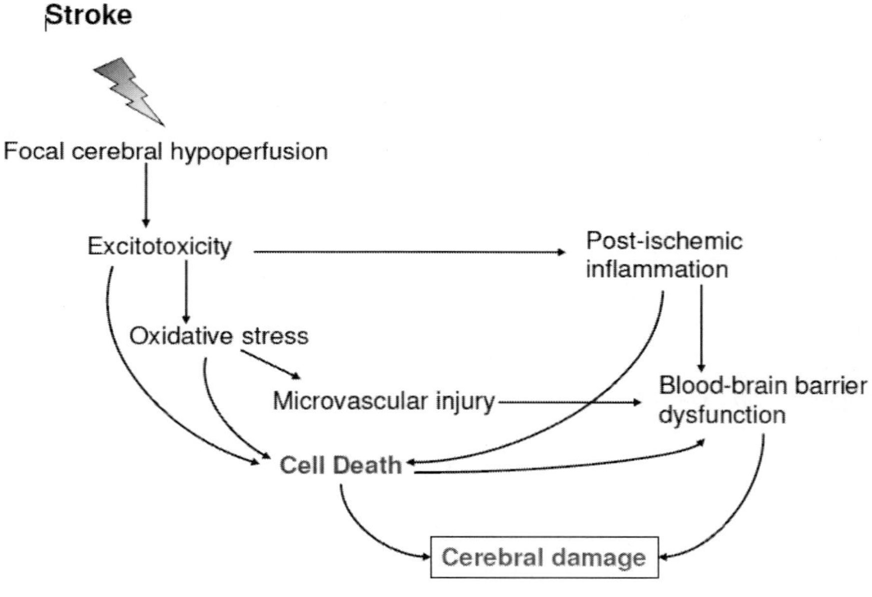

Figure 1. Ischemic cascade leading to cerebral damage: Ischemic stroke leads to hypo-perfusion of a brain area that initiates a complex series of events. Excitotoxicity, oxidative stress, microvascular injury, blood-brain barrier dysfunction and post-ischemic inflammation lead ultimately to cell death of neurons, glia and endothelial cells. The degree and duration of ischemia determine the extent of cerebral damage.

Mechanisms of Neuronal Injury

Cerebral ischemia results in a number of hemodynamic, biochemical, and neurophysiology alterations (Ostrowski RP 2006). A series of complex acute, subacute and chronic events occur after the incidence of stroke and reperfusion (Jean WC 1998). Ischemic injury involves energy failure, loss of cell ion homeostasis, acidosis, increased intracellular calcium excitotoxicity, free radical-mediated toxicity, and pathological permeability of the blood-brain barrier (BBB). Free radicals, specifically reactive oxygen species (ROS) that are generated soon after ischemia, as well as in later stages of ischemic reperfusion (e.g., by inflammatory cells), are the fundamental mediators of reperfusion injury.

The development of hypoxic-ischemic neuronal injury is significantly influenced by the release of excitatory neurotransmitters, primarily glutamate and aspartate in the brain. This process is called excitotoxicity and is activated by depletion of cellular energy stores. Glutamate, normally stored inside the synaptic terminals, is released into the extracellular space in a depleted energy state, which then results in the opening of calcium channels associated with N-methyl- D asapartate (NMDA) and alpha-amino-3-hydroxy-5-methyl-4-isoxanole propionate (AMPA) receptors. This leads to an influx of calcium, sodium and chloride ions and efflux of potassium ions. (Siesjo BK 1989, Hademenos GJ 1997, Garcia JH 1994). The influx of calcium is responsible for the activation of a series of destructive enzymes such as proteases, endonucleases, and lipases that allow release of cytokines and other inflammatory mediators, resulting in the loss of cellular integrity (Siejo BK 1981, Becker KJ 1998). Inflammatory mechanisms play an important role in tissue injury by inducing the rapid production of many different inflammatory mediators. Within 30 minutes after ischemia and reperfusion, leukocytes recruited to the ischemic area activate mediators of inflammation such as oxygen free radicals, cytokines, and nitric acid.

Ischemia causes brain damage by activating the ischemic cascade, which progresses to local depletion of oxygen or glucose, causing failure of production of high energy phosphate compounds, like adenine triphosphate (ATP). This adversely affects energy-dependent processes necessary for tissue cell survival, and sets off a series of interrelated events culminating in cellular injury and death. The extent of damage usually depends on duration, severity, and location of ischemia. Neuron, owing to its role in impulse transmission, requires a constant supply of glucose and oxygen, in order to maintain the ionic gradients across its membrane, and is most susceptible to hypoxia changes. The various mechanisms involved in tissue injury/neuroprotection are:

- **Failure of mitochondria leads to depletion of cellular energy store:** This causes further energy depletion and may trigger cell death due to apoptosis. Ischemia also causes loss of potassium and ATP, which are essential for energy exchange. It has been observed that energy failure do not precipitate immediate cell death, but 5–10 min of occlusion may lead to irreversible brain injury. Most of the ischemic strokes do not usually cause complete occlusion of blood supply, however even a partial occlusion for prolonged period may cause harmful effect due to deterioration of ion gradient and by-products (like lactic acid, hydrogen ions) of anaerobic metabolism (Karaszewski JM 2009).
- **Loss of membrane ion pump function and its deleterious effects:** Ischemia, leading to inadequate energy supply at the cellular level, leads to malfunction of ion gradient, which results in loss of potassium in exchange of sodium, chloride, and calcium ions. This is accompanied by an inflow of water, resulting in rapid swelling of neurons and glia (cytotoxic edema).
- **Release of excitatory neurotransmitters:**
    - *Glutamate*: Ischemic cascade stimulates release of excitatory neurotransmitters in the brain, viz. glutamate and aspartate. Glutamate is vital for neuronal plasticity; however an uncontrolled release in ischemic areas mediate excitotoxic

synaptic transmission via activation of N-methyl-d-aspartate (NMDA), 2-amino-3-hydroxy- 5-methyl-4-propionate (AMPA) or kainite receptors, which allows Na+ and Ca^{2+} influx. This has disastrous effect on the neuronal membrane, due to: (i) utilization of already depleted ATP in maintaining calcium balance; and (ii) causing disordered activation of a wide range of enzyme systems (proteases, lipases, and nucleases). These enzymes and their metabolic products, such as oxygen free radicals, damage cell membranes, genetic material, and structural proteins in the neurons, ultimately leads to cell death (Nakanishi N 2009). Understanding of these steps has triggered a search for potential blocking agents (Brouns R 2009). Release of excitatory neurotransmitter, glutamate, to modulate activity in nearby neurons occur through six known mechanisms: (i) reversal of uptake by plasma membrane glutamate transporters (Szatkwoski M 1990), (ii) anion channel opening induced by cell swelling (Kimelberg HK 1990), (iii) Ca^{2+}-dependent exocytosis (Parpura V 1994), (iv) glutamate exchange via the cystine–glutamate antiporter (Warr O 1999), (v) release through ionotropic purinergic receptors (Duan S 2003), and (vi) functional unpaired connexons, 'hemichannels', on the cell surface (Ye ZC 2003). Though these various mechanisms of glutamate release have been elucidated, ambiguity still persists in terms of which of these mechanisms operate during normal physiological settings and which come into play during pathological settings like ischemia or stroke, since the latter may require conditions like cell swelling or a low extracellular Ca^{2+} concentration (Malarkey EB 2008).

- *Synaptosomal-associated protein 25* (*SNAP-25*): It is a neuron-specific protein, primarily localized in nerve endings and axons and involved in synaptic vesicle exocytosis, axonal outgrowth and transmitter release. Studies have shown that SNAP-25 is differentially regulated in ischemic stroke. Marti et al. (Marti E 1998) has demonstrated an increase in SNAP-25 mRNA levels in the infarct and penumbra of stroke patients, mainly during the first 6 days after stroke. The Ca^{2+}-dependent controlled exocytosis mechanism of glutamate release by the astrocytes is regulated by a complex of proteins, the soluble N-ethyl maleimide-sensitive fusion protein attachment protein receptor (SNARE) complex (Montana V 2004), which includes synaptobrevin 2, Syntaxin 1 and synaptosome-associated protein of 23 kDa (SNAP-23) (Parpura V 1995, Crippa D 2006) along with a Ca2+ sensor Synaptotagmin 4. Cultured astrocytes have been shown to exhibit expression of synaptobrevin II, cellubrevin and syntaxin but not SNAP-25 (Parpura V 1995). Astrocytes have also been observed to contain certain proteins which are important for sequestration of glutamate into vesicles. These proteins include: vacuolar type H+-ATPase (V-ATPase), which is responsible for creating the proton concentration gradient necessary for glutamate transport into vesicles (Araque A 2000, Bezzi P 2001) and the three known isoforms of vesicular glutamate transporters (VGLUT): 1, 2 and 3, which use the proton gradient created by V-ATPases to package glutamate into vesicles (Freneue RT Jr 2002, Anlauf E 2005). The glutamergic exocytosis of astrocytes has been noted to be potential targets for various pharmacological agents and molecular biological manipulations (Montana V 2004).

- **Production of oxygen free radicals and other reactive oxygen species:** These react with and damage a number of cellular and extracellular elements, of which vascular endothelium is particularly important. It may also act by means of redox signalling to initiate the apoptotic pathway.
- **Apoptosis**: In contrast to necrosis causing cell death in the ischemic core, apoptosis (programmed cell death) occurs in the peripheral neurons. Ischemic damage causes an early response in gene expression of Bcl-2 and p53, followed by release of proapoptotic molecules such as cytochrome c and apoptosis-inducing factor from mitochondria. This leads to the activation of caspases and other genes that augment cell death (Joza N 2001, Ekshyan O 2004). The caspase cascade can be activated either by an extrinsic or death receptor-dependent route; and an intrinsic or death receptor-independent (mitochondrial) pathway (Eldadah BA 2000). Ischemia also activates various other signalling pathways which ultimately culminate in cell death. Prominent among these, include p53 (Mihara M 2003), JNK (of MAPK family (Gupta S 1995)), c-jun (Hayashi T 2000), p38 (Barone FC 2000) and cyclin dependant kinase 5 (cdk-5) (Green SL 1997), which are potential targets for therapeutic intervention.
- **Neuroprotection:** Ischemic cascade also activated various neuroprotective mechanisms as a defense against apoptotic and necrotic cell death. These include:
    - *Bcl-2* gene family: Includes antiapoptotic and proapoptotic counter molecules. Antiapoptotic members suppress release of sequestered proteins; and can also modulate calcium fluxes and caspase activation in the ER and inhibit the active form of Bax in mitochondria (Thominius MJ 2003).
    - Heat shock protein 70 (HSP70): HSP 70 is one of the earliest to be released. Its mRNA is expressed within 1–2 h of ischemia, with subsequent deregulation in 1–2 days. In animal models, HSP70 inducer, geranylgeranylacetone, has shown efficacy in limiting infarct volume. It also acts by increasing *Bcl-2* expression and inhibiting monocyte/macrophage activation (Gifard RG 2004, Yasuda H 2005).
    - Prion protein (PrPc): PrP mRNA is upregulated during hypoxia, and it inhibits Bax-induced cell death in neurons. Studies have observed that PrPc deletion results in reduced post-ischemic Akt phosphorylation, enhanced caspase-3 activation, with resultant exacerbation of ischemic neuronal injury in animals (Weise J 2006).
    - Neurotrophin-3 (NT-3): Neurotrophins are growth factors, especially essential for the survival and maintenance of neurons, where NT-3 expression may be important in defining neuronal survival after brain ischemia. Animal studies have suggested that altered NT-3 expression following ischemia may be part of a physiological neuroprotective response after excitotoxic or ischemic damage (Yang JT 1998). Interestingly, continuous low-dose treatment with NT-3 protected against striatal neuronal loss in mild neonatal hypoxic/ischemic brain injury (Galvin KA 2003), suggesting that it might possibly be of therapeutic benefit in ischemic brain injury in man.
    - Granulocyte-colony stimulating factor (G-CSF): The initial studies by Schabitz et al. (Shabitz WR 2003) have unraveled the neuroprotective potential of the

potent haematopoietic factor G-CSF in an acute stroke model. Further studies have demonstrated the role of G-CSF in activating multiple cell survival pathways, reduction of infarct volume after stroke and possible role in improving long term behavioral outcome and plasticity after cerebral ischemia in animal models (Schenieder A 2005), while it has also been noted to offer protection to human cerebral neurons following *in vitro* ischemia (Jung KH 2006).

- Interleukin-10: IL-10 gene expression is elevated in association with most major diseases in the CNS and aids survival of neurons and glial cells by blocking the effects of proinflammatory cytokines and promoting expression of cell survival signals (Strle K 2001). Studies have also been suggested that following a cerebral ischemic attack, IL-10 may have a neuroprotective role (Spera PA 1998). It has also been reported that there is a significant reduction in serum IL-10 levels of stroke patients soon after an acute event, indicating that the anti-inflammatory response is subsequently downregulated in this subset of patients (Perini F 2001).

Knowledge of these mechanisms is vital in order to salvage brain tissue undergoing ischemic damage. Neuroprotective drugs that scavenge reactive oxygen species, inhibit excitotoxic neurotransmitters or inhibit apoptosis, if used during the ongoing phase of ischemic injury may help act to achieve this goal. Deep barbiturate coma, and recently described, NXY-059, the disulfonyl derivative of the radical-scavenging spintrap phenylbutylnitrone, is reported to be neuroprotective in stroke (Fernandez Gomez 2008).

Concept of Ischemic Penumbra

Cerebrovascular tissue undergoing ischemia has two layers: (a) outer layer of less severe ischemia (penumbra), supplied by collaterals, and contain cells which can be retrieved by timely therapeutic intervention; and (b) inner core of severe ischemia with blood flow below 10–25%, displaying necrosis of both neuronal as well as supporting glial elements. Following an ischemic injury, the center of the core is perfused at 10–12 ml/100 g/min or less, while the ischemic area around it (surrounded by the penumbra) is critically hypo-perfused at less than 18–20 ml/100 g/min and is at risk of dying within hours. In contrast, the penumbra is perfused at least likely at approximately 60 ml/100 g/min and is less likely to die (Heusman PU 2003). Neurons in the penumbra are mostly dysfunctional, but may recover if reperfused in time. This forms the basis of current protocols which favor early pharmacological intervention for re-canalization of occluded vessel, since it will not only salvage neuronal and glial cells from the penumbra, but also glial cells from the central ischemic core zone, thereby markedly limiting the size of infarcted tissue (Turner R 2007). (See below figure 2 of Ischemic pnembura)

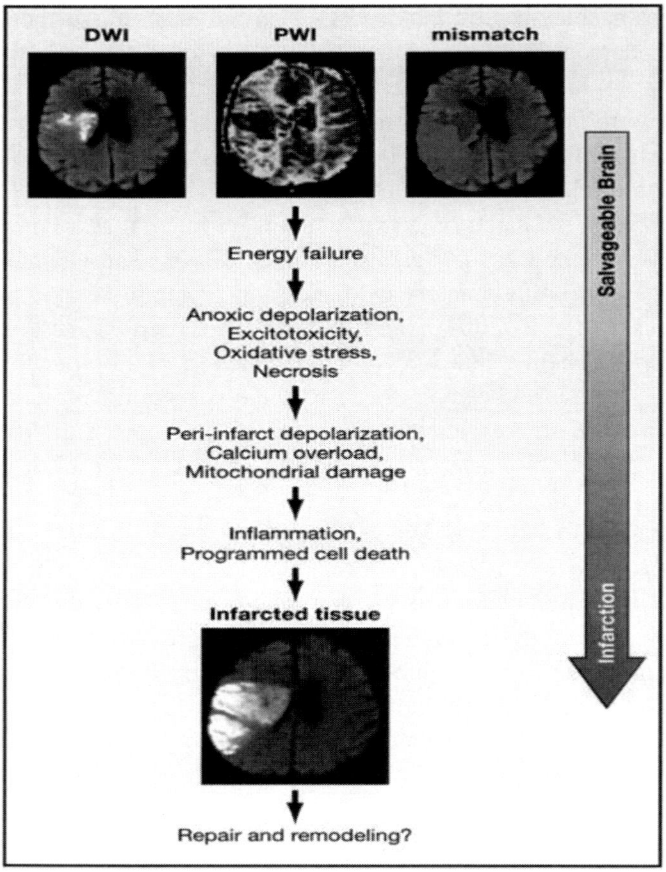

Figure 2. The Ischemic Penumbra: The ischemic penumbra represents compromised, but viable brain tissue lying distal to an occluded blood vessel. The top three MR images in this figure were taken in the same patient early after occlusion of the middle cerebral artery. The images are shown in the horizontal plane passing through the lateral ventricles. ''Stunned, but not dead tissue'' is detected by magnetic resonance imaging (MRI) techniques that assess (1) the spatial extent of the perfusion or blood flow deficit that presents as red and yellow areas on perfusion-weighted imaging (PWI, top middle image) and (2) severely damaged tissue in the ischemic core that presents as high-intensity areas on diffusion-weighted imaging (DWI, top left image) (Ebinger et al., 2009). In this patient, the perfusion deficit is larger than diffusion lesion. The top right image depicts the mismatch between core areas with a diffusion lesion (dark blue) and the larger areas with low perfusion (light blue-green). Over hours to days (see text), the core territory expands due to the complex cascades involving excitotoxicity, oxidative stress, programmed cell death mechanisms, and inflammation, as the initial trigger of energy failure ultimately progresses to infarcted tissue. The resulting infarct is shown in the image at the bottom of the figure and is about the size of the initial perfusion deficit in this untreated patient. In later stages, some patients may also partially recover, in part due to endogenous mechanisms of repair and remodeling (Chopp et al., 2007). MRI scans courtesy of G. Alberts, Stanford.

Cerebral Edema and Its Effects

This is of primary concern since it accounts for much of the death and disability. An understanding of the underlying mechanism, is important since management over the years have primarily addressed the effect without targeting the cause, which probably is attributable to the effects of neurogenic inflammation, mediated via neuropeptides, such as substance P. Klatzo classified edema as:

- Cytotoxic/cellular edema (Klatzo I 1987, Fishman RA 1992): Evolves within minutes to hours and are potentially reversible. It is characterized by swelling of all the cellular elements of the brain, including neurons, glia, and endothelial cells, due to failure of ATP-dependent ion (sodium and calcium) transport, as well as release of oxygen-derived free radicals.
- Vasogenic edema (Klatzo I 1987, Fishman RA 1992): Occurs over hours and days and are irreversible. It causes increased permeability of brain capillary endothelial cells to macromolecular serum proteins (e.g., albumin), resulting in an increase in extracellular fluid volume along with increased intracranial pressure (ICP).

This may displace the brain hemisphere; or shift one compartment of the brain, thereby compressing neurons, nerve tracts, and cerebral arteries. A sustained increase in pressure causes persistent ischemia; irreversible damage to brain cells; and, when severe may lead to cerebral herniation and potentially death. Initially acute hypoxia causes cytotoxic edema, which gives way to vasogenic edema with progression of infarction. This probably suggests that time is needed for the defects in endothelial cell function and permeability to develop.

Effects of Ischemia on Structural Integrity of Brain

- Apart from the deleterious effect on brain cells, hypoxia also causes loss of structural integrity of brain tissue and blood vessels, partly through the release of proteases like matrix metalloproteases (MMP). Loss of vascular structural integrity results in the breakdown of the protective blood–brain barrier, manifesting as cerebral edema, along with secondary progression of brain injury (Adibhatla RM 2008). Studies have shown alterations of vascular endothelial receptor expression in ischemic stroke. Enhanced expression of vascular endothelial receptors is possibly mediated by both protein kinase C (PKC) and mitogen activating protein kinase (MAPK) which are the basis of treatment with PKC and MAPK inhibitors to limit the infarct volume (Edyinsson L 2009).
- Brain ischemia also tends to activate the immune mechanism, which in some cases may be the cause for the exacerbation of damage and clinical deterioration of the patient. Experimental studies have shown that inhibition of the inflammatory process has led to the control of the extent of injury, an aspect which has gained paramount importance in understanding stroke and management of cases thereof (Ross R 1999, Ten Essecu R 2008, Adibhatla RM 2008).
- *Angiogenesis*: Extent of angiogenesis within the penumbra of ischemic stroke correlated with patient's survival time. This is mediated by either: (a) hypoxia inhibiting degradation of hypoxia-inducible factor-1 (HIF-1), which stimulates VEGF, which is essential for angiogenesis; (b) angiogenic growth factor secreted by inflammation-associated infiltrates (leukocytes, macrophages, damaged blood platelets) (Krupinski J 1994).

Hemorrhagic Stroke

This form of stroke occurs due to a blood vessel rupture in the brain. Its harmful effects are a resultant of: (a) hypoxia due to disrupted vascular supply; (b) irritant effect of releasing blood on brain parenchyma and vasculature; and (c) raised ICP due to continued bleeding, which may further restrict cerebral blood flow. In this respect, hemorrhagic strokes are more dangerous than ischemic strokes. There are two types of hemorrhagic stroke: intra-cerebral hemorrhage (generally occurs in small arteries or arterioles and is commonly due to hypertension, trauma, bleeding disorders, amyloid angiopathy, illicit drug use like amphetamines or cocaine, and vascular malformations), and sub-arachnoid hemorrhage (due to rupture of aneurysms from the base of the brain and bleeding from vascular malformations near the pial surface). It constitutes only 10–15% of all strokes (Escudero D 2008).

Atherosclerosis and Stroke

Atherogenesis is a decade-long process which involves luminal obstruction by cellular and extracellular substances. The pathogenetic process from onset of atherosclerotic changes in cerebrovascular or extracranial circulation to precipitation of acute ischemic stroke with its consequent cell damage is complex and many of the intermediary steps are not fully understood. Changes may manifest in the form of: (a) *fatty streak*, earliest lesions seen as yellowish areas of discoloration of intima, due to accumulation of lipid-filled macrophages (foam cells) in approximately 30% children below 5 years (Stary HC 1987); (b) *more advanced lesions with massive extracellular lipid* at the branching points of arterial vessels, in late childhood and early adolescence (Ip JH 1990); (c) *complicated fibrous plaques*: central acellular area of lipid covered by a cap of smooth muscle cells and collagen, seen in the third decade of life (IP JH 1990). Persons with risk factors for atherosclerotic disease (e.g., hypertension, hypercholesterolemia, cigarette smoking) tend to have clinically advanced atherosclerotic lesions with increased frequency. Sequence of events in atherogenesis is:

***(1) Injury to arterial wall*:** In his "response-to-injury" theory, Ross had hypothesized that, atherosclerosis is the effect of the complex interplay among monocytes, lipoproteins, platelets, lymphocytes, and smooth muscle cells in the intimal layer (Ross R 1999). Ip et al. In 1990 put forth a three-tier pathophysiologic classification system:

- *Type I injury*: Chronic minimal injury with functional alterations of endothelial cells without significant morphological changes, primarily caused by the turbulence of blood flow. Other contributory factors being hypertension, hypercholesterolemia, circulating vasoactive amines, immunocomplexes, viral infections, and tobacco smoke.
- *Type II injury*: Endothelial denuding and superficial internal injury, possibly due to toxic products released by accumulating macrophages in the intima. These changes may be accompanied by platelet deposition with or without thrombus formation, and subsequent thrombus incorporation.
- *Type III injury*: Manifested by deep intimal and medial damage, accompanied by marked platelet aggregation and mural thrombosis, generally following plaque rupture.

(2) Role of monocytes and T-lymphocytes in foam cell transformation:
The next important events are:

- *Circulating monocyte adhesion*: Abnormal shear stress at atherosclerotic lesion-prone sites in the circulatory system enhances the production of certain transcription factors, which promotes the expression of endothelial vascular cell adhesion molecule (VCAM), which is imperative for monocyte binding to endothelial cells (Gimbrone MA Jr 1995).
- *Monocytes insinuation* between the tight junctions of the endothelial cells to enter the subendothelial space.
- *Activation of immune mechanism*: In the form of T-lymphocyte activation, in both early fatty lesions and in advanced fibrous lesions, which helps monocytes migration and its transformation into "foam cell".

(3) Oxidation of LDL-cholesterol: Oxidation of LDL cholesterol induced by free radicals produced by macrophages, endothelial cells, or smooth muscle cells, participates by:

a) Formation of foam cells;
b) Cytotoxic properties promoting endothelial injury;
c) Chemoattractant for circulating monocytes; and
d) Inhibiting egress of macrophages from plaques (Adibhatla RM 2008).

(4) Smooth muscle cell migration and proliferation: A number of molecular factors may play a role in this vital plaque-forming process. They include growth factors (e.g., platelet-derived growth factor, or PDGF, a polypeptide released from blood platelets and endothelial cells that may attract smooth muscle cells to the intima and encourage them to divide); eicosanoids (which can stimulate the hydrolysis of cholesterol ester, producing free cholesterol); certain cytokines (e.g., tumor necrosis factor, interleukin-1 and interferon); and nitric oxide which acts to dilate blood vessels.

(5) Role of platelet: Platelet aggregation and adhesion promoted by toxic products released by macrophages and by moderate damage to the internal surface with denudation of the epithelium have vital roles in the progression of atherosclerosis (Ip JH 1990).

***(6) Plaque fissuring and thrombus formation**:* The process of plaque destabilization (fissuring and rupture, followed by thrombus formation) is not fully understood.

- **Plaque fissuring is possibly due to:**
  a) Loss of an internal lattice of collagen supporting the cap of the plaque., making it vulnerable to circumferential stress during systole;
  b) Infiltration of the cap tissue with foam cells, which possibly weakens the tissue by passively distorting the spatial arrangement of the connective tissue matrix or by actively destroying connective tissue matrix protein by lyric mechanisms (Slager CJ 2005).

- **Thrombus formation occurs by:**
  - o *Platelet activation*: On coming in contact with the sub-endothelial collagen, exposed by way of plaque rupture, circulating platelets get activated, and

subsequently aggregate and adhere, through interaction with platelet surface receptors (most important being GP-Ib-IX) and sub-endothelial protein ligand von Willebrand factor (VWF). An association between elevated vWF concentrations and arterial thrombosis has been described (Jansson JH 1991).

- *Platelet activation and blood flow*: Under high fluid shear-stress conditions, as in atherosclerosis, there is evidence that platelet aggregation depends on the binding of VWF to platelet GPIIb/IIIa, blockade, of which inhibits platelet aggregation and thrombus formation without disturbing the initial platelet adhesion (Stoll G 2008).
- *Activation of the coagulation cascade*: Endothelial injury constitutes the primary impetus for the initiation of the extrinsic pathway of the coagulation cascade. Activated platelets, apart from forming the backdrop of the clotting process, also acquire enhanced capacity to catalyze interactions between activated coagulation factors (which normally circulate as inactive precursors: *zymogens*). Factor Xa, is the active catalytic component of the "prothrombinase" complex, which converts prothrombin to thrombin. Thrombin cleaves fibrinopeptides (FPA, FPB) from fibrinogen, allowing the resultant fibrin monomers to polymerize, and converts Factor XIII to XIIIa, which crosslinks (XL) the fibrin clot. Thrombin accelerates the process by its potential to activate Factors V and VIII, while a number of natural plasma inhibitors retard clotting, including C1-inhibitor (C1 INH), tissue factor pathway inhibitor (TFPI), and antithrombin II (ATIII). The fibrin molecules aggregate together, trapping platelets, erythrocytes, and leukocytes to form the thrombus. Subsequently, there is a tendency for the clot to enlarge as blood flow slows around it, resulting in enlargement of size ("*propagating thrombus*").

- **Physiologic-subtypes of thrombosis related ischemic stroke:**

Ischemic stroke with different etiologies, possibly have a link based on the process of thrombosis:

- Atherothrombotic occlusion of larger arteries (e.g., carotid, middle cerebral, basilar): Most common causes of primary large vessel occlusive cerebrovascular disease, and also is the most common cause of stroke.
- Embolism is the second most common cause of stroke. Most are due to cerebral arterial atherothrombosis; or may also arise from other cardiogenic sources and deep vein thrombosis.
- Microatheroma of an influx of fat-like materials (lipohyalinosis) affects small vessels; and most prominently causing lacunar strokes.

(7) The potential outcomes of plaque fissuring: It includes:

a. Sealing of the fissure with fibrosis of incorporating thrombus; or
b. Mural intra-intimal and intra-luminal thrombosis, resulting in partial or transient reduction in blood flow (precipitating transient ischemic attacks: TIA). It may progress to occlusive thrombosis, which, if persistent due to absence of collateral flow, can lead to ischemic stroke (IP JH 1990).

(8) Evolution of cerebral atherothrombosis: Thrombosis may evolve over a few minutes, or take hours or even days. A stroke that is actively progressing as a direct result of increasing occlusion and ischemia is termed '*stroke in evolution*' or '*progressing stroke*'. A large blood vessel may evolve over a longer period of time, as compared to a smaller vessel, and there may be warning signs like TIA. Damage in ischemic stroke may result not only from infection, but also from edema, which generally peaks in 2–5 days. (*I*) *Hemorrhagic conversion*: Natural consequence of reperfusion of blood through damaged blood–brain barrier, in ischemic stroke, generally has 'bland' infarction associated with secondary bleeding. This is referred to as hemorrhagic conversion or hemorrhagic transformation (HT), and is characterized by gross parenchymal hematoma with possible intraventricular extension, midline shift and herniation; along with widespread leukocyte infiltration and macrophage invasion (Teal PA 1992). HT may be seen as hemorrhagic infarction (HI) or, less commonly, parenchymatous infarction (PH). Though both have different incidences, pathogenesis, and clinical outcome, but distinguishing HI and PH on CT may be difficult. On CT, HI appears as a discontinuous heterogeneous mixture of high and low densities occurring within the vascular territory of the infarct. In contrast, PH appears as a discrete, homogeneous collection of blood that often exerts mass effect and may extend beyond the original infarct boundaries or even into the ventricles (Teal PA 1992).

Recent studies have suggested the role of an abnormal expression of some matrix metalloproteinases (MMPs) which can degrade almost all components of the extracellular matrix and basal lamina such as laminins, fibronectin, or type IV collagen, weakening brain microvessels and predisposing them to rupture and increasing the risk of cerebral hemorrhage and precipitate hemorrhagic transformation events after stroke (Gasche Y 1992). Previous animal models (Heo JH 1999, Rosenberg GA 1996) have demonstrated an abnormal expression of MMP-2 (Galatians A) or MMP-9 (Galatians B) after cerebral ischemia and in lipopolysaccharide-injured brains (Mun-Bryce S 1998), contributing to brain injury and BBB breakdown. Further, Asahi et al. 2001 and Sumii et al. 2002 reported that pharmacological or genetic inhibition of MMP-9 has caused a significant reduction in size of the infarct, as well as the risk of hemorrhagic complications, while Wang et al. 2003 and Tsuji et al. 2005 noted tissue plasminogen activator-associated hemorrhage and edema appeared to be correlated to MMP-9 dysregulation. Investigations dealing with ischemic stroke in human subset have revealed high MMP-9 levels in peripheral blood, with MMP-9 levels showing correlation with poor neurological outcome, infarct growth, and hemorrhagic transformation events (Montaner A 2001, 2003). Rossel et al. 2008 have reported a strong neutrophil infiltration in the infarcted and hemorrhagic areas with local high MMP-9 content closely related to basal lamina collagen IV degradation and blood–brain barrier breakdown. Hemorrhagic infarction (HI) occurs regularly in the natural evolution of acute embolic stroke and is usually asymptomatic. Autopsy studies of HI may vary from patchy petechial bleeding to more confluent hemorrhages, with an occurrence rate ranging from 51% to 71% of recent embolic strokes (Teal PA 1992). According to another estimate (Leonard AD 1992), approximately 20% of patients with cardioembolic stroke have hemorrhagic transformation in the infarcted zone, usually occurring within 48 h, and is rare in the first 6 h. HI has been often explained as a result of reperfusion of the vascular bed of the infarct, such as would occur after fragmentation and distal migration of an embolus or after early reopening of a large vessel occlusion in the setting of a large infarction; the full pressure of arterial blood into hypoxic capillaries results in a diapedesis or red cells through their hypoxic walls (Mohr JP 1992).

It has been observed that HI may develop in areas distal to a persisting occlusion, suggesting that reperfusion is not always a prerequisite for this phenomenon. Many studies have found strong correlation with risk factors like:

1) One or more surges of arterial hypertension;
2) Associated hyperglycemia; and
3) Restoration of blood flow to ischemic territories.

Possible mechanism for this is marked tissue energy depletion accompanied by acidosis damaging brain vessels, causing leakage of edema fluid and red blood cells.

Parenchymatous infarctions (PH) occur less frequently, but are often symptomatic due to extension and mass effect beyond the original infarct territory (Teal PA 1992). In contrast to HI, it has been proposed that the pathogenesis of PH may involve "ischemic necrosis resulting in the rupture of small penetrating vessels analogous to hypertensive hemorrhage, leading to massive bleeding". Trials of thrombolytic therapy for acute ischemic stroke, has revived interest in this, since PH appears to be associated with anticoagulation therapy (Adhi bhatla RM 2008, Pandian JD 2009).

Free Radicals in Cerebral Damage

A vast amount of data implicates oxygen-derived free radicals (especially superoxide and hydroxyl radicals) and high-energy oxidants (such as peroxynitrile) as mediators of inflammation in ischemia/reperfusion injury (Cuzzocrea S 2001). Free radicals are highly reactive molecules generated predominantly during cellular respiration and normal metabolism. Imbalance between cellular production of free radicals and the ability of cells to defend against them is referred to as oxidative stress (Valko M 2007). After brain injury from ischemic stroke, the production of ROS dramatically increases, leading to tissue damage via several different cellular, molecular pathways, and mechanical pressure (Figure 3).

ROS can cause damage to cellular components such as lipids, protein, and nucleic acids, leading to subsequent cell death (Janardhan V 2004). Damage can become more widespread due to weakened cellular antioxidant defense systems in ischemia. ROS are the major stimulators of inflammatory cytokine production (such as interleukin-1, tumor necrosis factor-α, and interferon-γ) and protease secretion by microglia, leukocytes, and resident cells of the neurovascular unit (Haddad JJ 2002). As these neuroinflammatory mechanisms become activated, alterations in cytokine profiles, adhesion-molecule expression, and tight-junction components mediate further vascular leakage. Significant evidence exists suggesting that ROS are involved in every fundamental physiological step that leads to neuronal death (Cao W 1988) and thus are considered an important target in developing an effective stroke therapy (Juurlink BH 1997).

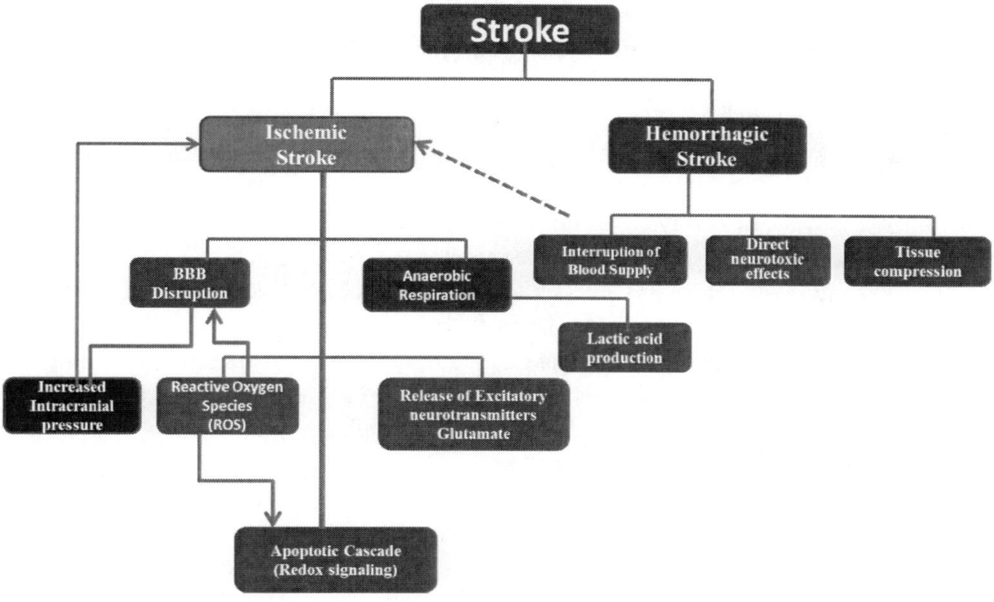

Figure 3. Schematic showing different types of stroke and cascade of events following ischemia.

Oxidative and Nitrosative Stress Oxidative and nitrosative stress are also powerful mediators of ischemic injury. In one scenario, the redox environment of cells modulates signal transduction cascades that tip the balance between prodeath and prosurvival pathways (Crack and Taylor, 2005). In the second scenario, ROS and perhaps reactive nitrogen species, including peroxynitrite, act directly as executioners of cell death (Chan, 2001). The brain appears particularly vulnerable to radical-mediated attack because of its limited antioxidant defenses (Adibhatla and Hatcher, 2010). Until recently, it was accepted that during ischemia ROS were generated principally by mitochondria, a well-known ROS source during electron transport and oxidative phosphorylation. However, it was recently shown that NADPH oxidase generates the majority of superoxide anion produced in vivo and in vitro during NMDA receptor activation and ischemia (Brennan, 2009; Girouard, 2009). Thus, the mitochondrion does not appear to be the major source of radicals following NMDA receptor activation. However, the close proximity of NADPH oxidase to neuronal mitochondria (Girouard, 2009) raises the possibility that this enzyme generates ‘‘kindling’’ ROS that promote mitochondrial uncoupling, triggering a secondary ROS surge from mitochondria (Figure 3). These observations point to NADPH oxidase as a potentially important therapeutic target in stroke but also highlight the need for a better understanding of the interaction among the different ROS sources and the relative contribution of vascular versus neuronal sources. In this regard, a surprising finding has been that activation of NMDA receptors increases ROS both in neurons and vascular cells (Girouard, 2006), suggesting a role of vascular ROS in excitotoxic brain damage. Although this observation emphasizes the close relationships between vessels and neurons (see Protecting the Neurovascular Unit), it has not been established how vascular oxidative stress may contribute to tissue outcome in excitotoxic brain injury.

NO and related oxidation products are key players in excitotoxicity. Reactive nitrogen species have important cellular effects, such as inhibition of key mitochondrial enzymes, facilitating mitochondrial transition pore formation, DNA damage, PARP activation, and activation of Ca2+-permeable TRPM7 channels (Aarts and Tymianski, 2005; Pacher,2007). As a potential second mechanism, NO modifies protein groups by covalently attaching two cysteine residues forming an S-nitrosothiol derivatives. This posttranslational modification significantly impacts cell survival by altering, for example, the function of critical regulatory proteins such as campuses, metalloproteases (GU et al., 2002), and the glycolytic enzyme GAPDH (Nakamura and Lipton, 2009). As NO has the potential to target a number of specific cysteine residues to alter protein function, the impact of S-nitrosylation is (largely) underexplored in the ischemic process. Taken together, the experimental evidence implicating oxidative and nitrosative stress in stroke is strong. But the translation of these fundamental concepts into clinical applications has proven to be challenging. Most recently, a nitrone-based radical spin trap failed in the final phase 3 clinical trial for acute ischemic stroke (Shuaib, 2007). And more broadly, the history of antioxidant therapies in clinical trials for neurodegeneration has been littered with many disappointments (Kamat, 2008). Overproduction of reactive nitrogen and oxygen species are surely damaging to brain cells. But at lower, homeostatic levels, radicals are critical signaling molecules participating in normal neuronal and vascular function (Faraci, 2006). Finding novel ways to scavenge or suppress deleterious radicals without interfering with endogenous signaling will be important to design effective therapies. As discussed above for excitotoxicity, a desirable strategy would be to develop drugs that only become activated by the pathological state intended for inhibition, i.e., during oxidative stress (Lipton, 2007b). Another approach would be to test antioxidant molecules with pleiotropic properties, such as activated protein-C (APC). APC blocks ROS generation, suppresses postischemic inflammation, and blocks apoptosis in neurons and endothelial, thereby providing both parenchymal and vascular protection (Yamaji, 2005; Cheng, 2006; Liu,2004). APC as well as other pleiotropic agents with a broad spectrum of activity in experimental stroke are undergoing clinical trial testing (Ginsberg, 2009).

Excitotoxicity

Cerebral ischemia initiates a cascade of detrimental events including glutamate associated excitotoxicity, membrane lipid degradation, DNA damage, formation of reactive oxygen species and acute inflammation, which lead to the disruption of cellular homeostasis and structural damage of ischemic brain tissue. Excitotoxicity and calcium overload are major factors contributing to the early stages of ischemic cell death. The canonical pathway asserts that glutamate, the most abundant neurotransmitter, accumulates into the extracellular space as a consequence of energy and ion pump failure, as well as the failure of re-uptake mechanisms (Choi and Rothman, 1990). The glutamate overload leads to prolonged stimulation of AMPA and NMDA ionotropic receptor subtypes to dramatically enhance the influx of calcium, sodium, and water into neurons. Massive calcium influx activates catabolic processes mediated by proteases, lipases, and nucleases (Ankarcrona, 1995). In addition, activation of nNOS, PLA2, and other Ca2+-dependent enzymes leads to production of NO, arachidonic acid metabolites, and superoxide, which act as additional triggers of cell death

(Dirnagl, 1999; Lo et al., 2003). For these and other reasons, oxidative phosphorylation becomes uncoupled; leading to further ATP depletion, ROS production, and release of stored Ca2+ from mitochondria, further accelerating a series of catastrophic events that lead to acute cell death. Despite the validation of glutamate toxicity in the laboratory setting and its enormously positive impact on the quest for new therapeutics in neuroscience, numerous clinical trials targeting NMDA and AMPA receptors have failed to improve outcome in stroke patients (Ginsberg, 2009). Although replete with shortcomings in trial design and implementation, the failure to translate has reinforced the notion that the glutamate hypothesis may have oversimplified the complexity of the cell death process and underestimated the diversity of expressing cell types as well as the heterogeneity of glutamate responses following receptor overstimulation in stroke. Moreover, it is likely that NMDA-AMPA pathways comprise only a subset of routines disrupting ionic imbalance following glutamate receptor activation. As originally conceived, the NMDA-AMPA model did not consider the delayed and invariably fatal glutamate-independent calcium influx following oxygen-glucose deprivation or the failure of the glutamate receptor blockade to halt cell death after very intense oxygen-glucose deprivation (Aarts, 2003).

Equally importantly, it could not account in an obvious way for the death of non-neuronal cell types such as abstracts, vascular cells, or microglia in ischemic tissue. An alternative viewpoint is that the drugs tested in clinical trials were poorly chosen, because many of them block all receptor functions (Lipton, 2007a). As a result, the dosing may have been suboptimal, due to the development of untoward side effects that prevented dose escalation to neuroprotective levels. A more suitable approach would be to use therapeutic agents that selectively target excessive channel opening (e.g., uncompetitive inhibitors with a relatively fast offrate, such as mountain (Orgogozo, 2002; Mobius and Stoffler, 2002; Lipton, 2006; Kavirajan and Schneider, 2007), thereby retaining normal receptor functions (Lipton, 2007a).

To add to the complexity, it is now known that NMDA receptor location and subunit composition differently regulate neuronal survival or death, although the strength of the calcium signal may specify the fate of neurons best following NMDA over-activation (Stanika, 2009). With notable exceptions, selective enhancement of synaptic receptors (in which NR2A peptide subunits predominate over NR2B) promotes neuronal survival, whereas activating extra synaptic receptors (in which NR2B peptide subunits predominate over NR2A) promote cell death (Chen,2007), in part, by activating death-associated protein kinase 1 (Tu,2010). Turning CREB-dependent signaling and BDNF expression up or down is critical for cell fate determination during NMDA receptor activation. The MAP kinase family members P38 and ERK1/2 participate, most likely by phosphorylation-dependent regulation of sub-membrane scaffolding proteins and NR2A and NR2B receptor subunits (Hardingham, 2002). Under ischemic conditions, the vulnerability to cell death is reduced when postsynaptic scaffolding proteins are modified, and PSD-95 binding is prevented (Cui, 2007). Moreover, successfully targeting the glutamate receptor complex early on would also diminish the opening of the downstream channels, e.g., transient receptor potential channels (TRP) and acid-sensing ion channels, as well as suppress the frequency of cortical spreading depolarizations (see below), ongoing within the ischemic penumbra. Hence, understanding and leveraging the repertoire of diverse responses and mediators at the receptor and second messenger level can only enhance possibilities for successfully targeting excitotoxicity for the treatment of ischemic injury.

Calcium Dysregulation

It is also known that increased calcium influx from glutamate receptor overactivation combined with release of Ca2+ from mitochondria and other stores (e.g., endoplasmic reticulum) may not fully account for the irreversible buildup of intracellular Ca2+ after excitotoxic stimulation. Other channels and ion pumps activated during ischemia in addition to glutamate receptors have been implicated in the Ca2+ accumulation. These include the Na+/Ca2+ exchange (Bano, 2007) hemichannels (Contreras, 2004), acid-sensing ion channels (Xiong et al., 2004), volume-regulated anion channels (Kimelberg et al., 2006; Simard, 2007), and TRP channels (Aarts and Tymianski, 2005). In particular, ASIC1a, activated by ischemia-induced acidosis, is involved in the Ca2+ influx and its inhibition is neuroprotective (Simon, 2006). ASICs are stimulated within the pH range commonly found in ischemic brain tissue, thus explaining the well-established link between acidosis and worsening of ischemic outcome in animals and humans. Failure of Ca2+ efflux mechanisms, especially the Na+/Ca2+ exchanger also contributes to the Ca2+ accumulation. Prostaglandin E2 EP1 receptors have a role in the failure of the Na+/Ca2+ exchanger during ischemia, and their inhibition is markedly neuroprotective (Abe, 2009; Kawano, 2006). Therefore, targeting Ca2+ influx-efflux mechanisms may be a valuable approach to counteract Ca2+ dysregulation and associated injury in conjunction with novel drugs targeting glutamate receptors.

Cortical Spreading Depolarizations

In addition to excitotoxic events at the molecular and cellular level, massive release of glutamate and ionic imbalance negatively impact the evolution of ischemic injury at the tissue level. Cortical spreading depolarization (CSD), a high energy consuming phenomenon akin to the cortical spreading depression of Leao, is triggered by high levels of extracellular glutamate and K^+ and is characterized by slowly propagating massive depolarization of neurons and astrocytes along with drastic disruption of ionic gradients (Somjen, 2001). Electrophysiological and imaging data convincingly demonstrate CSD in patients with ischemic stroke (Dohmen, 2008). In experimental animals, a single cortical spreading depolarization expands the area of severe hypoperfusion by more than 20% (Shin, 2006). In fact, it appears that a greater frequency, but more importantly, duration of DC shifts correspond to accelerated infarct maturation and core expansion (Mies, 1993; Back, 1996). The infarct expansion is probably due to mismatch between high metabolic demand to support membrane re-polarization and marginal tissue perfusion due to constrained penumbral blood flow (Back, 1996). Hence, suppressing CSD may prove worthwhile for reducing infarct maturation. Notably, the noncompetitive NMDA receptor antagonist ketamine markedly suppressed CSD frequency in head injury patients (Sakowitz, 2009), but it is unclear whether it improved clinical outcome. By contrast, irreversible depolarizations resistant to NMDA receptor antagonists (anoxic depolarization) developments in the ischemic core territory (Nellgiad and Wieloch, 1992) and are probably terminal events contributing to severe ionic imbalance and tissue failure.

Inflammation

Focal ischemia evokes a robust inflammatory response that begins within a few hours of onset and typifies the secondary or delayed response to ischemia. It involves the activation of microglia and astrocytes as well as an influx of hematogenous cells recruited by cytokines, adhesion molecules, and chemokines across the activated blood vessel wall. Stimulated brain cells and blood vessels then communicate with one another through a complex network of paracrine and autocrine signaling. The highly choreographed response evolves over many days, with multiple signals and targets triggering expression of novel proteins and secondary infarct expansion (Kleinig and Vink, 2009). Innate and adaptive immune systems participate as well. At least early on, inflammation amplifies the ischemic lesion, but, as discussed later, it may set the stage for tissue repair in the late post-ischemic period. A number of therapeutic trials designed to target the inflammatory response have failed to show clinical benefit (Sughrue, 2004), underscoring the need to clarify further the complexities of acute and delayed postischemic inflammatory signaling within the brain. As noted above, cerebral blood vessels are the first to be exposed to the ischemic insult, and their reaction to injury sets the stage for the inflammatory response. Early on, production of cytokines, such as TNF-α and IL1b, in vascular cells and perivascular microglia-macrophages upregulates adhesion molecule expression (e.g., ICAM-1, P and E-selectin) and, along with integrins, promote leukocyte rolling and sticking to the vessel surfaces (Zhang 1998). Neutrophils are the first blood-borne cells to be recruited into the brain, followed by monocytes and, starting on days 1–2, lymphocytes. As the brain's primary immune cell, activated microglia transform into macrophages and accumulate at the border zone along with blood-borne macrophages to clear debris and dead cells and produce pro-inflammatory mediators and toxic molecules (Schilling, 2003). Molecules released from injured or dying brain cells also contribute to the inflammatory response. In particular, products from cells undergoing oxidative stress and necrosis, for example lipopeptides, advanced glycation end-products (AGE), modified lipids, heat shock proteins, hyaluronic acid, and the nuclear protein HMGB1, lead to activation of the innate immune system by engaging toll-like receptors (TLRs). TLRs are expressed in multiple cells and, in conjunction with CD36, receptors for AGE (RAGE), and other scavenger receptors, may serve to detect ''danger signals'' triggering NFkb-dependent inflammatory signaling (Oppenheim and Yang, 2005; Wang, 2007). PARP activity appears to function as an NFkb coactivator (Chiarugi and Moskowitz, 2003), with therapeutic potential for delayed administration of PARP-1 inhibitors (Kauppinen, 2009). Besides NF-kB, other transcriptional activators, including activator protein-1, STAT-3, interferon regulatory factor 1, and C/EBP beta, exert a proinflammatory effect (Kapadia, 2006; Iadecola, 1999), while PPARgamma acts as a negative modulator of postischemic inflammation (Kapadia, 2008). In addition to neutrophils and monocytes, T cell subsets have recently been implicated as modulators of secondary infarct progression. Treg cells express the antinflammatory cytokines IL10 and TGF-β and normally dampen the immune response by suppressing T cell effector activity (Liesz, 2009). Secondary infarct progression is impacted by a second subset of invading T lymphocytes, gamma-delta T cells, a source of the proinflammatory cytokine IL-17. After deletion of IL-17, infarct size decreases (Shichita, 2009).

These findings support the notion that taming post-ischemic inflammation may block secondary events that extend brain injury. However, as noted below, during the later stages in the injury process, inflammation promotes critical events necessary for tissue repair. Therefore, therapeutic interventions targeting post-ischemic inflammation should be mindful of temporal considerations by minimizing the destructive potential of inflammation in the acute phase while enhancing its beneficial contributions to tissue repair in the late stages of cerebral ischemia. Necrosis, Necroptosis, and Autophagy: The Execution Necrosis and apoptosis are the principal mechanisms of cell death after ischemic injury, and the details of both have been mentioned (Yuan, 2006, 2009). Depending in part upon the magnitude, type of stimulus, and cell type, a number of cell death triggers promote necrosis or apoptosis, although cellular features of apoptosis and necrosis are sometimes found together in dying ischemic cells. Probably due to its ATP dependence, apoptotic cell death is prominent after milder injury and is more delayed (Bonfoco, 1995), although severe ischemia is associated with early-onset of caspase cleavage, enzyme activation, and acute cleavage of substrate proteins (Namura et al., 1998).

Apoptosis and necrosis can be induced by multiple triggers, such as Ca2+ overload or oxidative stress. Mitochondria play an essential role in both (Schinzel, 2005), serving as a reservoir for proapoptotic and antiapoptotic proteins and cytochrome C. One such protein apoptosis-inducing factor (AIF) is released from the outer membrane of mitochondria in response to activation of the nuclear protein PARP and generation of a PAR polymer, its toxic product (Yu, 2006). AIF then translocates to the nucleus to promote a caspase-independent form of cell death, in part by promoting DNA fragmentation and chromatin condensation. Release of mitochondrial proteins sets in motion (or suppresses) multiple caspase-dependent and -independent processes to dismantle critical homeostatic and repair mechanisms. Despite the expression of executioner procaspases, activated caspases, and caspase cleavage products, classic apoptotic morphology is rarely found in humans within the adult ischemic brain. However, it does appear more prominently in the ischemic brains of neonates (Ferriero, 2004).

Until now, necrotic cell death was defined as unregulated, unprogrammed, and lacking cell signaling events. It is the predominant form of ischemic cell death. It was recently shown that certain cells, including those within the brain, possess a molecular switch that determines whether cells die by necrosis or apoptosis in a TNF-dependent way (Holler, 2000). In this cell death variation, necrosis are triggered by two kinases, RIP 1 and RIP 3, reciprocally interacting, often in the presence of an apoptosis inhibitor (Cho, 2009). Activated RIP3 is capable of stimulating enzymes such as the glycogen-degrading enzyme, glycogen phosphorylase, to steer TNF-induced apoptosis toward necrosis, in part through bursting energy metabolism and ROS generation (Zhang, 2009). Nec-1, a small-molecule inhibitor of RIP-1, decreases ischemic cell injury in models of ischemia-reperfusion and improves neurological outcome, suggesting RIP-1 as a potential therapeutic target (Degterev, 2005). Autophagy, an energy-dependent process implicated as a cell death mechanism, is used by eukaryotes to degrade and recycle subcellular organelles. Its precise role in the death process is controversial because autophagic activity may be cytoprotective, at least in some disease models, e.g., polyglutamine expansions or in aging models (Levine and Kroemer, 2009). In other disease models, such as in neonatal hypoxia-ischemia, autophagy reportedly promotes cell death (Puyal, 2009). Precisely how this is accomplished remains for further study.

Inflammation and Stroke

Currently there is increasing evidence that some form of inflammatory mechanism plays a role in the development and progression of stroke, especially in the setting of cerebral ischemia due to subarcahnoid hemorrhage, head injury or cardiac arrest. It has been reported that low grade inflammation with raised levels of C-reactive protein (CRP) is an independent risk factor for stroke and TIA (Di Napoli M 2001). In pediatric population, inflammation without significant atherosclerosis has been associated with stroke. Novel imaging techniques have been adopted to facilitate *in vivo* observation of the dynamic effects of inflammation in causing brain tissue damage and neurologic outcome.

Inflammatory conditions associated with stroke

Stroke has been associated with a wide range of systemic inflammatory conditions. It may be associated with primary vasculitis, like giant cell arteritis, primary angitis of CNS, Takayasu's arteritis; vasculitis secondary to SLE, progressive systemic sclerosis, rheumatoid arthritis; and other inflammatory conditions like inflammatory bowel disease (IBD) and sarcoidosis. Fortunately the majority of these are rare, with stroke being an unusual complication in most cases (Emsley HC 2002, Hu Z 2000).

Infective Conditions Associated with Stroke

A number of acute and chronic infective conditions have been observed to precede a stroke. Most often these are of respiratory and bacterial origin, occurring within the previous month. These cases tend to present with more neurological deficit as compared to ones without infection (Campbell LA 2000, Grayston JT 1990, Tarnacka B 2002). Of the chronic infections *Chlamydia pneumoniae* has been known to affect macrophages/monocytes, endothelial cells, and vascular endothelium and thus having a pivotal role in atherogenesis. Evidence to this regards have been in the form of demonstration of the organism in atherosclerotic plaques of coronary artery and middle cerebral artery (Campbell LA 2000), and seropositivity in more than 50% individuals in their sixth decade (Grayston JT 1990). Currently, an acute recrudescence of infection (diagnosed by immunoglobulin M titers) is associated with acute stroke and TIAs. Similarly, increased serum levels of immune complexes containing chlamydial lipopolysaccharide have also been associated with increased stroke incidence and worse clinical outcome (Tarnacka B 2002). *Helicobacter pylori* have also been implicated in stroke pathogenesis, with one report emphasizing association with small vessel occlusion. However, seropositivity for *H. pylori* may be an independent risk factor for ischemic stroke (Emsley HC 2002, Grau AG 2001). Recurrent or chronic respiratory infection (independent from acute episodes), herpes virus, periodontal infection (gingivitis or periodontitis) has been suggested to be independent risk factors in ischemic stroke (Emsley HC 2002, del Zeppo G 2000). Neurological complications, though, are common in human immunodeficiency virus infections, associated with stroke remains unclear. It has been suggested to conduct randomized intervention studies, especially in cases of *C. pneumoniae*, in order to resolve the uncertainty over the temporal sequence of infection and stroke.

Inflammatory Mediators in Acute Stroke

The onset of ischemic cascade heralds the initiation of various processes, including inflammation, excitotoxicity, nitric oxide production, free radical damage, and apoptosis, all of which play a role in tissue injury. The molecular consequences of brain ischemia include temporal changes in cell signaling, signal transduction, metabolism, and gene regulation/expression. Currently these are potential therapeutic targets to minimize tissue loss and neurologic deficit by lessening the proportion of penumbral tissue recruited into the infarcted core. Inflammation occurs both by the molecular and cellular components at the blood-microvascular endothelial cell interface (Tan asesco 2008, Adibhatla 2008). With the onset of brain ischemia, microglia, astrocytes, endothelial cells, and neurons are known to release a number of cytokines, like interleukin-1β (IL-1β) and tumor necrosis factor-α (TNF-α), which enables leukocyte recruitment, activation, and the final adhesion to the endothelium of the cerebral microvasculature. These activated leukocytes obstruct the vascular channel, followed by transmigration in the infected areas along with monocytes/macrophages. Similarly, reperfusion, and systemic inflammatory processes, both before and after acute stroke, may also stimulate the inflammatory response, thus hampering the efficacy of thrombolytic therapy.

Inflammatory Gene Expression

Cerebral ischemia is known to upregulate the expression of a number of proinflammatory genes like transcription factors, heat shock proteins, cytokines, chemokines, and adhesion molecules. Among this transcription factor, nuclear factor (NF)-κB, has been demonstrated to regulate expression of TNF-α, IL-1β, IL-6, nitric oxide synthase (NOS), cycloxygenase-2 (COX-2) and intercellular adhesion molecule-1 (ICAM-1) during *in vitro* conditions (Tan asesco 2008, Adibhatla 2008, del Zoppo G 2000). In the periphery (NF) - κB, was expressed by activating macrophages, monocytes, lymphocytes, endothelial cells, fibroblasts, platelets, while in cerebral infarctions (NF)-κB has been seen to be induced in activated microglia and glial cells (Terai K 1996).

Cytokines

These are polypeptides associated with inflammation, immune activation, and cell differentiation or death. In systemic setting these are produced by activating macrophages, monocytes, lymphocytes, endothelial cells, fibroblasts, platelets, and many other cell types, whereas in CNS their source are activated microglia. Proinflammatory cytokines like TNFα, IL-1β lead to parenchymal damage, while IL-10 and IL-1 receptor antagonist (IL-1ra) have an anti-inflammatory and neuroprotective role.

- *Tumor necrosis factor-* α: Permanent or focal MCAO has been associated with induction of TNF-α mRNA. The effects of this proinflammatory cytokine have been controlled by administration of soluble TNF-receptor 1 (sTNF-R1) or anti-TNF-α monoclonal antibody. The TNF - a expression appears sequentially in ischemic core, periinfarct areas, adjacent brain, followed by remote areas. CSF and blood levels have been elevated in most ischemic stroke patients, within first 6–12 and 24 h of onset. In lacunar infarcts, elevated levels have been associated with early neurologic deterioration and poor functional outcome. Elevated sTNF-RI and sTNF-RII concentrations are associated with carotid atherosclerosis, while sTNF-RI concentrations are increased in patients with acute ischemic stroke and infection (Adibhatla RM 2008, Emsley HC 2002, Buttini M 1996, Elkind MS 2002).

- *Interleukin-1*: Experimental studies have proved its proinflammatory property, which have been neutralized by IL-1ra administration (Emsley HC 2005). In contrast, neutralizing antibody to IL-1ra has resulted in enhancing the effects of brain ischemia. Increased IL-1 messenger RNA (mRNA) expression in peripheral mononuclear cells have been seen 1–3 days after onset of symptoms and reducing to normal levels by 20–31 days (Kostulas N 1999). Elevated plasma IL-1ra levels have been seen in patients with acute ischemic stroke within 4±2 days (Beamer NB 1995, Emsley HC 2002, Adibhatla RM 2008).
- *Interleukin-6*: Cerebral ischemia is a potential bioactivator of IL-6 mRNA, especially in middle cerebral artery occlusion (MCAO) in animal models. Intracerebroventricular injection of anti-inflammatory IL-6 has been associated with significant reduction in ischemic damage. In a clinical study, circulating IL-6 levels were found to increase significantly, reaching a plateau between 10 h and 3 days, before returning to baseline by 7 days. It also correlated with volume of computed tomography of brain lesion, as well as, poor functional and neurologic outcome. Similar correlation in CSF studies has also been noted. However, IL-6 may also have a proinflammatory role, as in advanced atherosclerosis.
- *Transforming growth factor*-β: Increased expression of TGF- β 1 RNA and protein expression has been seen after an ischemic stroke, especially in infarct border zones (Krupinski J 1996). Its expression in penumbra and in recovery phase of some CNS diseases suggests a neuroprotective function.
- *Interleukin-10*: In ischemic and hemorrhagic stroke cases, peripheral blood mononuclear cells are seen to secrete this neuroprotective cytokine (Van Exel E 2002). Studies have shown that lower IL-10 levels are associated with increased risk of stroke.
- *High mobility group protein*-1 (*HMG*-1): It is a ubiquitous and abundant nuclear and cytoplasmic protein and a chromatin component in eukaryotic cells; which acts by binding to DNA, in addition to facilitating gene transcription and stabilizing the nucleosome structure. It is released and secreted by activated innate immune cells, macrophages, monocytes and astrocytes, and can act as a proinflammatory mediator, and also acts to promote the release of other proinflammatory mediators (Kumar A 2008). Experimentally antiHMG1 antibodies have been used to counter its effect on ischemic injury.
- *Other cytokines*: Limited studies and evidence are available with interferon-γ (IFN-γ), IL-2, IL-4, IL-16, IL-17, and granulocyte-macrophage colony stimulating factor (GM-CSF) (Emsley HC 2002).

Chemokines

These polypeptides are generally smaller than cytokines, and have a role in cellular communication and inflammatory cell recruitment in host defense. Of these, IL-8 and monocyte chemo-attractant protein-1 (MCP-1), of the CXC and CC chemokine families, respectively, have been implicated in cerebral ischemia (Mennicken F 1999):

- *IL-8*: Studies have noted that patients with ischemic stroke have IL-8 mRNA expressing mononuclear cells in blood and elevated IL-8 in plasma, which possibly has a proinflammatory role in recruiting neutrophils. Overall, CSF levels are higher than plasma level, indicating its site of production in CNS (Kostulas N 1999). Interestingly, CSF levels of IL-8 tend to increase initially and then fall rapidly in large infarcts or gray matter infarcts suggesting a proinflammatory role, in contrast to constant elevated levels (for 3 months) in small white matter lesions suggesting a neuroprotective function (Tarkwoski E 1999).
- *MCP-1*: Significant rise in acute ischemic stroke (proinflammatory) has been associated with monocyte/ macrophage infiltration (Losy J 2001).
- *Interferon-γ-inducible protein-10* (*IP-10*): In a recent study by Canoui-Poitrine et al. (Canoui Poitrine F 2009), it was observed that in healthy middle-aged men, higher systemic levels of chemokines like IP-10 and RANTES are most likely independent predictors of future ischemic stroke.
- *CC chemokine ligand-5* (*CCL-5*)/*Regulated on Activation Normal T Cell Expressed and Secreted* (*RANTES*): Aggregates of RANTES, a member of the CC chemokine family, that form on the cell surfaces have been reported to mediate through its receptor (CCR5), and act as powerful activators of leukocytes for promoting the directed migration of leukocytes into damaged or inflamed tissue (Appay V 2001, Backon KB 1995, Canoui Poitrine F 2009). It is produced by a variety of cells, including T-lymphocytes, platelets, endothelial cells, smooth muscle cells, and glial cells. A study by Terao et al. (Terao S 2008) strongly implicated this chemokine in the pathogenesis of experimental ischemic stroke, and suggested that the RANTES that mediates the cerebral inflammation, blood–brain barrier dysfunction, and tissue infarction is largely derived from circulating blood cells.

Nitric oxide and cycloxygenase-2 (COX-2) Three NOS isoforms exist (Del Zoppo G 2000):

- Neuronal NOS: Harmful effects on ischemic stroke.
- Endothelial NOS: Beneficial effect, since it causes vasodilatation.
- Inducible or immunologic NOS (iNOS): Contributes to ischemic injury. Inhibition of iNOS reduces infarct volume in middle cerebral artery obstruction (MCAO), and it has been demonstrated in neutrophils and blood vessels in patients who died within 24 h of ischemic stroke (Forester C 1999).

Experimental cerebral ischemia have shown elevated COX-2 mRNA and protein, as well as toxic prostanoids and reactive oxygen species, secreted by microglia, at the border of the ischemic territory, and thought to exacerbate the effects of ischemia (del Zoppo G 2000).

Matrix Metalloproteinases (MMPs)

These are a family of proteolytic enzymes involved in extracellular matrix modeling, but may contribute to the neuroinflammatory response. Upregulation of MMP-9 in the acute phase, as compared to MMP-2 in chronic recovery stage reflects both deleterious and beneficial effects (Adibhatla RM 2008, Mun-Bryce S 1998). MMP, especially MMP-9 levels, have been associated with poor neurological outcome, infarct growth, and hemorrhagic transformation events (Montanner J 2001 and 2003, Ross A 2008).

Adhesion Molecules

Leukocyte interaction with vascular endothelium is mediated by three main groups of cell adhesion molecules: selectins (comprising P-selectin, E-selectin, and L-selectin); integrins (e.g., lymphocyte function-associated antigen-1, and Mac-1); and the immunoglobulin superfamily (which includes ICAM-1 and vascular adhesion molecule-1: VCAM-1) (DeGraba TJ 1998). These molecules not only enable leukocyte infiltration during acute stroke, but also have a role in pathogenesis of atherosclerosis and changes in atheromatous plaque. In the human brain, the expression of ICAM-1, VCAM-1, and E-selection of cerebral microvascular endothelial cells is increased by IL-1β, TNF-α, and lipopolysaccharide. Localized ICAM-1 type is expressed in histologically normal human carotid bifurcation, a high-risk region for the development of atherosclerotic plaque, whereas endothelial ICAM-1 expression is increased in symptomatic versus asymptomatic carotid plaque. Serum levels of sICAM-1 (and E-selectin) are elevated in cerebrovascular (large and small vessel) diseases; becomes high after cerebral ischemia; and attains peak levels in 24 h of acute ischemic stroke. In contrast, sVCAM-1 elevates between days 1 and 5, and peaks at 5 days (Emsley HC 2002).

Neuropeptides

A number of neuropeptides have been implicated in the genesis of neurogenic inflammation, including substance P (SP), calcitonin gene-related protein (CGRP) and neurokinin A (Karaszeski B 2009). Stimulation of the neuronal C-fibers by vanilloids, histamine or prostaglandins, among others, leads to neuropeptide release.

- *Neuropeptide Y* (*NPY*): This modulates the immune cell distribution, T helper cell differentiation and natural killer cell activation. Studies have shown that NPY and its receptor Y1 partly mediate ischemic/reperfusion injury via upregulation of nNOS and eNOS, the effects of which can be controlled by NPY-Y1 receptor inhibition. NPY levels, in experimental studies, were found to be increased at 6 h in the peri-ischemic region and peaked at around 3 days, decreasing at 10 days (Askalan R 2001).
- *Substance P*: Most potent of the neuropeptides. Is a member of the tachykinin family that also includes neurokinin A (NKA), neurokinin B (NKB) and neurokinin? (NK?) (Turner R 2007). These peptides are produced from preprotachykinin genes 1 and 2 (Campos MM 2000) SP potentially binds to three receptors (NK1, NK2, NK3) but has a higher affinity for the neurokinin 1 (NK1) receptor, which results in neurogenic inflammation, manifesting as increased vascular permeability, vasodilatation, tissue swelling and cell migration. Release of SPmaybe one of the earliest pathophysiological events associated with injury to the brain, leading to release of inflammatory cytokines, free radical and endothelial nitric oxide (Persson MG 1991). SP is capable of regulating the action of other neurotransmitters, including dopamine and acetylcholine, and the opening of inward cation channels, in particular calcium. Levels of SP has been observed to be raised in ischemic stroke, while administration of an SP antagonist (SR-140333, nolpitantium besilate) significantly reduced infarct

volume and improved neurological function measured at 24 h following ischemia (Karaszeski B 2009).

Cellular Arm

The key components of this arm are blood derived leukocytes, which have a role in secondary brain damage in ischemic and reperfusion stages; while microglial cells, are the major CNS source of cytokines and other mediators, and also become phagocytes when fully activated by neuronal death.

Leukocytes

Elevated total leucocyte counts, independent of smoking, have been associated with higher incidence of vascular diseases and cerebral infarction. Various studies have shown that neutrophil accumulation starts within 6–12 h of onset, increases for 24 h, peaks in 48–72 h, and finally replaced by mononuclear cells in 4–6 days. This also correlates with CSF neutrophil levels (Akopoy SE 2006).

Microglia

Generally microglia is in a resting phase and constitutes 5% to 20% of glial population. During ischemia, depending on the time and extent, these get activated, and undergo substantial morphological and metabolic transformation, along with rapid and profound genetic upregulation. Subsequently they transform into the principal CNS source of cytokines like IL-1β, TNF-α, and TGF- β (Gregerson R 2000).

Acute Phase Reactants and Body Temperature

In the normal condition body tends to respond to various tissue injury, including inflammatory and infective conditions, by means of cytokines, primarily IL-6 and IL-1. The classic acute phase reactants in cerebrovascular ischemia are C-reactive proteins (CRP), serum amyloid A protein, and fibrinogen.

C-reactive Protein

Healthy person normally has a median CRP concentration of approximately 1 mg/L, while during any tissue injury, inflammation or infection it tends to undergo 100-fold or more increase. Elevated CRP levels have been demonstrated to predict the risk of: (a) first ischemic stroke among apparently healthy men; (b) future ischemic stroke and TIA in the elderly; and (c) fatal stroke in the elderly. Studies have shown a very early increase (within 3 h) in patients with acute stroke with or without infection, and are an independent predictor of survival or nonfatal vascular event after ischemic stroke (Hu Z 2000, Rost NS 2001).

Erythrocyte Sedimentation Rate And Fibrinogen (ESR)

In cases of ischemic stroke, elevated ESR is an independent predictor of poor outcome within the first month, and early stroke recurrence (Belestrino M 1998). In contrast, fibrinogen, is an independent risk factor for stroke and significant hyperfibrinoginemia occurs in patients with acute cerebral infarction in association with leukocytosis and an increase in leukocyte aggregation (D'Erasmo E 1991, Belch J 1998).

Body Temperature

Studies on animal models revealed hypothermia of the brain and body had profound influence on stroke outcome, since it tends to reduce infarct size, unlike hyperthermia, which enhances neuronal damage (Yenari M 2008, Mi'nembres E 2008). Subsequent clinical studies have shown that body temperature has been independently and significantly related to initial stroke severity, lesion size, mortality, and outcome in survivors. Elevated body temperature in patients with acute stroke, possibly due to infections, has been associated with increased morbidity and mortality.

Role of Neuroimaging in Evaluation of CNS Inflammation in Stroke

Newer imaging techniques have enabled *in vivo* evaluation of cerebral inflammation, and subsequent correlation with neurologic outcome and brain tissue damage. These include gamma camera imaging of reinjected 111indium-labeled leukocytes (Pozzili C 1985) demonstrating neutrophilic infiltration within 24 h of acute cerebral infarcts; and technetium-99m hexamethylpropyleneamine oxime (99mTc HMPAO)-labeled leukocyte brain single-photon emission computed tomography (Wang PY 1993), showing neutrophilic accumulation with infected areas. PK11195 is a specific ligand for the peripheral benzodiazepine binding site. After cerebral ischemia, increased binding of PK11195 is colocalized with invading the cells of mononuclear-phagocytic lineage, in and around infarcted tissue. Presence of activated microglia can be demonstrated for weeks after onset of ischemic injury (Gerhard A 2000).

Proposed Interactions Unifying Various Pathophysiologic Mechanisms

A wide range of mechanisms has been proposed for unifying and linking inflammation, infection, atherosclerosis and vascular risk factors in the pathogenesis of stroke.

Inflammatory Mechanisms

Apparently inflammation, marked by raising CRP levels, is the pivotal point, which not only contributes to atherogenesis, but also contributes to plaque rupture, precipitating acute thromboembolic phenomenon, culminating in acute stroke. However, the interactions between these multiple factors are quite complex. CRP may be elevated in a number of cardiovascular risk factors like increasing age, smoking, body mass index, lipid levels, and hypertension, while hypertension it may have a proinflammatory role mediated by sICAM-1 and IL-6 (Pasceri V 2000).

It may also be elevated in response to other infective etiologies, and have a proinflammatory effect by modulating expression of adhesion molecules on vascular endothelium, with subsequent recruitment of monocytes and other immune cells. These, along with activated T-cells release various growth factors and cytokines, like TNF-α and IL-1, leads to advanced phase of atherosclerosis (Barath P 1990, Galia J 1996).

Procoagulant State

A prothrombotic state in various inflammatory and infectious conditions, with altered immune function, predisposing thelarge vessel to atherothrombosis and stroke. Modulation occurs due to reduced circulating antithrombotic activated protein C (APC), elevated C4b-binding protein, and a low ratio of tissue plasminogen activator to plasminogen activator inhibitor, or due to increased fibrin D-dimer levels, Cardiolipin immunoreactivity, and fibrinogen levels (Kumar A 2008, Ameriso SF 19991).

Evidence of continued endothelial damage is reflected by increased levels of vWF, while acute episodes are represented by raising CRP levels, which act in tandem with proinflammatory cytokines, like IL-6, to produce a procoagulant state, which act by the extrinsic pathway (Di Napoli M 2001). Procoagulant state precipitating occlusive cerebrovascular disease is encountered in a number of disease process:

(a) SLE: Antiphospholipid antibodies like anticardiolipin antibodies and lupus anticoagulant acts by inhibition of prostacyclin formation, causing platelet aggregation; inhibition of prekallikrein, alterations of antithrombin III, decreased fibrinolysis, decreased release of plasminogen activator, inhibition of protein C activation, and the induction of endothelial injury and thrombotic thrombocytopenic purpura (Kumar A 2008, Kitagawa Y 1990).
(b) Inflammatory bowel disease: Affected by hypercoagulability-related thrombosis, vasculitis, and consumption coagulopathy leading to hemorrhagic events (Lossos A 1995).
(c) Bacteriemia and septicemia: Incidence of thromboembolism in infective endocarditis and in septicemia is 20% and 10%, respectively. Mechanisms of thrombosis responsible include reduced levels of antithrombin III, proteins C and S, increased platelet aggregation and adhesion, impaired fibrinolysis, and antiphospholipid antibody formation; apart from the effects of endotoxins,

Other bacterial toxins, and proinflammatory cytokines such as IL-1 and TNFα (Veltonen V 1993).

Vasculitis and Altered Circulation

Though atherothrombosis and atherothrombotic embolism are the commonest mechanisms for cerebrovascular occlusion, other less frequent causes include inflammatory vasculitis, like giant cell arteritis, Takayasu arteritis and Wegener granulomatosis; and infective pathology due to Mycoplasma infection, varicella zoster and neurosyphilis (Emsley HC 2002, Eskalan R 2001).

Vascular supply may be compromised in cervical artery stenosis, due to preexisting anomalies of extracellular matrix; or due to cardioembolism in a setting of systemic lupus erythmatosus (SLE) with valvular heart disease.

For the above considerations and more, there is a compelling need to accelerate efforts to interrogate the stroke process and define the links that exist with other conditions such as vascular and neurodegenerative dementia. It is also crucial to expand the narrow repertoire of therapeutic opportunities for these devastating conditions. To accomplish this, novel approaches are required that expand upon our evolving mechanistic understanding of the fundamentals of cell survival and death processes as well as tissue repair. The future depends upon how successful we are in deciphering these mechanisms and bringing clarity to the complex interactions between the multiplicity of cell and tissue types within the brain (Lo, 2003). Armed with this knowledge and its successful therapeutic application, the field of stroke could be transformed.

Keeping in view this spirit, we will now try to address the selected issues fundamental to the science of ischemic stroke and vascular dementia. It begins with posing questions about stroke risk factors followed by a discussion of key cell and tissue mechanisms that render brain susceptible as well as tolerant to ischemic injury, including those promoting tissue protection and repair. The chapter ends by highlighting promising treatment strategies, inspired by these endogenous mechanisms, which present the opportunity to open new avenues in stroke therapy.

Stroke Risk Factors and Triggers

A stroke risk factor is a characteristic of an individual that increases the risk for stroke compared to someone without that characteristic (Hankey, 2006). Some risk factors cannot be modified, such as a family history of cerebrovascular diseases, older age, male sex, and Hispanic or Black race (Allen and Bayraktutan, 2008; Hankey, 2006). Other risk factors are modifiable, and their correction reduces the chance of having a stroke (Table 1). These factors, which often coexist, have been estimated to account for 60%–80% of stroke risk in the general population (Allen and Bayraktutan, 2008; Hankey, 2006). Genome-wide association studies are increasingly being employed to identify susceptibility genes for stroke (Hegele and Dichgans, 2010). Although several loci have been identified, the need for independent replication and the modest effect sizes have precluded the full assessment of the clinical relevance of these findings (Hegele and Dichgans, 2010).

Table 1. Major Modifiable Risk Factors for Ischemic Stroke

Classification	Risk Factor	References
Casuals	Hypertension	Lawes et al., 2004a
	Diabetes	Lawes et al., 2004b
	Hypercholesterolemia	Amarenco et al., 2006
	cigarette smoking	Bonita et al., 1999
	atrial fibrillation	Hart et al., 1999
	valvular heart disease	Kizer et al., 2005
	ischemic cardiomyopathy	Loh et al., 1997
	carotid stenosis	Rothwell et al., 2003
Probable	Hyperhomocysteinemia	Wald et al., 2002
	increased inflammatory markers (WBC, CRP, infection)	Di Napoli et al., 2005
	elevated plasma fibrinogen	Rothwell et al., 2004
	Dyslipidemia	Holme et al., 2009
	patent foramen ovale	Nedeltchev et al., 2008
	obstructive sleep apnea	Culebras, 2009
	body mass index	Hu et al., 2007
	lack of exercise	Hu et al., 2005
	low fruit and vegetable diet	Dauchet et al., 2005
	psychosocial stress	Simons et al., 1998

[a] Factors demonstrated in randomized clinical trials to reduce stroke risk if corrected, or for which a strong, consistent, and independent association with stroke has been established (Hankey, 2006).

[b] Factors for which the association with stroke is less firm and/or no causative role has been established.

WBC, white blood cells; CRP, C-reactive protein.

Risk Factors and Propensity to Stroke?

Risk factors have profound effects on the structure and function of blood vessels and on their interface with circulating blood. Many of the established risk factors alter the vascular structure by promoting atherosclerosis and stiffening of the arteries and by inducing narrowing, thickening, and tortuosity of arterioles and capillaries (Allen and Bayraktutan, 2008; Iadecola and Davisson, 2008). With the brain, these morphological changes are often associated with reductions in resting cerebral blood flow (CBF) and marked alterations in CBF regulation. Thus, aging, hypertension, diabetes, and hypercholesterolemia impair vital adaptive mechanisms that assure that the brain is adequately perfused (Arrick, 2007; Iadecola and Davisson, 2008; Iadecola, 2009; Kitayama, 2007). The ability of the endothelium to regulate microvascular flow is compromised, while the increase in blood flow evoked by neural activity is suppressed, resulting in a mismatch between the brain's energy supply and demand (Arrick, 2007; Iadecola and Davisson, 2008; Iadecola, 2009; Zou, 2004a).

Some risk factors, like hypertension and diabetes, impair protective vascular mechanisms that keep CBF stable during reductions in blood pressure (cerebrovascular autoregulation), facilitating the occurrence of ischemia if intravascular pressure drops (Immink,2004; Kim,2008). These vascular alterations increase the brain's vulnerability to ischemia after arterial occlusion because they compromise the development of collateral flow arising from adjacent nonischemic vascular territories, which is vital to the survival of the ischemic perinfarct zone (see Parenchymal Failure Section). In addition to their vascular effects, some risk factors, like aging and diabetes, may enhance the intrinsic susceptibility of brain cells to injury, amplifying the tissue damage produced by ischemia (Biessels,2002), but the biological bases of this effect are not well understood. Little is known about the interaction among the different stroke risk factors and whether their vascular effects are additive or synergistic. Furthermore, the relative contribution of parenchymal and vascular factors to stroke risk remains to be determined.

Cerebral Blood Vessel Alteration by Risk Factors?

Many cardiovascular risk factors increase the production of reactive oxygen species (ROS) and promote inflammation in systemic and cerebral blood vessels. The predominant vascular sources of ROS are the superoxide-producing enzyme NADPH oxidase, xanthine oxidase, mitochondrial enzymes, and uncoupling of nitric oxide synthase (NOS), a state in which this enzyme generates superoxide instead of NO (Faraci, 2006) (Figure 4).

Many of the damaging effects of oxidative stress on blood vessels are related to the biological inactivation of NO by the free radical superoxide, which reduces NO bioavailability and prevents its beneficial effects (Pacher, 2007; Schulz, 2008). Thus, loss of the vasoregulatory effects of endothelial NO leads to vasoconstriction and reduced NO-dependent vascular responses, with a negative impact on the regulation of microvascular flow (Schulz, 2008). Loss of the antiaggregant, antiproliferative, and anti-cell adhesion effects of NO promotes platelet aggregation, leukocyte adhesion to endothelial cells, and smooth muscle proliferation, key steps in vascular inflammation (Pepine, 2009; Zou, 2004b).

In addition, ROS can directly promote inflammation by increasing blood-brain barrier (BBB) permeability through upregulation of vascular endothelial growth factor (VEGF) and by inducing the expression of cytokines, matrix remodeling enzymes, including metalloproteases, and proinflammatory genes through NFkb activation (Marchesi, 2008). One such NFkb-dependent gene product, inducible nitric oxide synthase, produces large amounts of NO, which alter vascular structure and function through nitration and nitrosylation of critical proteins (Gunnett, 2005; Guzik, 2003; Lima, 2010).

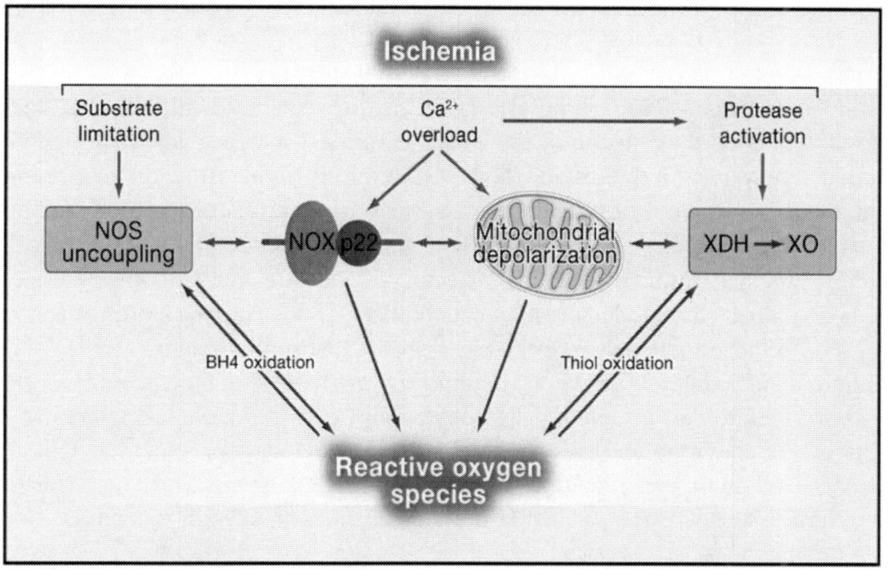

Figure 4. Major Sources of ROS in Brain and Blood Vessels. Stroke risk factors and ischemia lead to the activation of several ROS-generating enzymatic systems. In ischemia, the increase in cytosolic Ca2+ activates the superoxide-producing enzyme NADPH oxidase (NOX), through PKC and NO derived from neuronal NOS (Brennan, 2009; Girouard, 2009). Mitochondria become depolarized by the Ca2+ overload (Nicholls, 2008) and, possibly, by ROS derived from NADPH located near the mitochondria (Girouard, 2009) producing large amounts of superoxide. The Ca2+-induced activation of proteases and/or the pro-oxidant environment convert xanthine dehydrogenase (XDH) to xanthine oxidase (XO) (Abramov, 2007), a superoxide-generating enzyme involved in purine degradation. Finally, the substrate deprivation induced by ischemia and the oxidative inactivation of essential cofactors like tetrahydrobiopterin (BH4) uncouple L-arginine oxidation from NO formation by NOS, resulting in superoxide production (NOS uncoupling) (Förstermann, 2010). Other potential sources of ROS include enzymes for arachidonic acid or catecholamine metabolism, but their participation in stroke-induced oxidative stress remains in question (Adibhatla and Hatcher, 2010; Kunz, 2007a).

Peroxynitrite, a potent nitrating agent produced by the reaction of NO with superoxide, alters vasomotor reactivity by inactivating critical endothelial and smooth muscle enzymes and by activating the DNA repair enzyme poly-ADP-ribose polymerase (PARP), which leads to ATP depletion and vascular ion channel dysfunction (Pacher, 2007). Whereas ROS may set the stage for inflammation, vascular inflammation, in turn, leads to ROS production, creating a vicious circle that enhances vascular damage. Activation of the plasminogen system by oxidative stress and inflammation promotes matrix remodeling, smooth muscle cell migration, and intimal hyperplasia (Nicholl, 2006), factors that promote atherosclerosis and alterations in vascular structure. Thus, oxidative stress and vascular inflammation are major pathways through which risk factors exert their deleterious effects on blood vessels. However, it remains to be determined how individual risk factors trigger the activation of one or both of these processes. This is a critical question for targeting preventive strategies in patients with specific risk factors.

Role of Stroke Triggers

While vascular risk factors increase the likelihood of stroke in affected individuals, precipitating factors that act as ''stroke triggers'' must also be postulated. In some patients, the specific event responsible for the arterial occlusion can be identified, e.g., neck trauma leading to dissection and occlusion of the Table 1. In most instances the factors precipitating the ischemic event cannot be established. Although systemic infections, pregnancy and puerperium, use of illicit drugs, and mental stress often trigger a stroke (Elkind, 2007), precisely how these factors exert their effect remains unclear. Exacerbation of vascular inflammation and activation of the coagulation cascade are likely to play a role (Welsh, 2009). For example, the added vascular dysfunction and blood clotting abnormalities, superimposed on those induced by stroke risk factors, could precipitate vascular occlusion or hemodynamic insufficiency. This view is supported by the fact that acute stroke often occurs in the setting of increased circulating leukocytes and elevated plasma markers of systemic inflammation and vascular activation, which also predict a poor outcome (Elkind, 2007; Welsh, 2009). Thus, our understanding of stroke triggers is limited, and mechanistic studies addressing these issues would be valuable in the identification of high-risk cases.

Parenchymal Failure: Brain Death during Ischemia?

Because of its high intrinsic metabolic activity and large concentrations of the neurotransmitter-excitotoxin glutamate (Choi, 1992), the brain is especially vulnerable to ischemic insult. This can develop either as a consequence of thrombosis in situ or following embolic occlusion of a cerebral blood vessel, the latter usually arising from the heart or atherosclerotic plaques in the carotid artery and aortic arch. Although neurological dysfunction occurs within seconds to minutes of vessel occlusion, the evolution of ischemic injury and cell death continues in stages for minutes, hours, and even days, depending, in part, upon the vulnerability of the particular brain region, its cellular constituents, and the extent of residual perfusion.

The responses of blood vessels and their perfusion are important to the outcome as well. For example, a deficiency of vasodilating molecules such as endothelial NO enlarges the stroke size (Huang, 1996). Early restoration of blood flow by clot lysis and reperfusion decreases ischemic injury, and this may be achievable by giving recombinant tissue plasminogen activator (tPA), the only FDA-approved treatment for reestablishing flow and salvaging brain tissue. However, tPA is used in <10% of patients and even less frequently after 3 hr because of the risk of hemorrhage into ischemic tissue (NINDS tPA Study Group, 1995). Moreover, tPA may have other unintended risks (Kaur, 2004), such as injury to the blood-brain barrier by activating matrix metalloproteinases (Wang, 2003) or excitotoxicity in experimental models (Nicole, 2001). Combination therapies that ameliorate these effects may extend the TPA's therapeutic window while mitigating the untoward effects of reperfusion and plasminogen activation (Liu, 2004; Cheng, 2006; Murata, 2008). Theoretically, that could prolong tissue viability for hours or even longer, depending upon the rapid delivery of drug to the compromised brain (Ginsberg, 2008). Whether or not the vulnerable brain tissue can be rescued or protected after a protracted time period in the absence of partial or complete restoration of blood flow is an unanswered question. In all likelihood, areas of vulnerable brain do remain viable for hours after vessel occlusion, at least in some instances. For example, the hemiparesis that follows middle cerebral artery occlusion in the baboon was reversed in 73% of animals with reperfusion at 2–4 hour, compared to 33% and 17% in animals with reperfusion at 8 and 16–24 hour, respectively (Marcoux, 1982; Crowell, 1981; Jones, 1981). The challenge then is to restore adequate blood flow quickly after vessel occlusion and to protect viable tissue from unleashing mechanisms that lead to cell and tissue demise.

Salvageable versus Non-salvageable Tissue as Target for Therapy: Tissue distal to an occluded blood vessel is often heterogeneous, meta-stable, and differentially susceptible to ischemic injury. This meta-stable zone, termed the ischemic penumbra or the perinfarct zone (Astrup, 1981), is characterized by significantly depressed tissue perfusion that is barely sufficient to support basal ATP levels and oxygen metabolism as well as normal ionic gradients in the presence of electrical silence and suppressed protein synthesis. The ischemic penumbra, then denotes an "at risk" region that is functionally impaired but potentially salvageable. However, unless perfusion is improved or calls made relatively more resistant to injury, the tissue at risk dies within a few hours (Lo, 2008a, 2008b). The ischemic core by contrast, refers to the irreversibly damaged tissue distal to an occluded blood vessel, characterized by <20% of baseline blood flow levels, depleted ATP stores, and irreversible failure of energy metabolism (Lo, 2008b). With time, the infarct core expands into the ischemic penumbra, and therapeutic opportunity is lost. Therefore, detecting a penumbra in patients can help to identify those who might benefit most from acute treatments that restore blood flow (thrombolysis or endovascular clot retrieval) or treatments for the future that render viable brain more resistant to ischemic injury. For this purpose, magnetic resonance imaging methods such as perfusion-weighted and diffusion-weighted imaging are most often used. Perfusion-weighted imaging measures the spatial extent of blood flow compromise, whereas diffusion-weighted imaging is thought to detect the region of attenuated diffusion of water, a putative surrogate marker for severely damaged brain tissue. The difference is thought to reflect the ischemic penumbra (Figure 2) (Ebinger, 2009). Although the predictive value of this method is still debated, perfusion-diffusion mismatch provides a useful first attempt to define the tissue at risk.

Prominent Mechanisms Leading to Cell and Tissue Demise in Stroke?

Within the ischemic penumbra, multiple mechanisms have been identified over the past few decades that irreversibly damage brain tissue (Figure 5). Understanding the contribution of each informs us about potential therapeutic opportunities and treatment targets. In the area of severely limited blood supply, ATP utilization continues in the presence of minimal synthesis and levels drop, leading to acidosis and loss of ionic homeostasis. As a consequence, cells swell and membranes rupture. However, ischemic cell death cannot be equated with limited ATP availability; rather, tissue death develops as a consequence of numerous ionic, biochemical, and cellular events that impose overwhelming stresses upon already compromised tissue (Dirnagl, 1999; Lo, 2003).

Causes of White Matter Damage Underlying Vascular Cognitive Impairment VCI?

In the cerebral autosomal-dominant arteriopathy with subcortical infarct sandleuko-encephalopathy (CADASIL syndrome), amonogenic disease associated with dementia, extensive white matter damage is caused by notch-3 mutations in vascular smooth muscle leading to vascular insufficiency (Chabriat,2009).

In common forms of lacrosse, however, the mechanism of the white matter damage remains unclear, although family history, hypertension, diabetes, and chronic smoking are well established risk factors (Selnes and Vinters, 2006). The white matter lesions consist of demyelination, axonal loss, enlarged perivascular spaces, astrogliosis, and microglial activation (Fernando, 2006; Pantoni and Garcia, 1995). The wall of arterioles is thickened by accumulation of hyaline material (lipoialinosis) or completely disrupted (fibrinoid necrosis), leading to microhemorrhages (Fisher, 1968; Pantoni and Garcia, 1995). Capillary density, resting CBF, and cerebrovascular reactivity is reduced both in normal and affected white matter (Brown, 2007; Mandell, 2008; O'Sullivan, 2002).

Disruption of the arteriolar wall by amyloid, as observed in genetic or sporadic forms of cerebral amyloid angiopathy and in AD, is also associated with white matter lesions (Weller, 2009). Hypoxia-inducible genes and markers of endothelial activation are unregulated, suggesting hypoxia-ischemia (Fernando, 2006).

A causative role of hypoxia-ischemia is also suggested by the fact that the blood supply to the subcortical and basal ganglia white matter is provided by terminal arterioles located on the watershed between two vascular territories: perforating arteries from the neocortex and penetrating branches arising from larger arteries at the base of the brain (Iadecola, 2009). Therefore, these areas may be particularly susceptible to vascular insufficiency, especially if the structure of the arterioles and their vasomotor function are altered. On the other hand, energy and blood flow requirements of white matter are much lower than those of gray matter, rendering the tissue, in theory, less vulnerable to anorexia-ischemia (Hertz, 2008). Therefore, alternative mechanisms leading to an increased intrinsic vulnerability to injury may also play a role. For example, risk factors for dementia could enhance white matter susceptibility to anorexia, as aging has been described to do (Baltan et al., 2008). Disruption of the BBB, an early event in leukoaraiosis, could lead to injury by producing perivascular edema, microhemorrhages, and inflammation, contributing to demyelination (Farrell and Wardlaw, 2009). Demyelinated axons may be more susceptible to ischemic injury due to their heightened metabolic requirements caused by loss of energy-efficient salutatory conduction and leaky sodium channels (Trapp and Stys, 2009). Furthermore, dysfunction within the endothelium may compromise the trophic effect that these cells exert on neurons and glia, contributing to brain dysfunction and damage (see section on repair mechanisms). Aging, inflammation, hypoxia and, possibly, other risk factors can also reduce the repair potential of the damaged white matter by impairing oligodendrocyte progenitor recruitment and differentiation (Back, 2002; Pang, 2010; Sim, 2002). Therefore, the mechanisms underlying leukoaraiosis might be distinct from those of ischemic cell death and are a fertile ground for new investigations.

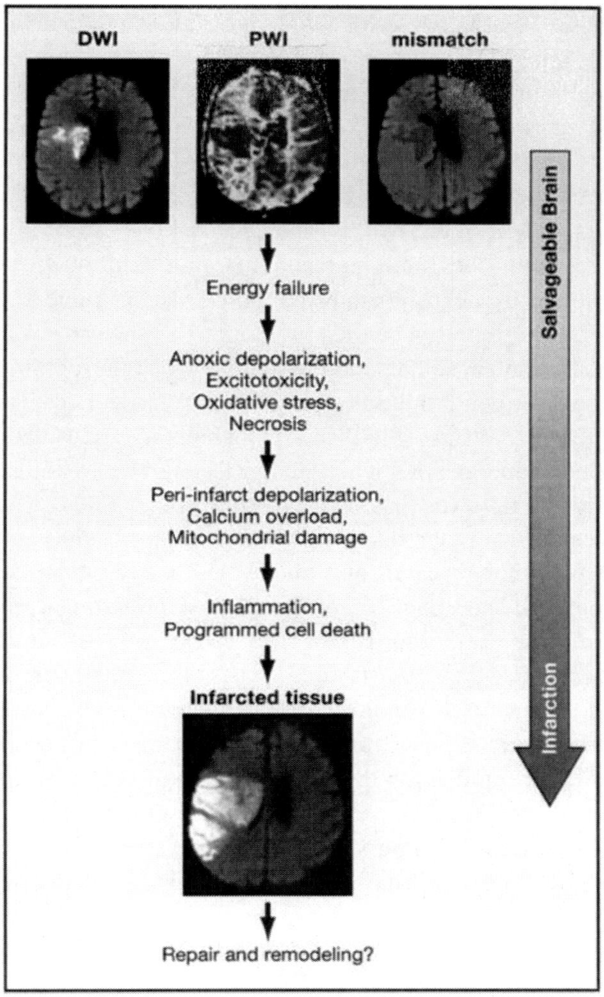

Figure 5. The Ischemic Penumbra. The ischemic penumbra represents compromised, but viable brain tissue lying distal to an occluded blood vessel. The top three MR images in this figure were taken in the same patient early after occlusion of the middle cerebral artery. The images are shown in the horizontal plane passing through the lateral ventricles. ''Stunned, but not dead tissue'' is detected by magnetic resonance imaging (MRI) techniques that assess (1) the spatial extent of the perfusion or blood flow deficit that presents as red and yellow areas on perfusion-weighted imaging (PWI, top middle image) and (2) severely damaged tissue in the ischemic core that presents as high-intensity areas on diffusion-weighted imaging (DWI, top left image) (Ebinger,2009). In this patient, the perfusion deficit is larger than diffuse lesion. The top right image depicts the mismatch between core areas with a diffusion lesion (dark blue) and the larger areas with low perfusion (light blue-green). Over hours to days (see text), the core territory expands due to the complex cascades involving excitotoxicity, oxidative stress, programmed cell death mechanisms, and inflammation, as the initial trigger of energy failure ultimately progresses to infarcted tissue. The resulting infarct is shown in the image at the bottom of the figure and is about the size of the initial perfusion deficit in this untreated patient. In later stages, some patients may also partially recover, in part due to endogenous mechanisms of repair and remodeling (Chopp, 2007). MRI scans courtesy of G. Albers, Stanford.

Stroke and Dementia?

The major mechanisms of tissue dysfunction and death cited above develop as a consequence of acute vessel occlusion and the attendant activation of endogenous mechanisms of cell injury and tissue demise. More subtle and less well understood mechanisms are beginning to define a new research frontier linking cerebrovascular dysfunction and small strokes to the development of vascular cognitive impairment (VCI) and Alzheimer's disease (AD), the most common causes of dementia (Fotuhi, 2009). AD and ''vascular'' dementia have traditionally been considered distinct entities (Iadecola, 2004). Thus, AD, the most prevalent of the two, is characterized pathologically by deposition of the amyloid b peptide (Ab) in the brain parenchyma (amyloid plaques) and blood vessels (amyloid angiopathy) and by neurofibrillary tangles (Querfurth and LaFerla, 2010). On the other hand, cerebrovascular diseases can lead to cognitive impairment in different ways. For example, a single stroke can cause dementia by damaging brain regions critical for cognition (strategic infarct dementia), while multiple strokes can cause stepwise cognitive deterioration through cumulative brain damage (multi-infarct dementia) (Leys, 2005; Pinkston, 2009). Most often, VCI has been due to small white matter lesions (leukoaraiosis) that are thought to interrupt neural pathways involved in cognition (Pinkston, 2009). A recent realization has been that AD and cerebrovascular diseases coexist in up to 60% of cases (Leys, 2005; Pinkston, 2009). Thus, although cases of ''pure'' AD and vascular dementia can exist, in most cases the cognitive decline can be attributed to overlapping cerebrovascular and AD pathologies (Querfurth and La-Ferla, 2010). The causes of leukoaraiosis and the overlap between AD and cerebrovascular diseases are discussed in the next sections. Stroke doubles the risk of developing dementia (Leys et al., 2005). Although, as discussed above, location, size, and number of ischemic lesions, as well as leukoaraiosis can account for the cognitive impairment in some cases, epidemiological and pathological evidence indicates that stroke also increases the risk for AD. Alzheimer pathology can facilitate the development of dementia in patients with ischemic injury, and, vice versa, ischemic injury can aggravate the cognitive deficits induced by AD (Fotuhi, 2009). These findings have suggested a previously unrecognized interaction between amyloid pathology and ischemic injury. This is not surprising, considering that Ab has powerful cerebrovascular effects. Ab constricts cerebral vessels, suppresses vascular reactivity, and impairs autoregulation, leading to vascular insufficiency and increased susceptibility to ischemic injury (Iadecola, 2004; Zhang, 1997).

Conversely, ischemia and hypoxia can induce Ab accumulation by promoting its cleavage from APP (Tesco, 2007) and by downregulating the lipoprotein-related receptor protein-1, a critical receptor in the vascular clearance of Ab (Bell et al., 2009; Tesco, 2007; Wu, 2005). Therefore, in a vicious cycle, the vascular effects of Ab aggravate ischemia, and, in turn, brain ischemia enhances Ab accumulation (Iadecola, 2004). Recent studies have also linked plasma Ab to the white matter damage underlying leukoaraiosis (Gomis, 2009; Gurol, 2006). The significance of this finding and its underlying mechanisms remain to be defined and placed in context with other findings showing that Ab could promote axonal injury directly through its cytotoxic effects (Querfurth and LaFerla, 2010) or indirectly by inducing vasoconstriction and ischemia (Iadecola, 2004). Therefore, the vascular dysfunction induced by circulating and parenchymal Ab may act in concert with the structural and functional vascular changes induced by the risk factors to amplify the vascular insufficiency in small white matter arterioles leading to white matter injury. However, factors other than Ab could also contribute to the interplay between AD pathology and cerebrovascular diseases. For example, cerebral arterioles of AD patients exhibit a tendency to constrict due to increased activity of transcription factors (serum response factor/myocardin) that control the expression of contractile proteins in smooth muscle cells (Chow, 2007). This finding may play a role in the increased vasoconstrictor tone and reduced CBF observed in AD (Iadecola, 2004). It remains to be established whether these changes in gene expression are related to Ab or to upstream molecular events independent of it.

Brain Repairment after Stroke

A well-known fact, in clinical stroke is that most patients show some degree of recovery over time. As the brain recovers, considerable reshaping of cortical areas takes place. Functional MRI studies demonstrate that peri-infarct areas are highly dynamic (Dijkhuizen, 2003; Chopp, 2007). Representational areas shift as latent networks are unmasked and parallel circuits are recruited adjacent to damaged regions (Murphy and Corbett, 2009). More recently, advanced optical imaging techniques combined with Electrophysiology demonstrated that this remodeling at a circuit level can be correlated with specific processes of dendritic and synaptic plasticity at a cellular level (Li and Murphy, 2008). Imaging of mitochondrial function (Liu and Murphy, 2009) and vascular dynamics (Schaffer, 2006) has provided new insight into how the brain responds to microvascular perturbations following ischemia. These powerful tools may eventually allow one to interrogate mechanisms of stroke recovery at a molecular and cellular level while testing pro recovery therapies and strategies (Murphy and Corbett, 2009; Zhang and Chopp, 2009). Repair and remodeling processes after stroke; A major advance within this past decade has been the realization that adult mammalian brains also exhibit focal areas of ongoing neurogenesis in the subventricular zone and subgranular zone. Under normal conditions, these newborn neurons migrate to olfactory regions and hippocampus. But after cerebral ischemia or hemorrhage; the birth of new cells seem to increase and neuroblasts reroute toward damaged brain tissue (Arvidsson, 2002; Parent, 2002); perhaps as part of an endogenous attempt by the brain to repair itself. However, whether these new neurons significantly contribute to functional recovery remains unclear. Neurogenic responses may persist for surprisingly long periods of time, but the majority of these newborn cells survive only for a few days (Arvidsson, 2002). Whether these cells develop normally, express neurotransmitters, or even integrate into existing neural networks remains to be fully elucidated. Future attempts to promote endogenous neurogenesis for therapeutic purposes will have to address ways to modify parenchymal microenvironments to enhance neuronal survival and integrate newly born cells into viable circuitry. In concert with neurogenesis and neural plasticity the brain recovering from stroke exhibits complex patterns of vascular remodeling. Angiogenesis and vasculogenesis in peri-infarct regions have been detected in rodent models of cerebral ischemia (Ding, 2008) as well as in human stroke (Krupinski, 1996). Indeed, it is now recognized that angiogenic and neurogenic responses are tightly coregulated after stroke and brain injury (Arai, 2009). This might not be surprising, because molecular mechanisms of neurogenesis and angiogenesis have been evolutionarily conserved so that similar mediators and pathways are involved in both phenomena (Carmeliet and Tessier-Lavigne, 2005). In the normal brain, the neurovascular niche defines these complex mechanisms of cell-cell signaling between cerebral endothelial and neural precursors in the subventricular and subgranular zones of ongoing neurogenesis. In the context of poststroke recovery, these close relationships between neurogenesis and angiogenesis are maintained. Neuroblasts migrate along perivascular routes (Thored et al., 2007). Promotion of neurogenesis enhances vascular regrowth and, conversely, angiogenic stimulation enhances neurogenesis (Ohab, 2006; Taguchi, 2004). Hence, it seems likely that brain recovery after stroke comprises interdependent neurovascular plasticity and remodeling processes that recruit multiple common mediators and signals (Snapyan, 2009). The new frontier of neurovascular repair may require a detailed exploration of how these multi-cell and multi-signal phenomena are regulated in the context of stroke. Recent experimental studies have suggested that pharmacological interventions such as EPO, statins, activated protein C, and phosphodiesterase inhibitors may promote functional recovery after cerebral ischemia (Wang, 2004; Zhang, 2006; Thiyagarajan, 2008; Chen, 2009). Ultimately, therapies that can augment these endogenous signals and substrates of neurovascular remodeling may have long therapeutic time windows in stroke (Zhang and Chopp, 2009).

Implications for Therapeutic Intervention beyond Thrombolytics

Current protocols of primary stroke management and secondary prevention focuses on modifiable vascular risk factors such as hypertension, smoking, carotid stenosis, atrial fibrillation, physical inactivity, diabetes mellitus, and dyslipidemia, with usage of drugs like antiplatelet agents, anti-hypertensive drugs, lipid-lowering agents, and anticoagulant drugs. A recent addition to this armamentarium was intravenous tissue plasminogen activator in cases of acute ischemic stroke, the efficacy of which is often limited by stroke severity, older age, systolic hypertension, location of arterial occlusion, collateral blood supply, and time from stroke onset to treatment, and reperfusion-associated inflammation (Pandian JD 2009, Adibhatla RM 2008 and 2009). The overall re-canalization rate in thrombolytic therapy varies from 46.2% during the first 6–24 h of intravenous administration, to 63.2% in intraarterial and 83.6% with mechanical reperfusion techniques (Pandian JD 2009). Current understanding of various patho-genetic mechanisms of stroke has paved the path for newer therapeutic approaches.

Currently Available Agents with Anti-Inflammatory Role

Commonly used agents like the anti-platelet agent acetylsalicylic acid (aspirin) and the lipid-lowering agent's β-hydroxy-β-methylglutaryl coenzyme A reductase inhibitors (statins) possess anti-inflammatory effects in addition to their traditionally accepted actions.

Aspirin: Apart from its well-established role in prevention of death, myocardial infarction, and stroke in high-risk patients, aspirin has a direct role in modifying CRP levels, thus raising the possibility of an anti-inflammatory action apart from its *anti-platelet* effect mediated via COX inhibition. Based on the findings of the Second European Stroke Prevention Study (ESPS-2), and European/Australian Stroke Prevention in Reversible Ischemia Trial (ESPRIT); a combination of aspirin and extended-release. Dipyridamole was found superior to aspirin alone in reducing the occurrence of the primary combined end point of vascular death, nonfatal stroke, nonfatal myocardial infarction, and major bleeding complications, and found favor with the most recent American Heart Association guidelines. This was partly attributed to the anti-inflammatory actions of this combination therapy (Weyrich AS 2009). Further, it is also thought to block NF-κB, which is the transcription factor for a host of proinflammatory mediators of ischemia. Since NF-κB also has a role in the resolution of inflammation, excessive modulation might create a problem during the recovery phase (Grilli M 1996).

Stations: *Lipid-lowering effect* of statins has already established its efficacy by significantly reducing the incidence of ischemic stroke in patients with coronary artery disease, both with and without elevated serum cholesterol concentrations (Crouse JR 1998).

Anti-inflammatory and/or neuroprotective properties of statins: Statins have found its base in their ability to reduce CRP levels, especially ones with high CRP levels (Di Napoli M 2001). Its efficacy has been demonstrated by measuring the intimal–medial thickness on carotid ultrasound, an indicator of atherosclerotic disease. It has also been reported that statins achieve atherosclerotic plaque stabilization or even regression by reducing macrophage activation within the vessel wall, inhibition of MMP-induced plaque rupture, and prevention of cytokine-mediated smooth muscle cell proliferation, whereas reduction in serum cholesterol encourages an antithrombotic state, by reducing platelet aggregation or by lowering plasminogen activator inhibitor-1 levels (Mohler ER 1999). It also has a neuroprotective action by upregulation of endothelial NOS and inhibition of iNOS, an effect associated with the augmented cerebral blood flow and reduced infarct size, reduction of leukocyte–endothelium interaction, modulation of CNS cytokine production, and antioxidant effects.

Recently, a Stroke Prevention by Aggressive Reduction in Cholesterol Levels study showed that treatment with high dose atorvastatin reduced risk of stroke in patients with recent stroke and transient ischemic attack and no known coronary artery disease (CAD) (Gedikli O 2008).

Angiotensin converting enzyme inhibitors and angiotensin II receptor blockers: The effects of these agents have been observed to reach beyond the known blood pressure lowering action mediated by the renin–angiotensin–aldosterone axis. Angiotensin II has proinflammatory effects via augmentation of expression of VCAM-1, MCP-1, and IL-6, and increased production of reactive oxygen species, which can be countered by angiotensin converting enzyme inhibitors or angiotensin II receptor blockers for having anti-inflammatory effect (Libby P 2001).

Novel Therapeutic Agents with Anti-Inflammatory Role

Neuroprotective agents: This includes a diverse range of drugs directed at restricting damage and salvaging the penumbral tissue. Though the small rim of penumbra acts as a barrier to the successful application of these drugs, their role can be vital in a setting where reperfusion obtained by combined thrombosis' and neuroprotective agent, is sufficient. These drugs act by modulating the excitatory amino acid system, controlling calcium influx, or can be metabolic activators, antiedema agents, inhibitors of leukocyte adhesion, and free radical scavengers.

Unfortunately, despite the safety and efficacy being proved by more than 100 clinical trials its translation into clinical practice remains awaited (Lebs Kind DS 2001).

- **Free radical scavenger:** Edaravone is the first clinical drug for neuroprotection in the world which has been used from 2001 in most ischemic stroke patients in Japan, and is especially useful in thrombolytic therapy with tissue plasminogen activator (tPA) (Abe K 2008).
- **Gene therapy:** Neural stem cell (Abe K 2008) could provide a future regenerative potential against ischemic brain damage at chronic stage.
- **Inhibiting apoptotic mechanism**: Brain parenchyma under threat of infarction contains neuronal cells, which undergo caspase-dependant (either by the caspase-3-dependant intrinsic pathway, originating from mitochondrial release of cytochrome c; or caspase-8-dependant extrinsic pathway, originating by the activation of cell surface death receptors) apoptosis, as well as non-neuronal cells which undergo non-caspase-dependent apoptosis. Current studies are directed towards therapeutic intervention of these potentially salvageable areas (Broughton BR 2009, Yuwan J 2009).
- **Ischemic preconditioning and inhibition of oxygen sensors; Ischemic postconditioning:** The rationale behind this strategy is downregulation of cellular and tissue metabolism (Yenari M 2008), which is similar to that of hypothermia (Minembres E 2008) to overcome the effects of ischemia. Further studies have described a new family of oxygen sensors—including prolyl hydroxylase domain-containing proteins 1-3 (PHD1-3)—which possibly has a role in balancing hypoxia tolerance, ischemic preconditioning and inflammation, and thus provide a novel setting for newer pharmacological interventions for ischemic and inflammatory diseases (Fraisl P 2009). Ischemic postconditioning was initially referred to a stuttering reperfusion and has been performed immediately after reperfusion, for preventing ischemia/reperfusion injury in both myocardial and cerebral infarction. It can be induced by a broad range of stimuli or triggers, and may even be performed as late as 6 h after focal ischemia and 2 days after transient global ischemia. Ischemic preconditioning or partial/gradual reperfusion, provides insights into the protective mechanisms of reperfusion injury and the acute, mitogen-activated protein kinase (MAPK), protein kinase C (PKC), and ATP-sensitive K+ (K(ATP)) channel cell signalling pathways (Edyinsson L 2009, Tanahashi N 2009).
- **Hyperbaric oxygen therapy:** Hyperbaric (HBO) or normobaric oxygen (NBO) therapy applied in acute ischemic stroke aims to salvage irreversible tissue damage by supplying oxygen to the ischemic area. Oxygen delivered at higher pressures (2.5–3 ATA) within initial few hours appears more promising for bridging of a transient ischemic period until reperfusion of the penumbra takes place, and has shown to reduce infarct size from 30–40%. Recent studies have demonstrated that physical oxygen therapy indeed improves oxygen supply of the ischemic penumbra as well as the cellular bioenergetic metabolism. In this mechanism, the mitochondria, including their role in apoptotic cell death pathways as well as the modification of the cellular hypoxia sensor HIF-1alpha are considered as potential "downstream pathways" of oxygen therapy (Poli S 2009).
- **Peroxisome proliferator-activated receptor-gamma (PPARγ):** PPARs are ligand-activated transcription factors that control lipid and glucose metabolism. These have a role in gene expression, as well as may modulate gene transcription by directly interfering with other transcription factor pathways in a DNA-binding independent

manner. Though all three isoforms (alpha, beta/delta, and gamma) are activated by the ischemic cascade, PPAR-γ, was shownto prevent post-ischemic inflammation and neuronal damage in several *in vitro* and *in vivo* models, and negatively regulating the expression of genes induced by ischemia/reperfusion (I/R). This may further be exploited for designing novel therapeutic targets (Collino M 2008).

- **Pituitary adenylate cyclase-activating polypeptide (PACAP) and vasoactive intestinal peptide (VIP):** Ischemic stroke not only leads to tissue degeneration, but also activates neuroprotective cellular mechanisms by releasing PACAP and VIP. These neuropeptides are widely distributed in both the central nervous system and peripheral organs of various vertebrates. They display pleiotropic biological activity and mediate via many intracellular pathways, with four categories of action: antiapoptotic, anti-inflammatory, metabolic, and modulation of gene expression. There are two structurally distinct receptors that recognize VIP peptides and PACAP with similar affinities (PACAP/VIPR-1, PACAP/VIPR-2), as well as a specific receptor for the PACAP peptide (PACAP-1). VIP has a wide physiological profile. In the periphery, VIP receptors are distributed throughout the gastrointestinal tract and genitourinary system, other smooth muscles and secretory glands and induce relaxation in smooth muscle. VIP inhibits secretion in certain tissues, but stimulates secretion in others; and modulates activity of cells in the immune system.

In the CNS, VIP receptors are found abundantly in the cortex, hippocampus and thalamus, and have a range of both excitatory and inhibitory actions. All VIP receptors activate adenyl cyclase (Wei Y 1996). Animal models confirm that the synthetic derivatives of these neuropeptides have considerable neuroprotective and anti-inflammatory potential, suggesting a possibility of their use as new therapeutic strategies in stroke management (Jo' zwaik-Bebenista M 2008).

- **Nuclear enzyme poly(ADP-ribose) polymerase 1 (PARP-1):** As discussed earlier, reactive oxygen and nitrogen species, including the reactive oxidant peroxynitrite, are generated in parenchymal, endothelial, and infiltrating inflammatory cells during ischemic stroke, and also during the reperfusion phase. These induce oxidative DNA damage and cause activation of the PARP enzyme family, which leads to depletion of its substrate NAD(+), slowing the rate of glycolysis, electron transport, andATP formation, eventually leading to functional impairment or death of cells, as well as upregulation of various proinflammatory pathways. Animal model studies have shown significant therapeutic benefits of PARP inhibitors, which have entered clinical development for the experimental therapy (Pacher P 2008).
- **Induced hypothermia** is another strategy gaining popularity since it may limit the final extent of cerebral infarct. Though paracetamol has shown to decrease body temperature in acute stroke, however its efficacy needs further validation (Mi nembres E 2008, Dippel DWJ 2001).
- **Minocycline in combination with tPA**: In an experimental study on spontaneously hypertensive rats, which were subjected to embolic focal ischemia using homologous clots and treated with combined minocycline at 4 h plus tPA at 6 h, it was noted that there was a decrease in plasma MMP-9 levels, reduction of infarction, and amelioration of brain hemorrhage. It was thus concluded that combination therapy

with minocycline may extend tPA treatment time windows in ischemic stroke (Murata Y 2008).

- ***Others*:** Other therapeutic strategies are based on the neuroprotective action of erythropoietin (Maise K 2008), melatonin (Reiter RJ 2007), estrogen (Lebesgue D 2009), NOS inhibitors (del Zoppo G 2000, Bath PM 2002), and anti-high mobility group box 1 (HMGB1) monoclonal antibody (mAb) by altering permeability of the blood–brain barrier, expression of TNF-α, iNOS and MMP-9 (Mori M 2009).

Antimicrobial drugs and vaccines: Antichlamydial antibiotics also act by suppressing reactivation of chronic inflammation within atherosclerotic plaques, and have a potential role in secondary prevention (Grayston JT 1999). Influenza vaccine has been reported not only to reduce viral infection, but also secondary bacterial infections. A recent study has found a negative association between influenza vaccine and brain infarction, particularly in under 75 years population (Lavalle P 2002).

Antileucocyte agents: The deleterious effects of leucocytes in an ischemic setting have prompted the use of monoclonal antibody to competitively block its adhesion to ICAM-1, and thus limit the extent of damage, and also extend the therapeutic window, during which thrombolytic therapy may be administered. Due to adverse outcome in the first human trial with anti-ICAM-1 murine monoclonal antibody, other strategies have been sought, viz. Antineutrophil serum and antineoplastic agents to achieve neutrophil depletion (Enlimomab Stroke Group 2001).

Cytokine targets: Dual, anti-inflammatory and proinflammatory, effects of TNF-α and of IL-6, have been the primary concern in using strategies directed against these *cytokines.* In contrast, IL-1ra directed against IL-1, has found favor with patients with rheumatoid arthritis, and also in cases of acute stroke (Kostulas M 1999, Emsley HC 2008).

Vitamins: Studies have shown that a diet rich in fruits and vegetables has a lower cardiovascular risk, possibly due to antioxidant nutrients: vitamin C, beta-carotene and vitamin E. These might reduce atheroma formation by inhibiting oxidation of LDL (Matsui T 2001). Homocysteine, a sulfur-containing amino acid, is a demethylation product of dietary methionine, which is converted to cysteine by cystathionine B-synthase (a vitamin B6-dependent enzyme), or is remethylated by methionine synthase. The latter reaction is vitamin B12 dependent and requires 5-methyl-tetrahydrofolate, a product of folic acid metabolism that uses methylene-tetrahydrofolate reductase (MTHFR). Defects of cystathionine B-synthase and MTHFR and deficiencies in folic acid, B12, and B6 can lead to raised levels of homocysteine, which have been associated with cardiovascular disease and stroke. Mechanism of homocysteine causing vascular damage include impairment of endothelial functions, endothelial desquamation, oxidation of LDL, increased monocyte adhesion to the vessel wall, impaired vascular response to nitric oxide, and thrombotic tendency mediated by activation of coagulation factors and platelet dysfunction (Matsui T 2001). Studies have shown a correlation between ischemic cerebrovascular disease withMTHFRgenotype and serum homocysteine concentration and an interaction with serum folate concentration. Others have also reported association of MTHFR A677V allele with severe carotid stenosis, a moderately elevated homocysteine after methionine loading with increased risk of ischemic stroke in young adults, a graded association of increasing plasma homocysteine with ischemic stroke caused by large-artery atherosclerosis and to a lesser extent small artery disease, an association with risk of silent brain infarction, an association with cervical artery dissection, and microvascular stroke (Sculz JB 1999). However, in contrast cross-sectional and case–control studies, prospective studies generally show less or no predictive ability for plasma homocysteine in coronary disease and stroke.

Predictive Role of Blood Biomarkers in Ischemic Stroke

A recent study reviewed the Medline and EMBASE from 1966 to January 2007 for studies of blood markers in patients with ischemic stroke and an assessment of outcome (death, disability, or handicap). Though cardiac markers showed the most consistent association with poor outcome, many studies were subject to bias. Although some markers had some predictive ability, none of the studies showed any added advantage of biomarkers over a validated clinical model. Thus the clinical usefulness for predicting prognosis in the setting of ischemic stroke is yet to be established, prior to being incorporated into any regimen (Whiteley W 2000).

Conclusion

The complex pathophysiology of a stroke encompasses various excitotoxicity mechanisms, inflammatory pathways, oxidative damage and ionic imbalances. Despite significant therapeutic advances in the form of carotid endarterectomy, thrombolytics, anticoagulant therapy, antiplatelet agents, neuroprotective agents, and treating associated risk factors such as hypertension and dyslipidemia have failed to reduce the burden of stroke. Current understanding of inflammation and ischemia has caused a paradigm shift in the perspective of stroke pathogenesis and outcome. It has also opened newer avenues in stroke management and prevention strategies, beyond the realms of antithrombotics. Though one needs to keep abreast with recommended protocols for stroke management, knowledge of the underlying patho-genetic process, aided by laboratory investigations and imaging, may usher in more therapeutic options. Well-designed clinical trials of novel therapeutic agents and strategies will be able to substantiate or refute their clinical usefulness, and confirm the possibility of being incorporated into evidence-based practice guidelines.

Several complex and overlapping pathways underlie the pathophysiology of cell death after ischemic stroke. While pharmaceutical agents can inhibit these pathways at various levels, resulting in effective neuroprotection in experimental models, no single agent intended for neuroprotection has been shown to improve outcome in clinical stroke trials. Refinements in patient selection, brain imaging, and methods of drug delivery, as well as the use of more clinically relevant animal stroke models and use of combination therapies that target the entire neurovascular unit, are warranted to make stroke neuroprotection an achievable goal. Ongoing trials assessing the efficacy of thrombolysis with neuroprotective agents and strategies aimed at extending the therapeutic window for reperfusion therapy promise to enhance the known benefits of reperfusion therapy. Most investigators agree that genomics and proteomics are the most promising recent developments impacting the future of stroke prevention, diagnosis, treatment, and outcome. Although many challenges lie ahead, an attitude of cautious optimism seems justified at this time.

References

Abe K, Neuroprotective therapy for ischemic stroke with free radical scavenger and gene-stem cell therapy, Rinsho Shinkeigaku 48 (2008) 896–898.

Ameriso SF, V.L.Y. Wong, F.P. Quismorio, M. Fisher, Immunohematologic characteristics of infection-associated cerebral infarction, *Stroke* 22 (1991) 1004–1009.

Asahi M, X. Wang, et al. Effects of matrix metalloproteinase-9 gene knock-out on the proteolysis of blood–brain barrier and white matter components after cerebral ischemia, *J. Neurosci.* 21 (2001) 7724–7732.

Aarts, M.M., and Tymianski, M. (2005). TRPMs and neuronal cell death. *Pflugers Arch.* 451, 243–249.

Aarts, M., Iihara, K., et al. (2003). A key role for TRPM7 channels in anoxic neuronal death. *Cell* 115, 863–877.

Abe, T., Kunz, A., Shimamura, M., et al. (2009). The neuroprotective effect of prostaglandin E2 EP1 receptor inhibition has a wide therapeutic window, is sustained in time and is not sexually dimorphic. *J. Cereb. Blood Flow Metab.* 29, 66–72.

Abramov, A.Y., Scorziello, A., and Duchen, M.R. (2007). Three distinct mechanisms generate oxygen free radicals in neurons and contribute to cell death during anoxia and reoxygenation. *J. Neurosci.* 27, 1129–1138.

Adams, H.P., Jr et al. (1996) Guidelines for thrombolytic therapy for acute stroke: a supplement to the guidelines for the management of patients with acute ischemic stroke – a statement for healthcare professionals from a Special Writing Group of the Stroke Council. American Heart Association. *Circulation* 94, 167–174.

Adibhatla, R.M., and Hatcher, J.F. (2010). Lipid oxidation and peroxidation in CNS health and disease: from molecular mechanisms to therapeutic opportunities. *Antioxid. Redox Signal.* 12, 125–169.

Allen, C.L., and Bayraktutan, U. (2008). Risk factors for ischemic stroke. *Int. J. Stroke* 3, 105–116.

Amarenco, P., Bogousslavsky, J., et al. Stroke Prevention by Aggressive Reduction in Cholesterol Levels (SPARCL) Investigators. (2006). High-dose atorvastatin after stroke or transient ischemic attack. *N. Engl. J. Med.* 355, 549–559.

Astrup, J., Siesjo¨, B.K., and Symon, L. (1981). Thresholds in cerebral ischemia -the ischemic penumbra. *Stroke* 12, 723–725.

Ankarcrona, M., Dypbukt, J.M., et al. (1995). Glutamate-induced neuronal death: a succession of necrosis or apoptosis depending on mitochondrial function. *Neuron 15,* 961–973.

Arai, K., and Lo, E.H. (2009a). Astrocytes protect oligodendrocyte precursor cells via MEK/ERK and PI3K/Akt signaling. *J. Neurosci. Res.* 88, 758–763.

Arai, K., and Lo, E.H. (2009b). An oligovascular niche: cerebral endothelial cells promote the survival and proliferation of oligodendrocyte precursor cells. *J. Neurosci.* 29, 4351–4355.

Adibhatla RM, J.F. Hatcher, Altered lipid metabolism in brain injury and disorders, Subcell. *Biochem.* 49 (2008) 241–268.

Adibhatla RM, J.F. Hatcher, Tissue plasminogen activator (tPA) and matrix metalloproteinases in the pathogenesis of stroke: therapeutic strategies, CNS Neurol. *Disord. Drug Targets* 7 (2008) 243–253.

Akopov SE, N.A. Simonian, G.S. Grigorian, Dynamics of polymorphonuclear leukocyte accumulation in acute cerebral infarction and their correlation with brain tissue damage, *Stroke* 27 (1996) 1739–1743.

Appay V, S.L. Rowland-Jones, RANTES: a versatile and controversial chemokine, *Trends Immunol.* 22 (2001) 83–87.

Askalan A, S. Laughlin, et al. Chickenpox and stroke in childhood: a study of frequency and causation, *Stroke* 32 (2001) 1257–1262.

Anlauf E, A. Derouiche, Astrocytic exocytosis vesicles and glutamate: a high-resolution immunofluorescence study, *Glia* 49 (2005) 96–106.

Araque A, N. Li, R.T. Doyle, P.G. Haydon, SNARE proteindependent glutamate release from astrocytes, *J. Neurosci.* 20 (2000) 666–673.

Barone FC, A.A. Parsons, Therapeutic potential of anti-inflammatory drugs in focal stroke, *Expert. Opin. Investig. Drugs* 9 (2000) 2281–2306.

Bezzi P, M. Domercq, et al. CXCR4-activated astrocyte glutamate release via TNF-α lpha: amplification by microglia triggers neurotoxicity, *Nat. Neurosci.* 4 (2001) 702–710.

Bath PM, Efficacy of nitric oxide in stroke (ENOS) trial, *Stroke* 33 (2002) 648–649.

Bezzi P, V. Gundersen, Astrocytes contain a vesicular compartment that is competent for regulated exocytosis of glutamate, *Nat. Neurosci.* 7 (2004) 613–620.

Barath P, M.C. Fishbein, et al. Detection and localization of tumor necrosis factor in human atheroma, *Am J Cardiol.* 65 (1990) 297–302.

Broughton BR, D.C. Reutens, C.G. Sobey, Apoptotic mechanisms after cerebral ischemia, *Stroke* 40 (2009) e331–e339, Epub 2009, January 29.

Bacon KB, B.A. Premack, P. Gardner, T.J. Schall, Activation of dual T cell signaling pathways by the chemokine RANTES, *Science* 269 (1995) 1727–1730.

Balestrino M, D. Partinico, C. Finocchi, C. Gandolfo, White blood cell count and erythrocyte sedimentation rate correlate with outcome in patients with acute ischemic stroke, *J. Stroke Cerebrovasc. Dis.* 7 (1998) 139–144.

Beamer NB, B.M. Coull, et al. Interleukin-6 and interleukin-1 receptor antagonist in acute stroke, *Ann. Neurol.* 37 (1995) 800–805.

Besancon, E., Guo, S., Lok, J., Tymianski, M., and Lo, E.H. (2008). Beyond NMDA and AMPA glutamate receptors: emerging mechanisms for ionic imbalance and cell death in stroke. *Trends Pharmacol.* Sci. 29, 268–275.

Biessels, G.J., van der Heide, et al. (2002). Ageing and diabetes: implications for brain function. *Eur. J. Pharmacol.* 441, 1–14.

Bonfoco, E., Krainc, D., et al. (1995). Apoptosis and necrosis: two distinct events induced, respectively, by mild and intense insults with N-methyl-D-aspartate or nitric oxide/superoxide in cortical cell cultures. *Proc. Natl. Acad. Sci. USA* 92, 7162–7166.

Bonita, R., Duncan, J., et al. (1999). Passive smoking as well as active smoking increases the risk of acute stroke. *Tob. Control* 8, 156–160.

Brennan, A.M., Suh, S.W., et al. (2009). NADPH oxidase is the primary source of superoxide induced by NMDA receptor activation. *Nat. Neurosci.* 12, 857–863.

Brown, W.R., Moody, D.M., et al. (2007). Vascular dementia in leukoaraiosis may be a consequence of capillary loss not only in the lesions, but in normal-appearing white matter and cortex as well. *J. Neurol. Sci.* 257, 62–66.

Belch J, M. Mclaren, et al. white blood cell and plasma fibrinogen in thrombotic stroke: a significant correlation, *Int. Angiol.* 17 (1998) 120–124.

Biswas A, A.K. Tiwari, R. Ranjan, et al. Prothrombotic polymorphisms, mutations, and their association with pediatric non-cardioembolic stroke in Asian-Indian patients, *Ann. Hematol.* 88 (2009) 473–478, Epub 2008, October 4.

Brouns R, P.P. De Deyn, The complexity of neurobiological processes in acute ischemic stroke, *Clin. Neurol. Neurosurg.* (May) (2009).

Buttini M, K. Appel, et al. Boddeke, Expression of tumor necrosis factor alpha after focal cerebral ischemia in the rat, *Neuroscience* 71 (1996) 1–16.

Campbell LA, M. Rosenfeld, C.C. Kuo, The role of Chlamydia pneumoniae in atherosclerosis—recent evidence from animal models, *Trends Microbiol.* 8 (2000) 255–257.

Canoui-Poitrine F, H.C. de Lyon, et al. Systemic chemokines levels and incident coronary heart disease and ischemic stroke events in asymptomatic middle-aged men: the Prime Study, *Circulation* 120 (2009) S428.

Campos MM, J.B. Calixto, Neurokinin mediation of edema and inflammation, *Neuropeptides* 34 (2000) 314–322.

Crippa D, U. Schenk, et al., Synaptobrevin2-expressing vesicles in rat astrocytes: insights into molecular characterization, dynamics and exocytosis, *J. Physiol.* 570 (2006) 567–582.

Collino M, N.S. Patel, C. Thiemermann, PPARs as new therapeutic targets for the treatment of cerebral ischemia/reperfusion injury, *Ther. Adv. Cardiovasc. Dis.* 2 (2008) 179–197.

Carmeliet, P., and Tessier-Lavigne, M. (2005). Common mechanisms of nerve and blood vessel wiring. *Nature* 436, 193–200.

Chabriat, H., Joutel, A., Dichgans, M., Tournier-Lasserve, E., and Bousser, M.G. (2009). Cadasil. *Lancet Neurol.* 8, 643–653.

Chan, P.H. (2001). Reactive oxygen radicals in signaling and damage in the ischemic brain. J. Cereb. *Blood Flow Metab.* 21, 2–14.

Chen, Q., He, S., Hu, X.L., et al. (2007). Differential roles of NR2A- and NR2Bcontaining NMDA receptors in activity-dependent brain-derived neurotrophic factor gene regulation and limbic epileptogenesis. *J. Neurosci.* 27, 542–552.

Chen, J., Cui, X., Zacharek, A., Roberts, C., and Chopp, M. (2009). eNOS mediates TO90317 treatment-induced angiogenesis and functional outcome after stroke in mice. *Stroke* 40, 2532–2538.

Cheng, T., Petraglia, A.L., et al. (2006). Activated protein Activated protein C inhibits tissue plasminogen activator-induced brain hemorrhage. *Nat. Med.* 12, 1278–1285.

Crouse JR, R.P. Byington, C.D. Furberg, HMG-CoA reductase inhibitor therapy and stroke risk reduction: an analysis of clinical trials data, *Atherosclerosis* 138 (1998) 11–24.

DeGraba T, A.-L. Sirén, L. et al. Increased endothelial expression of intercellular adhesion molecule-1 in symptomatic versus asymptomatic human carotid atherosclerotic plaque, *Stroke* 29 (1998) 1405–1410.

Di Napoli M, Early inflammatory response in ischemic stroke, *Thromb. Res.* 103 (2001) 261–264.

Dippel DWJ, E.J. van Breda, etal. on behalf of the PAPAS Investigators, Effect of paracetamol (acetaminophen) on body temperature in acute ischemic stroke, *Stroke* 32 (2001) 1607–1612.

Duan S, C.M. Anderson, et al. P2X7 receptor-mediated release of excitatory amino acids from astrocytes, *J. Neurosci.* 23 (2003) 1320–1328.

del Zoppo G, I. Ginis, et al. Inflammation and stroke: putative role for cytokines, adhesion molecules and iNOS in brain response to ischemia, *Brain Pathol.* 10 (2000) 95–112.

Di Napoli, M., Schwaninger, et al. (2005). Evaluation of C-reactive protein measurement for assessing the risk and prognosis in ischemic stroke: a statement for health care professionals from the CRP Pooling Project members. *Stroke* 36, 1316–1329.

D'Erasmo E, M. Acca, F.S. Celi, G. Mazzuoli, Correlation between plasma fibrinogen levels and white blood cell count after cerebral infarction, *Stroke* 22 (1991) 1089.

Dohmen, C., Sakowitz, O.W., et al. Co-Operative Study of Brain Injury Depolarisations (COSBID). (2008). Spreading depolarizations occur in human ischemic stroke with high incidence. *Ann. Neurol.* 63, 720–728.

Dugas, J.C., Mandemakers, et al. (2008). A novel purification method for CNS projection neurons leads to the identification of brain vascular cells as a source of trophic support for corticospinal motor neurons. *J. Neurosci.* 28, 8294–8305.

Ebert, A.D., Yu, J., Rose, F., et al. (2009). Induced pluripotent stem cells from a spinal muscular atrophy patient. *Nature* 457, 277–280.

Edvinsson L, Cerebrovascular endothelin receptor upregulation in cerebral ischemia, *Curr. Vasc. Pharmacol.* 7 (2009) 26–33.

Ekshyyan O, T.Y. Aw, Apoptosis in neurodegenerative disorders, *Curr. Neurovasc. Res.* 1 (2004) 355–371.

Eldadah BA, A.I. Faden, Caspase pathways, neuronal apoptosis, and CNS injury, *J. Neurotrauma* 17 (2000) 811–829.

Enlimomab Acute Stroke Trial Investigators, Use of anti-ICAM-1 therapy in ischemic stroke: results of the Enlimomab Acute Stroke Trial, *Neurology* 57 (2001) 1428–1434.

Emsley HC, C.J. Smith, et al. Inflammation in acute ischemic stroke and its relevance to stroke critical care, *Neurocrit. Care* 9 (2008) 125–138.

Escudero Augusto D, L. Marqués Alvarez, F. Taboada Costa, Update in spontaneous cerebral hemorrhage, *Med. Intensiva* 32 (2008) 282–295.

Erren M, H. Reinecke, et al. Systemic inflammatory parameters in patients with atherosclerosis of the coronary and peripheralarteries, Arterioscler. *Thromb. Vasc. Biol.* 19 (1999) 2355–2363.

Elkind MS, J. Cheng, B. Boden-Albala, T. Rundek, J. Thomas, H. Chen, L.E. Rabbani, R.L. Sacco, Tumor necrosis factor receptor levels are associated with carotid atherosclerosis, *Stroke* 33 (2002) 31–38.

Elkind, M.S. (2007). Why now? Moving from stroke risk factors to stroke triggers. *Curr. Opin. Neurol.* 20, 51–57.

Emsley HC, C.J. Smith, et al. Acute Stroke Investigators, Arandomised phase II study of interleukin-1 receptor antagonist in acute stroke patients, *J. Neurol. Neurosurg. Psychiatry* 76 (2005) 1366–1372.

Emsley HC, P.J. Tyrrell, Inflammation and infection in clinical stroke, *J. Cereb. Blood Flow Metab.* 22 (2002) 1399–1419.

Forster C, H.B. Clark, M.E. Ross, C. Iadecola, Inducible nitric oxide synthase expression in human cerebral infarcts, *Acta Neuropathol.* 97 (1999) 215–220.

Ford GA, Clinical pharmacological issues in the development of acute stroke therapies, *Br. J. Pharmacol.* 153 (Suppl. 1) (2008) S112–S119.

Fishman RA, *Cerebrospinal Fluid in Diseases in the Nervous System*, 2nd Ed., W.B. Saunders Co., Philadelphia, PA, 1992, pp. 103–155.

Fernández-Gómez FJ, et al. Pharmacology of neuroprotection in acute ischemic stroke, *Rev. Neurol.* 47 (2008) 253–260.

Fremeau RT Jr., et al. The identification of vesicular glutamate transporter 3 suggests novel modes of signaling by glutamate, *Proc. Natl. Acad. Sci. U.S.A.* 99 (2002) 14488–14493.

Ferriero, D.M. (2004). Neonatal brain injury. N. Engl. J. Med. 351, 1985–1995. Fisher, C.M. (1968). The arterial lesions underlying lacunes. *Acta Neuropathol.* 12, 1–15.

Fraisl P, J. Aragonés, P. Carmeliet, Inhibition of oxygen sensors as a therapeutic strategy for ischemic and inflammatory disease, *Nat. Rev. Drug Discov.* 8 (2009) 139–152, Epub 2009, January 23.

Fernando, M.S., Simpson, J.E.et al. MRC Cognitive Function and Ageing Neuropathology Study Group. (2006). White matter lesions in an unselected cohort of the elderly: molecular pathology suggests origin from chronic hypoperfusion injury. *Stroke* 37, 1391–1398.

Fo¨ rstermann, U. (2010). Nitric oxide and oxidative stress in vascular disease. *Pflugers Arch.* 459, 923–939.

Fotuhi, M., Hachinski, V., and Whitehouse, P.J. (2009). Changing perspectives regarding late-life dementia. *Nat. Rev. Neurol.* 5, 649–658.

Gidday, J.M. (2006). Cerebral preconditioning and ischemic tolerance. *Nat. Rev. Neurosci.* 7, 437–448.

Ginsberg, M.D. (2008). Neuroprotection for ischemic stroke: past, present and future. *Neuropharmacology* 55, 363–389.

Ginsberg, M.D. (2009). Current status of neuroprotection for cerebral ischemia: synoptic overview. *Stroke* 40, S111–S114.

Galea J, J. Armstrong, et al. Interleukin-1 beta in coronary arteries of patients with ischemic heart disease, Arterioscler T hromb. *Vasc. Biol.* 16 (1996) 1000–1006.

Gimbrone Jr MA., M.I. Cybulsky, et al. Vascular endothelium. An integrator of pathophysiological stimuli in atherogenesis, *Ann N. Y. Acad. Sci.* 748 (1995) 122–131.

Gupta S, D. Campbell, B. Derijard, R.J. Davis, Transcription factor ATF2 regulation by the JNK signal transduction pathway, *Science* 267 (1995) 389–393.

Green SL, K.S. Kulp, R. Vulliet, Cyclin-dependent kinase 5 activity increases in rat brain following ischaemia, *Neurochem. Int.* 31 (1997) 617–623.

Galvin KA, D.E. Oorschot, Continuous lowdose treatment with neurotrophin-3 protects striatal medium spiny neurons from mild neonatal hypoxia/ischaemia, *Neuroscience* 118 (2003) 1023–1032.

Gasche Y, M. Fujimura, et a. Early appearance of activated matrix metalloproteinase-9 after focal cerebral ischemia in mice: a possible role in blood–brain barrier dysfunction, *J. Cereb. Blood Flow Metab.* 19 (1999) 1020–1028.

Gidday JM, Y.G. Gasche, et al. Leukocyte-derived matrix metalloproteinase-9 mediates blood–brain barrier breakdown and is proinflammatory after transient focal cerebral ischemia, *Am. J. Physiol. Heart Circ. Physiol.* 289 (2005) 558–568.

Giffard RG, M.A. Yenari, Many mechanisms for HSP70 protection from cerebral ischaemia, *J. Neurosurg. Anesthesiol.* 16 (2004) 53–61.

Gerhard A, B. Neumaier, et al. In vivo imaging of activated microglia using (11C)PK11195 and positron emission tomography in patients after ischemic stroke, *Neuroreport* 11 (2000) 2957–2960.

Gedikli O, M.Baykan, Statins in stroke prevention, *Anadolu Kardiyol Derg* 8 (2008) 217–222.

Grilli M, M. Pizzi, M. Memo, P. Spano, Neuroprotection by aspirin and sodium salicylate through blockade of NF-_B activation, *Science* 274 (1996) 1383–1385.

Grayston JT, Antibiotic treatment trials for secondary prevention of coronary artery disease events, *Circulation* 99 (1999) 1538–2159.

Gorelick PB, Stroke prevention therapy beyond antithrombotics: unifying mechanisms in ischemic stroke pathogenesis and implications for therapy: an invited review, *Stroke* 33 (2002) 862–875.

Grayston JT, L.A. Campbell, et al. A new respiratory tract pathogen: Chlamydia pneumoniae strain TWAR, *J. Infect. Dis.* 161 (1990) 618–625.

Grau AJ, F. Buggle, C. Lichy, T. Brandt, H. Becher, J. Rudi, Helicobacter pylori infection as an independent risk factor for cerebral ischemia of atherothrombotic origin, *J. Neurol. Sci.* 186 (2001) 1–5.

Gregersen R, K. Lambertsen, B. Finsen, Microglia and macrophages are the major sources of tumor necrosis factor in permanent middle cerebral artery occlusion in mice, *J. Cereb. Blood Flow Metab.* 20 (2000) 53–65.

Hacke, W. et al. (2004) Association of outcome with early stroke treatment: pooled analysis of ATLANTIS, ECASS, and NINDS rtPA stroke trials. *Lancet* 363, 768–774.

Hacke, W. et al. (2008) Thrombolysis with alteplase 3 to 4.5 hours after acute ischemic stroke. *N. Engl. J. Med.* 359, 1317–1329.

Hankey, G.J. (2006). Potential new risk factors for ischemic stroke: what is their potential? *Stroke* 37, 2181–2188.

Hassan A, H.S. Markus, Genetics and ischemic stroke, *Brain* 123 (2000) 1784–1812.

Heuschmann PU, K. Berger, et al. Frequency of thrombolytic therapy in patients with acute ischemic stroke and the risk of in-hospital mortality: the German Stroke Registers Study Group, *Stroke* 34 (2003) 1106–1113.

Hu Z, Q. Yang, S. Zheng, et al. Temporal arteritis and fever: report of a case and a clinical reanalysis of 360 cases, *Angiology* 51 (2000) 953–958.

Hu Z, Q. Yang, et al. Temporal arteritis and fever: report of a case and a clinical reanalysis of 360 cases, *Angiology* 51 (2000) 953–958.

Heo JH, J. Lucero, et al. Matrix metalloproteinases increase very early during experimental focal cerebral ischemia, *J. Cereb. Blood FlowMetab.* 19 (1999) 624–633.

Hayashi T, K. Sakai, et al. JNK and JIP response in rat brain after transient MCAO, *Neurosci. Lett.* 284 (2000) 195–199.

Ip JH, V. Fuster, L. Badimon, et al. Syndromes of accelerated atherosclerosis: role of vascular injury and smooth muscle cell proliferation, *J. Am. Coll. Cardiol.* 15 (1990) 1667–1687.

Jansson JH, T.K. Nilsson, O. Johnson, von Willebrand factor in plasma: a novel risk factor for recurrent myocardial infarction and death, *Br. Heart J.* 66 (1991) 351–355.

Jamorozik K, R.J. Broadhurst, et al. The role of lifestyle factors in the etiology of stroke. A populationbased case control study based at Perth, Western Australia, *Stroke* 25 (1994) 51–59.

Jó´zwiak-Bebenista, K. Bednarek, J.Z. Nowak, The neuroprotective effect of PACAP, VIP, and derivatives in brain ischemia, *Postepy Hig Med Dosw* (Online) 62 (2008) 478–489.

Joza N, S.A. Susin, E. et al. Essential role of the mitochondrial apoptosis-inducing factor in programmed cell death, *Nature* 401 (2001) 549–554.

Jung KH, K. Chu, et al. G-CSF protects human cerebral hybrid neurons against in vitro ischaemia, *Neurosci. Lett.* 394 (2006) 168–173.

Karaszewski, B J.M. et al. Early brain temperature elevation and anaerobic metabolism in human acute ischemic stroke, *Brain* 132 (2009) 955–964.

Kimelberg HK, S.K. Goderie, et al. Swelling-induced release of glutamate, aspartate, and taurine from astrocyte cultures, *J. Neurosci.* 10 (1990) 1583–1591.

Kumar A, S. Dogra, Pathophysiology and therapeutic strategies in the management of stroke: an update, *Drugs Today* (Barc.) 44 (2008) 757–766.

Krupinski J, P. Kumar, S. Kumar, J. Kaluza, Increased expression of TGF-_1 in brain tissue after ischemic stroke in humans, *Stroke* 27 (1996) 852–857.

Kamat, C.D., Gadal, S., et al. (2008). Antioxidants in central nervous system diseases: preclinical promise and translational challenges. *J. Alzheimers Dis.* 15, 473–493.

Kapadia, R., Tureyen, K., et al. (2006). Decreased brain damage and curtailed inflammation in transcription factor CCAAT/enhancer binding protein beta knockout mice following transient focal cerebral ischemia. *J. Neurochem.* 98, 1718–1731.

Kapadia, R., Yi, J.H., and Vemuganti, R. (2008). Mechanisms of anti-inflammatory and neuroprotective actions of PPAR-gamma agonists. *Front. Biosci.* 13, 1813–1826.

Kimelberg, H.K., Macvicar, B.A., and Sontheimer, H. (2006). Anion channels in astrocytes: biophysics, pharmacology, and function. *Glia* 54, 747–757.

Kitayama, J., Faraci, F.M., Lentz, S.R., and Heistad, D.D. (2007). Cerebral vascular dysfunction during hypercholesterolemia. *Stroke* 38, 2136–2141.

Kizer, J.R., Wiebers, D.O., et al. (2005). Mitral annular calcification, aortic valve sclerosis, and incident stroke in adults free of clinical cardiovascular disease: the Strong Heart Study. *Stroke* 36, 2533–2537.

Kitagawa Y, F. Gotoh, A. Koto, H. Okayasu, Stroke in systemic lupus erythematosus, *Stroke* 21 (1990) 1533–1539.

Kostulas N, S.H. Pelidou, et al. Increased IL-1beta, IL-8, and IL-17 mRNA expression in blood mononuclear cells observed in a prospective ischemic stroke study, *Stroke* 30 (1999)

Klatzo I, Pathophysiological aspects of brain edema, *Acta Neuropathol.* (Berl.) 72 (1987) 236–239.

Krupinski J, J. Kaluza, P. Kumar, S. Kumar, J.M. Wang, Role of angiogenesis in patients with cerebral ischemic stroke, *Stroke* 25 (1994) 1794–1798.

Kunz, A., Park, L., Abe, T., et al. (2007b). Neurovascular protection by ischemic tolerance: role of nitric oxide and reactive oxygen species. *J. Neurosci.* 27, 7083–7093.

Lawes, C.M., Bennett, D.A., Feigin, V.L., and Rodgers, A. (2004a). Blood pressure and stroke: an overview of published reviews. *Stroke* 35, 776–785.

Lawes, C.M., Parag, V., et al. Asia Pacific Cohort Studies Collaboration. (2004b). Blood glucose and risk of cardiovascular disease in the Asia Pacific region. *Diabetes Care* 27, 2836–2842.

Lossos A, Y. River, A. Eliakim, I. Steiner, Neurologic aspects of inflammatory bowel disease, *Neurology* 45 (1995) 416–421.

Lebesgue D, V. Chevaleyre, R.S. Zukin, A.M. Etgen, Estradiol rescues neurons from global ischemia-induced cell death: multiple cellular pathways of neuroprotection, *Steroids* 74 (2009) 555–561.

Lavallée P, V. Perchaud, et al. Association between influenza vaccination and reduced risk of brain infarction, *Stroke* 33 (2002) 513–518.

Libby P, Current concepts of the pathogenesis of the acute coronary syndromes, *Circulation* 104 (2001) 365–372.

Liebeskind DS, S.E. Kasner, Neuroprotection for ischemic stroke—an unattainable goal? *CNS Drugs* 15 (2001) 165–174.

Loddick SA, A.V. Turnbull, N.J. Rothwell, Cerebral interleukin-6 is neuroprotective during permanent focal cerebral ischemia in the rat, *J. Cereb. Blood Flow Metab.* 18 (1998) 176–179.

Losy J, J. Zaremba, Monocyte chemoattractant protein-1 is increased in the cerebrospinal fluid of patients with ischemic stroke, *Stroke* 32 (2001) 2695–2696.

Leonard AD, S. Newburg, Cardioembolic stroke, *J. Neurosci. Nurs.* 24 (1992) 69–76.

Lipton, S.A. (2006). Paradigm shift in neuroprotection by NMDA receptor blockade: memantine and beyond. *Nat. Rev. Drug Discov.* 5, 160–170.

Lipton, S.A. (2007a). Pathologically-activated therapeutics for neuroprotection: mechanism of NMDA receptor block by memantine and S-nitrosylation. *Curr. Drug Targets* 8, 621–632.

Lipton, S.A. (2007b). Pathologically activated therapeutics for neuroprotection. *Nat. Rev. Neurosci.* 8, 803–808.

Lo, E.H. (2008a). Experimental models, neurovascular mechanisms and translational issues in stroke research. *Br. J. Pharmacol.* 153 (Suppl 1), S396–S405.

Lo, E.H. (2008b). A new penumbra: transitioning from injury into repair after stroke. *Nat. Med.* 14, 497–500.

Lo, E.H., Dalkara, T., and Moskowitz, M.A. (2003). Mechanisms, challenges and opportunities in stroke. *Nat. Rev. Neurosci.* 4, 399–415.

Mennicken F, R. Maki, E.B. de Souza, R. Quirion, Chemokines and chemokine receptors in the CNS: a possible role in neuroinflammation and patterning, *Trends Pharmacol. Sci.* 20 (1999) 73–77.

Mi˜nambres E, M.S. Holanda, M.J. Domínguez Artigas, J.C. Rodríguez Borregán, Therapeutic hypothermia in neurocritical patients, *Med. Intensiva.* 32 (2008) 227–235.

Mori S, K. Liu, H.K. Takahashi, M. Nishibori, Therapeutic effect of anti-nucleokine monoclonal antibody on ischemic brain infarction, *Yakugaku Zasshi* 129 (2009) 25–31.

Murata Y, A. Rosell, et al. Extension of the thrombolytic time window with minocycline in experimental stroke, *Stroke* 39 (2008) 3372–3377.

Maiese K, Z.Z. Chong, J. Hou,Y.C. Shang, Erythropoietin and oxidative stress, *Curr. Neurovasc. Res.* 5 (2008) 125–142.

Mun-Bryce S, G.A. Rosenberg, Gelatinase B modulates selective opening of the blood–brain barrier during inflammation, *Am. J. Physiol.* 274 (5 Pt 2) (1998) R1203–R1211.

Malarkey EB, V. Parpura, Mechanisms of glutamate release from astrocytes, *Neurochem. Int.* 52 (2008) 142–154.

Marti E, I. Ferrer, J. Ballabriga, J. Blasi, Increase in SNAP-25 immunoreactivity in the mossy fibres following transient forebrain ischaemia in the gerbil, *Acta Neuropathol.* 95 (1998) 254–260.

Montana V,Y. Ni,V. Sunjara, X. Hua,V. Parpura. Vesicular glutamate transporter-dependent glutamate release from astrocytes, *J. Neurosci.* 24 (2004) 2633–2642.

Mihara M, S. Erster, A.et al. 53 has a direct apoptogenic role at the mitochondria, *Mol. Cell* 11 (2003) 577–590.

Mun-Bryce S, G.A. Rosenberg, Matrix metalloproteinases in cerebrovascular disease, *J. Cereb. Blood Flow Metab.* 18 (1998) 1163–1172.

Mohr JP, R.L. Sacco, Stroke in: H.J.M. Barnett, et al. (Eds.), *Pathophysiology, Diagnosis, and Management*, Churchill Livingstone, New York, 1992, p. 271.

Montaner J, J. Alvarez-Sabin, et al. Matrix metalloproteinase expression is related to hemorrhagic transformation after cardioembolic stroke, *Stroke* 32 (2001) 2762–2767.

Malarkey EB, V. Parpura, The role of TRPC1 in internal Ca2+ regulation in astrocytes, *Biophys. J.* 88 (2005) 84A–85A.

Matsui T, H. Arai, T. Yuzuriha, et al. Elevated plasma homocysteine levels and risk of silent brain infarction in elderly people, *Stroke* 32 (2001) 1116–1119.

Mohler ER, N. Delanty, D.J. Rader, E.C. Raps, Statins and cerebrovascular disease: plaque attack to prevent brain attack, *Vasc. Med.* 4 (1999) 269–272.

Montaner J, C.A. Molina, et al. Matrix metalloproteinase-9 pretreatment level predicts intracranial hemorrhagic complications after thrombolysis in human stroke, *Circulation* 107 (2003) 598–603.

Murphy, T.H., and Corbett, D. (2009). Plasticity during stroke recovery: from synapse to behaviour. *Nat. Rev. Neurosci.* 10, 861–872.

Nagai, M., Re, D.B., Nagata, T., et al. (2007). Astrocytes expressing ALS-linked mutated SOD1 release factors selectively toxic to motor neurons. *Nat. Neurosci.* 10, 615–622.

Nakamura, T., and Lipton, S.A. (2009). According to GOSPEL: filling in the GAP (DH) of NO-mediated neurotoxicity. *Neuron* 63, 3–6.

Namura, S., Zhu, J., Fink, K., et al. (1998). Activation and cleavage of caspase-3 in apoptosis induced by experimental cerebral ischemia. *J. Neurosci.* 18, 3659–3668.

Nakanishi N, S. Tu, Y. et al. Neuroprotection by the NR3A subunit of the NMDA receptor, *J. Neurosci.* 29 (2009) 5260–5265.

Nellga rd, B., and Wieloch, T. (1992). NMDA-receptor blockers but not NBQX, an AMPA-receptor antagonist, inhibit spreading depression in the rat brain. *Acta Physiol. Scand.* 146, 497–503.

Nicholl, S.M., Roztocil, E., and Davies, M.G. (2006). Plasminogen activator system and vascular disease. *Curr. Vasc. Pharmacol.* 4, 101–116.

Nicholls, D.G. (2008). Oxidative stress and energy crises in neuronal dysfunction. *Ann. N. Y. Acad. Sci.* 1147, 53–60.

O'Neill SM, W.S. Rubinstein, et al. M.T. Ruffin 4th, Family Healthware Impact Trial group, Familial risk for common diseases in primary care: the Family Healthware Impact Trial, *Am. J. Prev. Med.* 36 (2009) 506–514.

Persson MG, P. Hedqvist, L.E. Gustafsson, Nerve-induced tachykinin-mediated vasodilation in skeletal muscle is dependent on nitric oxide formation, *Eur. J. Pharmacol.* 205 (1991) 295–301.

Pacher P, C. Szabo, Role of the peroxynitrite-poly(ADP-ribose) polymerase pathway in human disease, *Am. J. Pathol.* 173 (2008) 2–13.

Pozzilli C, G.L. Lenzi, et al. Imaging of leukocytic infiltration in human cerebral infarcts, *Stroke* 16 (1985) 251–255.

Pandian JD, Re-canalization in acute ischemic stroke: the strategies, *Neurol. India* 57 (2009) 20–27.

Parpura V, T.A. Basarsky, et al. Glutamate-mediated astrocyte-neuron signalling, *Nature* 369 (1994) 744–747.

Pasceri V, J.T. Willerson, E.T.H. Yeh, Direct proinflammatory effect of C-reactive protein on human endothelial cells, *Circulation* 102 (2000) 2165–2168.

Pepine, C.J. (2009). The impact of nitric oxide in cardiovascular medicine: untapped potential utility. *Am. J. Med.* 122 (5, Suppl), S10–S15.

Pacher, P., Beckman, J.S., and Liaudet, L. (2007). Nitric oxide and peroxynitrite in health and disease. *Physiol. Rev.* 87, 315–424.

Poli S, R. Veltkamp, Oxygen therapy in acute ischemic stroke—experimental efficacy and molecular mechanisms, *Curr. Mol. Med.* 9 (2009) 227–241.

Parpura V, Y. Fang, T. Basarsky, R. Jahn, P.G. Haydon, Expression of synaptobrevin II, cellubrevin and syntaxin but not SNAP-25 in cultured astrocytes, *FEBS Lett.* 377 (1995) 489–492.

Perini F, M. Morra, et al. Temporal profile of serum anti-inflammatory and pro-inflammatory interleukins in acute ischemic stroke patients, *Neurol. Sci.* 22 (2001) 289–296.

Reiter RJ, D.X. Tan, L.C. Manchester, H. Tamura, Melatonin defeats neurally-derived free radicals and reduces the associated neuromorphological and neurobehavioral damage, *J. Physiol. Pharmacol.* 58 (Suppl. 6) (2007) 5–22.

Rao R, V. Tah, J.P. Casas, et al. Ischemic stroke subtypes and their genetic basis: a comprehensive meta-analysis of small and large vessel stroke, *Eur. Neurol.* 61 (2009) 76–86, Epub 2008, November 28.

Romanic AM, R.F. White, A.J. Arleth, E.H. Ohlstein, F.C. Barone, Matrix metalloproteinase expression increases after cerebral focal ischemia in rats: inhibition of matrix metalloproteinase-9 reduces infarct size, *Stroke* 29 (1998) 1020–1030.

Rosenberg GA, M. Navratil, F. Barone, G. Feuerstein, Proteolytic cascade enzymes increase in focal cerebral ischemia in rat, *J. Cereb. Blood Flow Metab.* 16 (1996) 360–366.

Rothwell, P.M., Howard, et al. (2004). Fibrinogen concentration and risk of ischemic stroke and acute coronary events in 5113 patients with transient ischemic attack and minor ischemic stroke. *Stroke* 35, 2300–2305.

Rosamond, W. et al. (2008) Heart disease and stroke statistics: 2008 update – a report from the American Heart Association Statistics Committee and Stroke Statistics Subcommittee. *Circulation* 117, 25–146.

Rosell A, E. Cuadrado, et al. Hemorrhagic transformation after human ischemic stroke breakdown and basal lamina type IV collagen degradation during MMP-9-positive neutrophil infiltration is associated to blood–brain barrier, *Stroke* 39 (2008) 1121–1126.

Rost NS, P.A. Wolf, et al. Plasma concentration of C-reactive protein and risk of ischemic stroke and transient ischemic attack: the Framingham study, *Stroke* 32 (2001) 2575–2579.

Ross R, Atherosclerosis—an inflammatory disease, *N. Engl. J. Med.* 340 (1999) 115–126.

Sumii T, E.H. Lo, Involvement of matrix metalloproteinase in thrombolysis-associated hemorrhagic transformation after embolic focal ischemia in rats, *Stroke* 33 (2002) 831–836.

Slager CJ, J.J.Wentzel, et al. The role of shear stress in the destabilization of vulnerable plaques and related therapeutic implications, *Nat. Clin. Pract. Cardiovasc. Med.* 2 (2005) 456–464.

Strle K, J.H. Zhou, et al. Interleukin-10 in the brain, Crit. Rev. Immunol. 21 (2001) 427–449.

Spera PA, J.A. Ellison, G.Z. Feuerstein, F.C. Barone, IL-10 reduces rat brain injury following focal stroke, *Neurosci. Lett.* 251 (1998) 189–192.

Schinzel, A.C., Takeuchi, O., et al. (2005). Cyclophilin D is a component of mitochondrial permeability transition and mediates neuronal cell death after focal cerebral ischemia. *Proc. Natl. Acad. Sci. USA* 102, 12005–12010.

Schulz, E., Jansen, T., et al. (2008). Nitric oxide, tetrahydrobiopterin, oxidative stress, and endothelial dysfunction in hypertension. *Antioxid. Redox Signal.* 10, 1115–1126.

Selnes, O.A., and Vinters, H.V. (2006). Vascular cognitive impairment. *Nat. Clin. Pract. Neurol.* 2, 538–547.

Schabitz WR, R. Kollmar, et al. Neuroprotective effect of granulocyte colony-stimulating factor after focal ischaemia, *Stroke* 34 (2003) 745–751.

Schneider A, C. Kruger, et al. The haematopoietic factor G-CSF is a neuronal ligand that counteracts programmed cell death and drives neurogenesis, *J. Clin. Invest.* 115 (2005) 2083–2098.

Schulz JB, M. Weller, M.A. Moskowitz, Caspases as treatment targets in stroke and neurodegenerative diseases, *Ann Neurol.* 45 (1999) 421–429.

Stary HC, Macrophages, macrophage foam cells, and eccentric intimal thickening in the coronary arteries of young children, *Atherosclerosis* 64 (1987) 91–108.

Szatkowski M, B. Barbour, D. Attwell, Non-vesicular release of glutamate from glial cells by reversed electrogenic glutamate uptake, *Nature* 348 (1990) 443–446.

Simard, J.M., Kent, T.A., et al. (2007). Brain oedema in focal ischaemia: molecular pathophysiology and theoretical implications. *Lancet Neurol.* 6, 258–268.

Simon, R.P. (2006). Acidotoxicity trumps excitotoxicity in ischemic brain. *Arch. Neurol.* 63, 1368–1371.

Simons, L.A., McCallum, J., Friedlander, Y., and Simons, J. (1998). Risk factors for ischemic stroke: Dubbo Study of the elderly. *Stroke* 29, 1341–1346.

Stoll G, C. Kleinschnitz, B. Nieswandt, Molecular mechanisms of thrombus formation in ischemic stroke: novel insights and targets for treatment, *Blood* 112 (2008) 3555–3562.

Shi C, X. Kang, Y.Wang, Y. Zhou, The coagulation factor V Leiden, MTHFRC677T variant and eNOS 4ab polymorphism in young Chinese population with ischemic stroke, *Clin. Chim. Acta* 396 (2008) 7–9, Epub 2008, June 15.

Stroke, (1989) Recommendations on stroke prevention, diagnosis, and therapy: report of theWHOTask Force on Stroke and other Cerebrovascular Disorders. *Stroke* 20, 1407–1431.

Tarkowski E, L. Rosengren, et al. Intrathecal expression of proteins regulating apoptosis in acute stroke, *Stroke* 30 (1999) 321–327.

Terao S, G. Yilmaz, K.Y. Stokes, et al. Blood cell-derived RANTES mediates cerebral microvascular dysfunction, inflammation, and tissue injury after focal ischemia–reperfusion, *Stroke* 39 (2008) 2560.

Tanahashi N, Thrombolysis by intravenous tissue plasminogen activator (t-PA)–current status and future direction, *Brain Nerve* 61 (2009) 41–52.

Teal PA, M.S. Pessin, Hemorrhagic transformation. The spectrum of ischemia-related brain hemorrhage, *Neurosurg. Clin. N. Am.* 3 (1992) 601–610.

Turner R, R. Vink, Inhibition of neurogenic inflammation as a novel treatment for ischemic stroke, *Timely Top. Med. Cardiovasc. Dis.* 11 (2007) E24.

Thomenius MJ, N.S. Wang, et al. Bcl-2 on the endoplasmic reticulum regulates bax activity by binding to BH3-only proteins, *J. Biol. Chem.* 278 (2003) 6243–6250.

T˘an˘asescu R, A. Nicolau, et al. An immunological approach to cerebral ischemia (I). Immune cells and adhesion molecules, *Rom. J. Intern. Med.* 46 (2008) 3–8.

Terai K, A. Matsuo, E.G. McGeer, P.L. McGeer, Enhancement of immunoreactivity for NF-_B in human cerebral infarctions, *Brain Res.* 739 (1996) 343–349.

Tarnacka B, G. Gromadzka, A. Członkowska, Increased circulating immune complexes in acute stroke: the triggering role of Chlamydia pneumoniae and cytomegalovirus, *Stroke* 33 (2002) 936–940.

Tsuji K, T. Aoki, et al. Tissue plasminogen activator promotes matrix metalloproteinase-9 upregulation after focal cerebral ischemia, *Stroke* 36 (2005) 1954–1959.

Valtonen V, A.Kuikka, J. Syrjänen, Thrombo-embolic complications in bacteraemic infections, *Eur. Heart J.* 14 (Suppl. K) (1993), 20–23.

van Exel E, J. Gussekloo, et al. Inflammation and stroke: the Leiden 85-plus study, *Stroke* 33 (2002) 1135–1138.

Weise J, R. Sandau, et al. Deletion of cellular prion protein results in reduced Akt activation, enhanced postischemic caspase-3 activation, and exacerbation of ischemic brain injury, *Stroke* 37 (2006) 1296–1300.

Wang X, S.R. Lee, et al. Lipoprotein receptor-mediated induction of matrix metalloproteinase by tissue plasminogen activator, *Nat. Med.* 9 (2003) 1313–1317.

Weyrich AS, E.J. Skalabrin, L.W. Kraiss, Targeting the inflammatory response in secondary stroke prevention: a role for combining aspirin and extended-release dipyridamole, *Am. J. Ther.* 16 (2009) 164–170.

Wei Y, S. Mojsov, Multiple human receptors for pituitary adenylyl cyclase-activating polypeptide and vasoactive intestinal peptide are expressed in a tissue-specific manner, *Ann. N. Y. Acad. Sci.* 805 (1996) 624–627.

Wang, Q., Tang, X.N., and Yenari, M.A. (2007). The inflammatory response in stroke. *J. Neuroimmunol.* 184, 53–68.

Welsh, P., Barber, M., et al. (2009). Associations of inflammatory and haemostatic biomarkers with poor outcome in acute ischemic stroke. *Cerebrovasc. Dis.* 27, 247–253.

Whiteley W, W.L. Chong, A. Sengupta, P. Sandercock, Blood markers for the prognosis of ischemic stroke: a systematic review, *Stroke* 40 (2009) e380–e389, Epub 2009, March 12.

Warr O, M. Takahashi, D. Attwell, Modulation of extracellular glutamate concentration in rat brain slices by cystine-glutamate exchange, *J. Physiol.* 514 (1999) 783–793.

Wang PY, C.-H. Kao, M.-Y. Mui, S.-J.Wang, Leukocyte infiltration in acute hemispheric stroke, *Stroke* 24 (1993) 236–240.

Wolpert, S.M. et al. (1993) Neuroradiologic evaluation of patients with acute stroke treated with recombinant tissue plasminogen activator: the rtPA Acute Stroke Study Group. Am. *J. Neuroradiol.* 14, 3–13.

Yasuda H, H. Shichinohe, et al. Neuroprotective effect of a heat shock protein inducer, geranylgeranylacetone in permanent focal cerebral ischaemia, *Brain Res.* 1032 (2005) 176–182.

Ye ZC, M.S. Wyeth, S. Baltan-Tekkok, B.R. Ransom, Functional hemichannels in astrocytes: a novel mechanism of glutamate release, *J. Neurosci.* 23 (2003) 3588–3596.

Yenari M, K. Kitagawa, P. Lyden, M. Perez-Pinzon, Metabolic downregulation: a key to successful neuroprotection? *Stroke* 39 (2008) 2910–2917, Epub 2008, July 24.

Yang JT, C.N. Chang, et al. Dexamethasone inhibits ischaemia-induced transient reduction of neurotrophin-3 mRNA in rat hippocampus neurons, *Neuroreport* 9 (1998) 3477–3480.

Yuan J, Neuroprotective strategies targeting apoptotic and necrotic cell death for stroke, *Apoptosis* 14 (2009) 469–477.

Zhang Q, M. Fukuda, et al. Synaptotagmin IV regulates glial glutamate release, *Proc. Natl. Acad. Sci. U.S.A.* 101 (2004) 9441–9446.

In: Recent Advances in Stroke Therapeutics
Editor: Manzoor Ahmad Mir

ISBN: 978-1-63117-754-5

Chapter III

Inflammation and Anti-Inflammatory Agents in Strokes

Abstract

Two important pathophysiological mechanisms involved during a stroke are oxidative stress and inflammation. Brain tissue is not well equipped with antioxidant defenses, so reactive oxygen species and other free radicals/oxidants, released by inflammatory cells, threaten the tissue viability in the vicinity of the ischemic core. In a stroke, cerebral blood vessels are the first to be exposed to the ischemic insult, and their reaction to injury sets the stage for the inflammatory response. Molecules released from injured or dying brain cells also contribute to the inflammatory response. Focal ischemia evokes a robust inflammatory response that begins within a few hours of onset and typifies the secondary or delayed response to ischemia. Hence there is a notion that taming post-ischemic inflammation may block secondary events that extend brain injury. However, as noted below, during the later stages in the injury process, inflammation promotes critical events necessary for tissue repair. Here in this chapter, we will discuss the molecular aspects of oxidative stress and inflammation in an ischemic stroke and potential therapeutic strategies that target neuroinflammation and the innate immune system. Currently, little is known about endogenous counter regulatory immune mechanisms. However, recent studies show that regulatory T cells are major cerebral-protective immunomodulators after stroke, suggesting that targeting the endogenous adaptive immune response may offer novel promising neuroprotectant therapies. New research has shown that brain ischemia and trauma elicit strong inflammatory reactions driven by both external and brain cells. The recognition of inflammation as a fundamental response to brain ischemia provides novel opportunities for new anti-inflammatory therapies. Hypertension, cardiovascular disease, arterial fibrillation, diabetes mellitus, smoking, and alcohol abuse are all risk factors for a stroke. Clinical observations suggest that inflammation is also a direct risk factor for a stroke. Recent studies have shown that plasma levels of inflammatory cytokines or soluble adhesion molecules are high in non-stroke patients, and anti-inflammatory therapy is effective at reducing the stroke incidence in not only animal models, but in humans as well. Statins have been shown to decrease the stroke incidence via anti-inflammatory effects that are both dependent and independent of their cholesterol-lowering effects. These reports suggest that inflammation might directly affect the onset of a stroke. Here in this chapter, we present the latest findings about the cellular and humoral aspects of immune and inflammatory reactions in the brain. They may have an impact on the treatment of neuro-injuries and ancillary brain diseases, and increase the understanding of the roles infections and immune reactions play in the brain milieu.

Introduction

Strokes are an important issue in public health due to their high rates of morbidity and mortality, and disability. A stroke is one of the most common causes of death and disability worldwide (Lyod Johnes D 2009). However, current therapeutic strategies for strokes have been largely unsuccessful. One possible explanation is that research and pharmacological management have focused on very early events in brain ischemia. New research has shown that brain ischemia and trauma elicit strong inflammatory reactions driven by both external and brain cells. The recognition of inflammation as a fundamental response to brain ischemia provides novel opportunities for new anti-inflammatory therapies. Hypertension, cardiovascular disease, arterial fibrillation, diabetes mellitus, smoking, and alcohol abuse are all risk factors for a stroke. Clinical observations suggest that inflammation is also a direct risk factor for a stroke. Stroke patients have high levels of inflammatory cytokines in plasma, and immune cells, such as macrophages and T-lymphocytes, are noted within stroke lesions. These inflammatory events are considered as a result of a stroke. However, recent studies show that plasma levels of inflammatory cytokines or soluble adhesion molecules are high in non- stroke patients, and anti-inflammatory therapy is effective at reducing stroke incidence in not only animal models, but in humans as well. Statins have been shown to decrease the stroke incidence via anti-inflammatory effects that are both dependent and independent of their cholesterol-lowering effects. These reports suggest that inflammation might directly affect the onset of a stroke. Microglial cells and blood-derived monocytes/macrophages play important roles in inflammation in both onset and aggravation of stroke lesions. Two important pathophysiological mechanisms involved during an ischemic stroke are oxidative stress and inflammation. Brain tissue is not well equipped with antioxidant defenses, so reactive oxygen species and other free radicals/oxidants, released by inflammatory cells, threaten the tissue viability in the vicinity of the ischemic core. This chapter will discuss the molecular aspects of oxidative stress and inflammation in ischemic strokes and potential therapeutic strategies that target neuroinflammation and the innate immune system. Currently, little is known about endogenous counterregulatory immune mechanisms. However, recent studies show that regulatory T cells are major cerebroprotective immunomodulators after a stroke suggesting that targeting the endogenous adaptive immune response may offer novel promising neuroprotectant therapies.

Here in this chapter, we present the latest findings about the cellular and humoral aspects of immune and inflammatory reactions in the brain. They may have an impact on the treatment of neuro-injuries and ancillary brain diseases, and increase the understanding of the roles infections and immune reactions play in the brain milieu. Although different mechanisms are involved in the occurrence and development of a stroke, inflammatory response is greatly involved in its sequence (Barone FC 2001). Inflammation is intricately related to the onset of a stroke and to subsequent stroke-related tissue damage. Focal ischemia evokes a robust inflammatory response that begins within a few hours of onset and typifies the secondary or delayed response to ischemia (Figure 3.1). Inflammation within the arterial wall plays a vital role in promoting atherosclerosis (Chomorro A 2004, Elkind MS 2002). Arterial thrombosis (usually associated with ulcerated plaques) is triggered by multiple processes involving endothelial activation, and proinflammatory and prothrombotic interactions between the vessel walls and circulating blood elements. An elevated stroke risk has been linked to high levels of serologic markers of inflammation such as C-reactive protein (Ridker PM 2000), ESR, interleukin-6, TNF-alpha, and soluble intercellular adhesion molecule (sICAM) (Tanne D 2000). These events are promoted in part by the binding of cell adhesion molecules from the selectin and immunoglobulin gene families expressed on endothelial cells to the glycoprotein receptors expressed on the neutrophil surface. As evidence, reduced ischemic infarction is observed in ICAM-1 knockout mice and infarction volumes are increased in mice that overexpress P-selectin (Connoly ES 1996 and 1997). The proinflammatory molecule P-selectin is expressed on vascular endothelial within 90 min after cerebral ischemia, ICAM-1 by 4 h, and E-selectin by 24 h (del Zoppo G 2000).

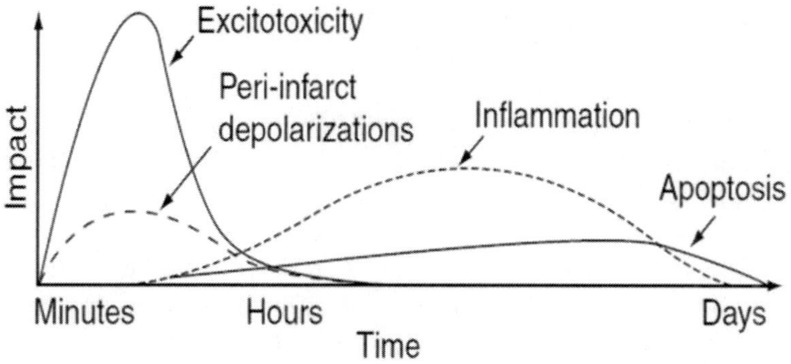

Figure 3.1. Inflammation Putative cascade of damaging events in focal cerebral ischemia.Very early after the onset of the focal perfusion deficit, excitotoxic mechanisms can damage neurons and glia lethally. In addition, excitotoxicity triggers a number of events that can further contribute to the demise of the tissue. Such events include peri-infarct depolarizations and the more-delayed mechanisms of inflammation and programmed cell death. The x-axis reflects the evolution of the cascade over time, while the y-axis aims to illustrate the impact of each element of the cascade on final outcome (courtesy of Dirnagl et al. 1999).

Inhibiting both selectin adhesion molecules and activation of complement reduces brain injury and suppresses neutrophil and platelet accumulation after focal ischemia in mice (Huang J 1999). In humans, neutrophil and complement activation significantly worsened outcomes in a clinical trial using humanized mouse antibodies directed against ICAM Enlimomab (Enlimomab 2000). Hence, the complexities of interactions between multiple pathways will have to be carefully considered for optimal translation to the clinic. Ischemic stroke-related brain injury itself triggers inflammatory cascades within the parenchyma that further amplify tissue damage (del Zoppo G 2000). As reactive microglia, macrophages, and leukocytes are recruited into ischemic brain, inflammatory mediators are generated by these cells as well as by neurons and astrocytes. Inducible nitric oxide synthase (iNOS), cyclooxygenase-2 (COX-2), interleukin-1 (IL-1), and monocyte chemoattractant protein-1 (MCP-1) are key inflammatory mediators, as evidenced by attenuated ischemic injury in mutant mice with targeted disruption of these genes (Barone FC 1999, Huggs PM 2002, Ledecolla C 2001, Boutin H 2001).

Initially after occlusion, there is a transient upregulation of immediate early genes encoding transcription factors (e.g., c-fos, c-Jun) that occurs within minutes. This is followed by a second wave of heat shock genes (e.g., HSP70, HSP72) that increases within 1–2 h and then decreases by 1–2 days. Approximately 12–24 h after a stroke, a third wave comprised of chemokines and cytokines is expressed (e.g., IL-1, IL-6, IL-8, TNF-alpha, MCP-1, etc.). Whether or not these three waves are causally related is not known. Nevertheless, therapies that seek to target these pathways need to be carefully timed to match the complex temporal evolution of tissue injury. Inflammatory Cascades stimulate both detrimental and potentially beneficial pathways after ischemia. For example, administering TNF-alpha neutralizing antibodies reduces brain injury after focal ischemia in rats (Nawashiro H 1997), whereas ischemic injury increases in TNF receptor knockout mice (Bruce AJ 1996). In part, these contrasting results may reflect signal transduction cascades activated by TNF-R1 and TNF-R2, with TNF-R1 augmenting cell death and TNF-R2 mediating neuroprotection (Fountaine V 2002). Similarly, the peptide vascular endothelial growth factor (VEGF) exacerbates edema in the acute phase of cerebral ischemia, but promotes vascular remodeling during stroke recovery (Zhang ZG 2000). Ultimately, the net effect of these mediators depends upon the stage of tissue injury or the predominance of a single signaling cascade among multiple divergent pathways.

In the early stage of cerebral ischemia, circulating leukocytes including neutrophils, macrophages, and lymphocytes migrate and adhere to the injured endothelial cells and infiltrate into the ischemic brain region *via* a dysfunctional blood–brain barrier (Lakhan SE 2009). The inflammatory response is also characterized by endogenous microglia activation following focal cerebral ischemia (Hellenbeck JM 1996, Morioka T 1993, Wang Q 2007). The infiltration of blood derived leukocytes and macrophages liberate toxic and inflammatory mediators involved in a "no reflow phenomenon" and amplify the ischemic brain injury (Yilmaz G 2010).

Post-ischemic reflow, either due to collateral circulation establishment or therapeutic recanalization, leads to the generation of reactive oxygen species (ROS), which then stimulates ischemic cells, including neurons and astrocytes to secrete inflammatory cytokines, chemokines and adhesion molecules (Ceulemans AG 2010). Once the inflammatory cascade is activated, inflammatory cells can release a variety of cytotoxic agents, including more cytokines, matrix metalloproteinases (MMPs), nitric oxide (NO) and induce more cell damage as well as disruption of the blood–brain barrier (BBB) and extracellular matrix (Denton GH 2003, Emsley HC 2002). Blocking various aspects of the inflammatory cascade was shown to attenuate ischemic brain injury from an experimental stroke (Han HS 2003) although this has yet to be demonstrated clinically (Becker K 2001). Exploration of ischemia-induced inflammatory related biomarkers therefore is important and necessary to understand the mechanism of ischemia-induced inflammatory brain injury.

During cerebral ischemia, inflammatory cytokines interleukin (IL)-1β, IL-6 and tumor necrosis factor (TNF), are extremely up-regulated (up to 40- to 60-fold) at least in the brain within the first 24 h of an experimental stroke model (Clausen 2005 and 2008, Hill JK 1999, Lambertsen 2005). These three cytokines are able to affect the volume of the ischemic induced tissue damage in a rodent experimental stroke model (Yang GY 1999). These cytokines also increase in cerebro-spinal fluid (CSF) and circulating blood after an ischemic stroke in humans (Allan SM 2005, Mccoy MK 2008 and Whiteley W 2009). Although IL-1β, IL-6, and TNFα are among the most investigated cytokines in CSF and blood in human stroke patients, their availability and mechanism of action in the human brain in the early phase after an experimental stroke remain unknown (Ginsberg MD 2008). Besides these three cytokines, other factors such as IL-8, IL-10, CD40L, IFNγ, IL-1α, IL-17, and TGFβ also participate in the inflammatory response after an ischemic stroke (Pang L 2001 and Smith CJ 2004). Understanding the cellular production of cytokines in normal brain, and the time profile and the cellular sources of these cytokines, and the possibilities of their transport in the ischemic territory in the early phase after the onset of a stroke is crucial to unveiling the mechanisms by which these cytokines potentially affect brain damage after an ischemic stroke. A panel of cytokines has been shown to vary their presence in the peripheral blood after cerebral ischemia, which is associated with changes of their levels in the brain tissue or the cerebral spinal fluid (CSF). However, the principal shortcoming including a high individual variance of circulating cytokine levels limited the establishment of clinical criteria for control groups. Using a modified method (mosaic ELISA kits), Zeng et al. has detected a cluster of cytokines in each sample at the same time. This novel method required less volume of a blood sample and significantly decreased biological error compared to other studies using single ELISA assay.

To establish a relevant control group is critical in clinical stroke studies. In most cases, studies are limited to the choice of healthy volunteer as a control group. Chronic disease such as diabetes, hypertension, hyperlipidemia also influence a chronic inflammatory response and result in the release of numerous circulating cytokines (Spraner J 2003 Greenberg AS 2006 and Wisse BE 2004). Stroke patients usually suffer a significantly higher frequency of cardiovascular risk factors compared to the healthy controls. Hence, the difference in circulating cytokine levels between the stroke group and the control group could not exclude the influence of cardiovascular risk factors. To eliminate this factor, Zeng et al. chose age, sex, cardiovascular risk factors matched normal controls to eliminate the influence of cardiovascular risk factors. As a result, they found that among the most studied panel of pro-inflammatory cytokines, IL-6 was the only one that was not up-regulated in plasma after cerebral ischemia but also correlated with the severity of neurological impairment.

Numerous studies have revealed a close relationship between pro-inflammatory cytokine release and post-stroke, inflammatory injury (Dnes A 2010, Lambertsen KL 2005 and Spalata G 2006). Although many studies focus on the clinical significance of individual cytokine, each source of circulating cytokines is unclear. A study on the source of cytokines in peripheral blood is useful to better understand the function of cytokine both in peripheral and brain inflammation. There are three major hypotheses:

(1) Cytokines are released into circulating blood by inflammatory cells in ischemic brain tissue *via* an impaired blood–brain barrier;
(2) Cytokines are secreted and released by activating leukocytes such as neutrophils, lymphocytes and monocytes;
(3) Cytokines are released by peripheral immune organs

However, some researchers (Planas Am 2006, Wang Q 2007, Tutolomonodo A 2008) did not find a positive relationship between plasma cytokine protein level and their RNA level in leukocyte. Therefore, the source of circulating cytokines needs to be further studied in the future. The interaction of cytokines is another important issue which is largely unknown. It is interesting that Zeng et al. adopted Bayesian network (BN) learning procedure in an attempt to understand the interactions (inter-influencing network) among the 8 cytokines in protein and mRNA level after an ischemic stroke. The BN method is used widely in many fields, including protein–protein interactions (Bradford JR 2006, Hack CE 2010), gene function analysis (Zhao B 2011), and brain functional connectivity using MRI (Burge J 2009). Zeng et al. used this method to explore the interaction among circulating pro-inflammatory cytokines in patients with acute ischemic stroke. Although the data need to be further confirmed by others, the original result revealed a suspected complex circulating pro-inflammatory cytokine network model with positive and negative feedback. Pro-inflammatory cytokine up-regulation in plasma and compensatory immunity, depression in leukocyte involve in peripheral inflammatory response to ischemic brain injury. IL-6 activation is a potential therapeutic target for stroke therapy to attenuate secondary inflammatory injury. The detailed cytokine network during ischemia development calls for further investigation with animal experiments *in vivo* and *in vitro*.

The most common cause of a stroke is the sudden occlusion of a blood vessel by a thrombus or embolism, resulting in an almost immediate loss of oxygen and glucose to the cerebral tissue. Although different mechanisms are involved in the pathogenesis of a stroke, increasing evidence shows that ischemic injury and inflammation account for its pathogenic progression (Muir KW 2007). Cerebral ischemia triggers the pathological pathways of the ischemic cascade and ultimately causes irreversible neuronal injury in the ischemic core within minutes of the onset (Dirnagl U 1999). However, a much larger volume of brain tissue surrounding this ischemic core, known as the penumbra, can be salvaged if cerebral blood flow is promptly restored. Thus, the original definition of the ischemic penumbra referred to areas of the brain that were damaged but not yet dead, offering the promise that if proper therapies could be found, one could rescue brain tissue after a stroke and reduce post-stroke disability. Despite advances in the understanding of the pathophysiology of cerebral ischemia, therapeutic options for acute ischemic stroke remain very limited (Donnan GA 2008). Only one drug is approved for clinical use for the thrombolytic treatment of acute ischemic stroke in the US and that is intravenous recombinant tissue plasminogen activator (rt-PA). When delivered within three hours after symptom onset, rt-PA reduces neurological deficits and improves the functional outcome of stroke patients. However, this improvement in recovery is achieved at the expense of an increased incidence in symptomatic intracranial hemorrhage, which occurs in ~6% of patients. Furthermore, since the large majority of patients with acute ischemic stroke do not go to the hospital within three hours of stroke onset most do not receive rt-PA treatment (Furlan AJ 2003). Consequently, the successful treatment of acute ischemic stroke remains one of the major challenges in clinical medicine. This chapter will provide a brief overview of the current understanding of the inflammatory mechanisms involved in an acute ischemic stroke and the neuroprotective agents that can curtail neuroinflammation and potentially show utility in the treatment of a stroke. Neuroprotective treatments or therapies block the cellular, biochemical, and metabolic elaboration of injury during exposure to ischemia. Of the more than 100 neuroprotective agents that reached randomized clinical trials in focal ischemic stroke, none has proven unequivocally efficacious, despite success seen in preceding animal studies (O'Collins VE 2006). However, the field trials of the past have greatly increased our understanding of the fundamental biology of ischemic brain injury and have laid a strong foundation for future advance. New anti-inflammatory targets continue to be identified, which is an important area of translational medicine in acute stroke. Overall, the prospects for safe neuroprotective therapies to improve stroke outcomes remain promising (De la Ossa NP 2007).

Immune Activation and Systemic Inflammation before a Stroke

The immune system plays a role in the development of atheromatous plaque and in plaque rupture (Koenig W 2007). The production of atheromatous plaque involves local inflammation within the wall of blood vessels (Croce K 2007, Hansson GK 2006). The cells in the plaque include macrophages, CD4 and CD8 T cells (Xu QB 1990, Jhonsson L 1990). One target of the immune attack in atherosclerosis is oxidized low density lipoprotein (oxLDL), which is highly immunogenic (Kobayashi K 2005). Some of the T cells in plaque are likely to be specific for oxLDL, as tolerance to oxLDL reduces the severity of atheroma through a mechanism involving regulatory T cells (Treg cells) (Mor A 2007, Van Pujvelde Gh 2006). The entry of leukocytes into tissue is mediated by endothelial expression of adhesion molecules, such as vascular cell adhesion molecule-1 (VCAM-1), intercellular adhesion molecule-1 (ICAM-1) and E-selectin and L-selectin (Moller F 2005, Galkina E 2006). Chemokines are members of a large superfamily of small molecules that have a role in the movement of leukocytes through tissues. This occurs through interaction with chemokine receptors on cells (Colobran R 2007). Chemokines play a role in the entry of lymphocytes into atheromatous plaque. For example, CXCR6 is required for the entry of CXC61 cells into atheromatous plaque (Galkina E 2007) and CXCL10 attracts effector T cells into plaque (Heller EA 2006). Another factor that regulates atherogenesis is an expression of CD40, which is a glycoprotein expressed on many cells including endothelial cells. Ligation of CD40 on endothelium results in endothelial activation. CD40 interacts with CD40 ligand (CD40L), which is expressed on CD41 T cells. CD40 is important in the entry of T cells into plaque and also in plaque activation (Mach F 1997) T cells that have entered an atheromatous plaque may release cytokines that lead to plaque rupture (Tedgui A 2006).

Systemic inflammation, measured as high levels of C-reactive protein (CRP) (Tanne D 2006) or fibrinogen (Zhu YC 2006), is a risk factor for a stroke (Elkind MS 2006). There is debate as to whether, in individual patients, there is a causal relationship between elevated levels of these proteins and stroke incidence. A recent study suggests that patients with echo-lucent plaques, that are likely to rupture, have higher levels of systemic inflammation than patients with plaques that are less likely to rupture (Withnoto AT 2006). Thus, inflammatory processes may predispose to stroke. Furthermore, in experimental animals, systemic inflammation induced by injection of lipopolysaccharide (LPS) causes exacerbation of damage through pathways involving interleukin-1 (IL-1) (McColl BW 2007). The brain is considered to be a site of relative immunological privilege, because of the relative lack of rejection of foreign tissue that has been transplanted into the brain (Simpson E 2006). Microglia, which are the resident antigen-presenting cells in the brain, are thought to provide constant surveillance of tissue injury (Nimerjhan A 2005) and become activated when injury occurs. However, for an adaptive immune response to occur, antigen- presenting cells must travel to draining lymph nodes. Microglia are thought to have little or no ability to travel to draining lymph nodes, which has been put forward as one reason for the relative immune privilege of the brain (Melchior B 2006). Nevertheless, there is immune surveillance of the brain and there are local immune responses to brain injury (Lucas SM 2006). As well as parenchymal microglia, the brain also has perivascular macrophages (Kim WK 2006) that are hematogenous in origin. Furthermore, in strokes, and in other pathological states, breakdown of the blood–brain barrier (Wang PY 1993) means that the injured tissue becomes relatively more exposed to immune processes with entry of blood-borne inflammatory cells. Macrophages of the brain are able to travel to draining lymph nodes to initiate adaptive immune responses (Fabreik BO 2005).

Post-Ischemic Inflammation

Although for many years the CNS was considered an immune-privileged organ, it is now well accepted that the immune and the nervous system are engaged in bidirectional crosstalk. Moreover, mounting data suggest that in the brain, as in peripheral organs, inflammatory cells participate in tissue remodeling after injury. Microglial cells are the resident macrophages of the brain and play a critical role as resident immunocompetent and phagocytic cells in the CNS. Ekdahl and colleagues (Ekdahl CT 2009) reported an increased number of activated microglial cells up to 16 weeks after two hours MCAO in rats. After activation by ischemia, microglia can transform into phagocytes and they can release a variety of substances, many of which are cytotoxic and/or cytoprotective. Microglia may exert neuroprotection by producing neurotrophic molecules such as brain-derived neurotrophic factor (BDNF), insulin-like growth factor I (IGF-I), and several other growth factors. There is substantial evidence that activated microglial cells in response to ischemia have the potential of releasing several pro-inflammatory cytokines such as TNF-α, IL-1β, and IL-6, as well as other potential cytotoxic molecules including NO, ROS, and prostanoids (Lucas SM 2006). Astrocytes, like microglia, are capable of secreting inflammatory factors such as cytokines, chemokines, and NO (Swanson RA 2004). Cytokines upregulate the expression of cell adhesion molecules (CAMs). Within four to six hours after ischemia onset, circulating leukocytes adhere to the vessel walls and migrate into the brain with subsequent release of additional pro-inflammatory mediators and secondary injury in the penumbra. Neutrophils are the earliest leukocyte subtype to show substantial upregulation in gene expression studies and to infiltrate areas of brain ischemia (see figure 3.2).

Recently, Shichita et al. (Shichita T 2009) demonstrated an infiltration of γdT cells 3 days after the onset of ischemia in a mouse model, along with a production of IL-17 which amplifies the inflammatory cascade. IL-23 from infiltrating macrophages appears to produce Il-23 which attracts the infiltrating γdT cells. Blocking a specific γdT cell receptor with an antibody effectively reduced three day infarct volumes, even when treatment was initiated at 24 hours after onset of cerebral ischemia. Targeting these γdT cells may offer a clinical opportunity with a longer therapeutic window to prevent the secondary inflammatory expansion of cerebral damage after a stroke. The described post-ischemic neuroinflammatory changes lead to dysfunction of the brain tissue. Therefore, therapeutic targeting of the neuroinflammatory pathways in acute ischemic strokes has become an important area of research in translational medicine.

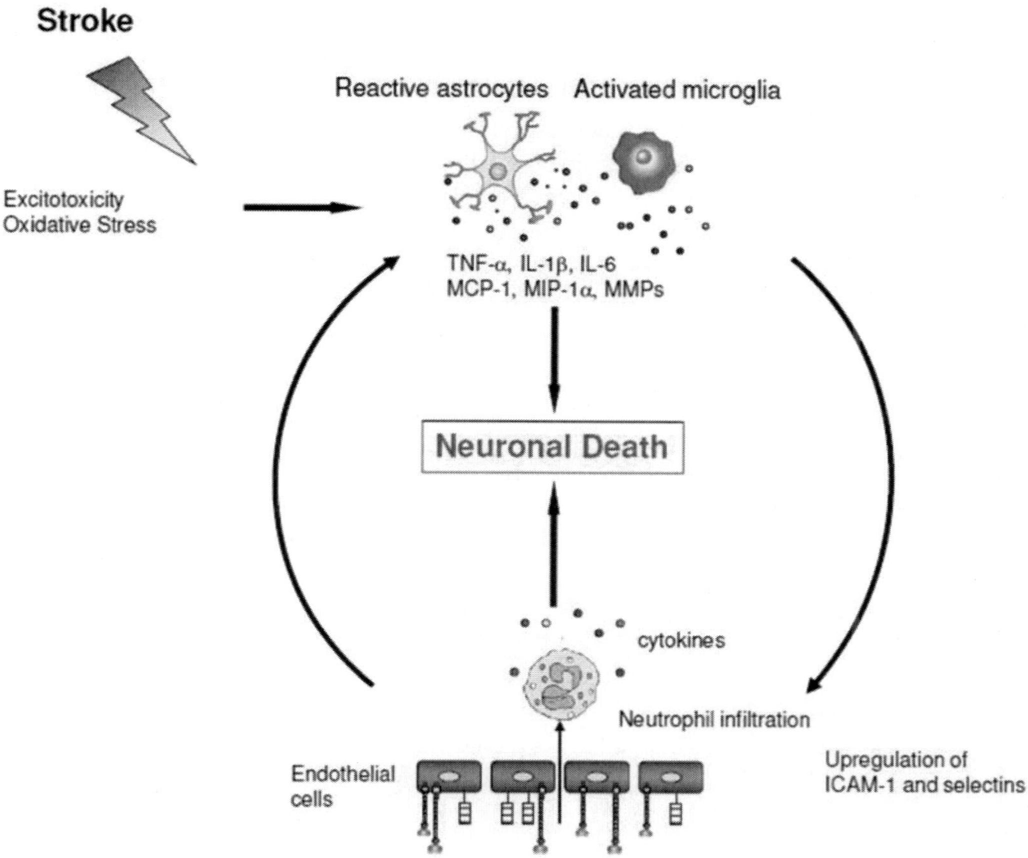

Figure 3.2. Postischemic inflammatory responses. Excitotoxicity and oxidative stress caused by the initial ischemic event activate microglia and astrocytes, which react by secreting cytokines, chemokines and matrix metalloproteases (MMP). These inflammatory mediators lead to an upregulation of cell adhesion molecules on endothelial cells, allowing blood derived inflammatory cells, mainly neutrophils, to infiltrate the ischemic brain area. Neutrophils themselves also secrete cytokines which cause a further activation of glial cells. These processes all result in neuronal cell death and enhance the damage to the ischemic brain.

Cytokines and Brain Inflammation

Cytokines are a group of small glycoproteins that are produced in response to an antigen and were originally described as mediators for regulating the innate and adaptive immune systems. Cytokines are thus upregulated in the brain in a variety of diseases, including strokes. In the brain, cytokines are expressed not only in the cells of the immune system, but are also produced by resident brain cells, including neurons and glia (Barone FC 1999). In addition, it has been shown that peripherally derived cytokines are involved in brain inflammation. Thus, peripherally derived mononuclear phagocytes, T lymphocytes, NK cells and polymorphonuclear leukocytes produce and secrete cytokines and might contribute to inflammation of the CNS (Ferrarese C 1999).

The most studied cytokines related to inflammation in an acute ischemic stroke are tumor necrosis factor-α (TNF-α), the interleukins (IL), IL-1β, IL-6, IL-20, IL-10 and transforming growth factor (TGF)-β. While IL-1β and TNF-α, appear to exacerbate cerebral injury, TGF-β and IL-10 may be neuroprotective (Zhu Y 2002, Spera PA 1998). Increased production of proinflammatory cytokines and lower levels of the anti-inflammatory IL-10 are related to larger infarctions and poorer clinical outcome. Elevated IL-1β mRNA expression occurs within the first 15-30 min after permanent MCAO and elevated IL-1β protein expression occurs a few hours later and remains elevated for up to 4 days (Caso JR 2007). There are studies that correlate an increase in the levels of IL-1β after ischemia with worsening of the infarct severity. For example, Yamasaki et al. (Yamasaki Y 1995) demonstrated that intraventricular injection of recombinant IL-1β after MCAO increases the formation of brain edema, the volume of the size and the influx of neutrophils. In addition, IL-1β deficient mice presented smaller infarcts in comparison with wild-type mice (Boutin H 2001). High circulating IL-1β elevates circulating IL-6, other well-known cytokine that is upregulated following cerebral ischemia (Clark WM 1999). Moreover, the serum level of IL-6 correlates with brain infarct volume (Acalovschi D 2003) and is a powerful predictor of early neurological deterioration (Vila N 2001). On the other hand, Clark et al. (Clark WM 2001) demonstrated that infarct size and neurological function were not different in animals deficient in IL-6 after transient CNS ischemia. This suggests that IL-6 does not have a direct influence on acute ischemic injury. IL-20 is induced when IL-1β modulates p38 MAPK and the NF-κB pathway. IL-20 in turn induces the production of IL-6. Inhibition of IL-20 by a specific mAb significantly ameliorated the brain ischemic infarction in rats following MCAO (Chen WY 2009). Several approaches are under investigation for managing IL-1 in a stroke (Table 1). IL-1 acts via membrane receptors (IL-1R), which can be blocked by a receptor antagonist (IL-1RA). In a randomized trial for an acute stroke, IL-1RA readily crossed the blood-brain barrier, was safe to use, and seemed to afford some benefit, particularly for patients with cortical infarcts (Gueorguieva I 2008). IL-10 is an anti-inflammatory cytokine that acts by inhibiting IL-1 and TNF-α, and by suppressing cytokine receptor expression and receptor activation as well. As a consequence, IL-10 could provide neuroprotection in acute ischemic strokes. Both central and systemic administration of IL-10 to rats subjected to MCAO significantly reduced infarct size 30 min to three hours post MCAO (30). In acute ischemic strokes, elevated concentrations of IL-10 in CSF have been found (Tarkowski E 1997). Moreover, patients with low plasma levels (<6 pg/ml) of IL-10 during the first hours after a stroke were three times more likely to have worsening neurological symptoms within 48 hours following the stroke (Vila N 2001). IL-10 also seems to mediate the reduction in infarct size by regulatory T cells.

Table 1. Clinical studies of agents targeting inflammatory pathways in acute ischemic strokes

S. No	Neuro-protective agent	Mode of action	Reference
1	Enlimomab	Anti-ICAM-1 monoclonal antibody	Enlimomab 2001
2	Cerovive (NXY-059)	Nitrone-based free radical trapping agent	Lyden PD et al. 2007 Shuyaib A et al. 2007
3	Recombinant human IL-1RA	Interleukin-1 receptor antagonist	Emsley HC et al. 2005

S. No	Neuro-protective agent	Mode of action	Reference
4	UK-279, 276	Neutrophil inhibitory factor	Krams M et al. 2003
5	Tirilazad	Lipid peroxidation inhibitor	Bath PM et al. 2001
6	Ginsenoside	Ca2+ channel antagonist	Liu X et al. 2009
7	Edaravone MCI-186	Free radical scavenger	Edaravone Study Group 2003
8	Acetaminophen (Paracetamol)	Anti-pyretic effect	Van Breda EJ et al. 2005
9	Minocycline	Anti-inflammatory	Lampl Y et al. 2007
10	ONO-2506 (Arundic Acid)	Astrocyte modulator	Pettigrew LC et al. 2006

Adapted from Shah et al., 2009.

Chemokines and Brain Inflammation

Chemokines, for example, monocyte chemoattractant protein 1, are a class of cytokines that guide the migration of blood borne inflammatory cells, such as neutrophils and macrophages, towards the source of the chemokine. Consequently, they play important roles in cellular communication and inflammatory cell recruitment. Expression of chemokines such as MCP-1, macrophage inflammatory protein-1α (MIP-1α), and fractakline following focal ischemia is thought to have a deleterious effect by increasing leukocyte infiltration (Kim JS 1995). The level of a variety of chemokines has been found to increase in animal models of ischemia and their inhibition or deficiency has been associated with reduced injury (Soriano S 2002, Huges PM 2002). Mice without the chemokine receptor CCR2 are protected against ischemia-reperfusion injury (Dimitrijevic OB 2007).

Cellular Adhesion Molecules

There is increasing evidence that cellular adhesion molecules (CAMs) play an important role in the pathophysiology of an acute ischemic stroke. CAMs are upregulated in the first days after a stroke by various cytokines and are responsible for the adhesion and migration of the leukocytes. Leukocytes roll on the endothelial surface and then adhere to the endothelial cells. The interaction between leukocytes and the vascular endothelium is mediated by three main groups of CAMs: the selectins, the immunoglobulin gene superfamily, and the integrins. Selectins, especially E- and P-selectins are upregulated and mediate leukocyte rolling and recruitment during the early stages of ischemia (Zhang, R 1998) Among the immunoglobulin family member, intercellular adhesion molecule-1 (ICAM-1) and vascular cell adhesion molecule-1 have been the most extensively investigated in cerebral ischemia. Within hours after the onset of s stroke, ICAM-1 expression increases upon stimulation by cytokines (Lindsberg PJ 1996). Patients with acute ischemic strokes had higher soluble intracellular adhesion molecule-1 (sICAM-1) levels compared to patients without cardiovascular disease. Moreover, sICAM-1 levels were significantly higher in patients who died compared to those who survived (Rallidis LS, 2009). High sICAM-1 levels on admission are associated with early death is ischemic middle-aged stroke patients, suggesting a pathogenic role of inflammation in the evolution of ischemic strokes.

A number of animal studies have shown that after transient and permanent focal ischemia the upregulation of CAMs, especially ICAM-1, P- and E-selectin, preceded the invasion of neutrophils into the brain. There is ample evidence from animal models of MCAO that expression of CAMs is associated with cerebral infarct size. Thus, genetic ablation of CAMs resulted in reduced infarct size, which could be mimicked by treatment with anti-CAM antibodies (Zhang RL 1994, Gossev AV 1998). Inhibition of leukocyte activation and infiltration into the ischemic cerebral tissue has, therefore, been an important area of neuroprotection research. Thus far, anti-CAM treatment has not been successful in patients with acute ischemic strokes. However, further translational research into the therapeutic targeting of CAM is ongoing. The spatiotemporal profile of CAMs is still largely unresolved, even though they are crucial for efficient anti-inflammatory therapies. More knowledge of the spatiotemporal profile of CAMs may lead the way to successful application and monitoring of promising anti-inflammatory treatment strategies after a stroke.

Matrix Metalloproteinases

MMPs are a family of proteolytic enzymes that are responsible for remodeling the extracellular matrix and that can degrade all its constituents. Expression of MMPs in the adult brain is very low to undetectable, but many MMPs are upregulated in the brain in response to injury (Montaner J 2001).

Neurons, astrocytes, microglia, and endothelial cells have all been shown to express MMPs after injury. A stroke is associated with a biphasic disruption of the blood brain barrier (BBB) leading to vasogenic edema and hemorrhage and experimental studies have shown that that BBB breakdown and hemorrhage results from the expression and activation of MMPs (Asaie M 2001). MMP-2 and MMP-9 have been implicated in cerebral ischemia. Elevated MMP-9 levels were found in brain tissue and in serum from patients with acute ischemic strokes and in animal models of strokes beginning at 12 h after permanent MCAO (Park KP 2009).

MMP-9 is normally absent and this is the major MMP associated with neuroinflammation. Early (day 1) MMP-9 inhibition reduced infarction of day 14. However, the benefit was lost when the treatment was delayed until day 3 and the stroke pathology was exacerbated when the administration was delayed until day 7. These studies all suggest that MMP inhibition could have a beneficial effect on the outcome of a stroke, but the effect will depend on the timing of treatment in relation to the stage of brain injury (Zhao BQ 2006).

Proinflammatory Cytokines in Strokes

A stroke is the third leading cause of death and a major cause of disability in industrialized countries. An ischemic stroke is the most common type of stroke, occurring in approximately 80% of all strokes. A less common type of stroke is a hemorrhagic stroke, which occurs due to a subarachnoid hemorrhage and/or an intracerebral hemorrhage. Hypertension, cardiovascular disease, arterial fibrillation, diabetes mellitus, obesity, smoking, and alcohol abuse are risk factors for a stroke (Goldstein LB 2011), even if there are slight differences in the influence of these factors between ischemic stroke and hemorrhagic stroke. However, some stroke patients do not have any of these risk factors, suggesting that other risk factors exist. For many years, clinical observations showed that plasma levels of inflammatory cytokines were increased after stroke onset, and immune cells, especially monocytes/macrophages and T-lymphocytes, existed in stroke lesions and related to exaggerate brain damage. In the clinical setting, elevated plasma levels of inflammatory cytokines, C-reactive protein (CRP), and chemokines are associated with future cardiovascular risk (Blake GJ 2002). Plasma levels of soluble intercellular adhesion molecule-1 (sICAM-1) and sE-selectin were observed to be increased both in large intracranial artery disease and small-artery disease (Fassbender K 1999), and plasma levels of ICAM-1 and monocyte chemoattractant protein-1 (MCP-1) were noted to be high in patients with ischemic stroke and myocardial infarction (Sánchez-Moreno C 2004, Arakelyan A 2005). Epidemiological studies have shown that elevated leukocyte count was associated with the risk for first-time myocardial infarction and ischemic stroke (Prentice RL 1982, Fawa M 1987, Gillum RF 1994) and the risk of recurrent myocardial infarction and ischemic stroke in a high-risk population (Grau AJ 2004). These observations indicate that inflammatory events occur in stroke patients and increase the risk of stroke recurrence. Recently, both clinical and animal studies revealed that these inflammatory events occurred prior to stroke onset. Plasma levels of soluble vascular cell adhesion molecule-1 (sVCAM-1), sICAM-1, sE-selectin, and MCP-1 were elevated in patients with essential hypertension in the absence of other diseases (Blann AD 1994, Madej A 2005, Desouza CA 1997). Anti-inflammatory strategies were shown to suppress the incidence of a stroke in both human and animal models. These reports suggest that inflammation might be a risk factor for a stroke. Atherosclerosis is one of the major risk factors for a stroke, and monocytes/macrophages affect the brain indirectly by inducing unstable plaques and plaque rupture in atherosclerotic lesions (Newby AC 2008). It is well recognized that atherosclerosis is an inflammatory disease and macrophages play important roles in the initiation and the progression of atherosclerotic lesion. Accumulation of monocytes/macrophages in the vascular wall occurs early during atherosclerosis (Ross R 1999). In addition to phagocytosis of oxidized low-density lipoproteins, macrophages secrete interleukin-1β (IL-1β), tumor necrosis factor-α (TNF-α), and transforming growth factor-β1 (TGF-β1). These inflammatory cytokines and growth factors induce endothelial dysfunction, smooth muscle cell migration and proliferation, and extracellular matrix production as fibrous plaques. During later disease stages, activated macrophages secrete several classes of neutral extracellular proteases, including serine proteases, cathepsins, and matrix metalloproteinases (MMPs) (Dollery AM 2006). Blood monocytes have already expressed low levels of a few MMPs (Bar-Or A 2003); however, contact with matrix leads to rapid upregulation of a broad spectrum of MMPs. Cell biology experiments identify mechanisms by which excessive MMP production can cause plaque rupture, either directly by destruction of extracellular matrix or indirectly through actions that promote death of macrophages (Johnson JL 2008) and vascular smooth muscle cells (Newbay AC 2006). Rupture of unstable plaques may lead to thrombotic stroke onset. Inflammatory cytokines, such as IL-1β, IL-6, and TNF-α, are secreted by activated microglial cells and macrophages in stroke lesions and induce the expression of chemokines, which recruit mois more circulatingonocytes/macrophages into lesions and lead to further brain damage. However, the role of each cytokine in a stroke is complicated.

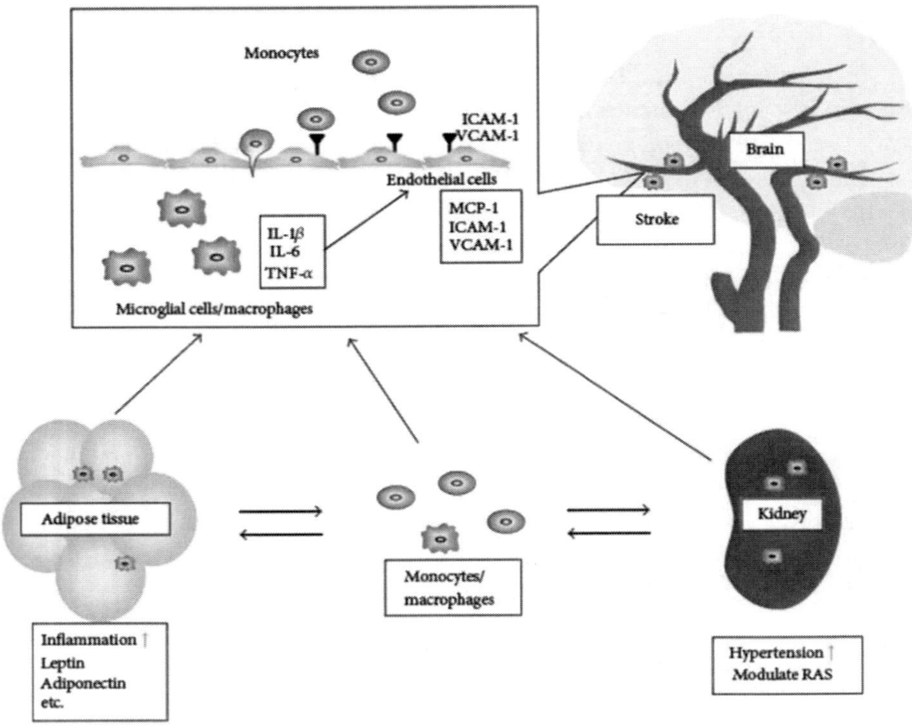

Figure 3.3. Inflammation: Monocytes/macrophages modulate adipose tissue and kidney functions and accelerate the onset of a stroke. Monocytes/macrophage infiltration into adipose tissue stimulates secretion of leptin and inflammatory cytokines and suppresses secretion of adiponectin, which induce systemic inflammation, endothelial cell dysfunction, and monocytes/macrophage activation. Monocytes/macrophages infiltration into kidney modulates renin-angiotensin system and increase blood pressure, which also induces endothelial cell dysfunction and monocytes/macrophages activation. Endothelial cells express MCP-1 and adhesion molecules, which induce monocytes chemotaxis, adhesion, and migration into subendothelial lesions. Microglial cells and infiltrated monocytes/macrophages in brain induce cerebrovascular damages and cause stroke onset.

Interleukin-1β

Recently, IL-1β has been considered a therapeutic target for a stroke. Chronic increases in IL-1β expression in the brain led to leukocyte infiltration and increased MCP-1 and ICAM-1 expressions in a mouse model, which is a phenotype also seen in stroke lesions. In addition, a number of studies have demonstrated that inhibiting the release or action of IL-1 markedly reduced ischemic cerebral damage in animal models. IL-1α and IL-1β double knockout mice exhibited dramatically reduced ischemic infarct volume compared with wild-type mice (Boutin H 2001). In a meta-analysis of animal model studies, IL-1 receptor antagonist (IL-1Ra), which represents the most advanced approach to modify IL-1 actions, reduced infarct volume in models of focal cerebral ischemia (Banwell V 2009). In humans, a phase II clinical trial of intravenous IL-1Ra compared with the placebo in patients with acute strokes is currently underway (Emsley HCA 2005). Further, IL-1Ra gene polymorphism represents a risk factor for an ischemic stroke (Olsson S 2012). These reports suggest that inhibition of IL-1β signals can prevent the onset of a stroke.

Interleukin-6

A prospective cohort study and systemic review revealed that plasma levels of IL-6 were associated with poor outcome after both ischemic and hemorrhagic strokes (Whiteley C 2009); however, it was not clear whether IL-6 increased before or after stroke onset. Animal models showed less association between IL-6 and strokes. IL-6 could not induce adhesion molecules and MCP-1 mRNA expressions in cerebrovascular endothelial cells derived from SHRSP. Mice deficient in IL-6 showed similar stroke lesion volume and neurological function as control mice in an acute ischemic injury model (Clark WM 2000). Furthermore, IL-6 mediates anti-inflammatory effects in addition to its proinflammatory role (Scheller A 2011). Therefore, its manipulation can have either detrimental or beneficial effects. Further studies are required to clarify the role of IL-6 in a stroke.

Tumor Necrosis Factor Alpha (TNF-α)

Increased serum and cerebro-spinal fluid levels of TNF-α have been found in patients 24 hours, 1 week, and 2 weeks after a stroke, and these increases correlate with infarct volume and severity of neurological impairment (Zaremba J 2001). However, previous reports suggest that TNF-α has a dual role in brain injury (Hallenbeck JM 2002). Blockade of TNF-α actions reduced infarct volume after permanent middle cerebral artery occlusion in BALB/C mice with the dimeric type I soluble TNF receptor, which binds to TNF-α and antagonizes its action (Nawashiro H 1997a). In contrast, TNF-α pretreatment was neuroprotective against permanent middle cerebral artery occlusion in BALB/C mice with reduction of infarct size, macrophages, and CD11b-positive neutrophils (Nawashiro H 1997b). In addition to these observations, pentoxifylline, an anti-inflammatory agent, attenuated damage of a stroke via the dual role of TNF-α. Pentoxifylline treatment increased serum levels of TNF-α, but not IL-1β and IL-6, and dose dependently prevented the occurrence of spontaneous brain damage by reducing macrophage infiltration into the lesion in SHRSP (Ban C 2004), suggesting a protective role of TNF-α. On the other hand, pentoxifylline reduced brain edema in a rat model of transient focal cerebral ischemia through a decline in TNF-α production (Vakili A 2011), suggesting aa deleteriousrole of TNF-α. Based on crucial evidence that implicate TNFa as a mediator of acute brain damage, a number of pharmacological strategies have been followed by di€erent investigators to either inhibit the synthesis or to neutralize the action of TNFa and to assess the e€ect of such treatments on the outcome of ischemia and trauma. The pharmacological approaches that have been applied to improve the outcome after brain injury were based on: (a) inhibition of TNFa synthesis of low molecular weight molecules; and (b) neutralization of the biological effect of TNFa by proteins such as specific antibodies or binding proteins. Although anti-TNF-α strategies have proved beneficial in other clinical settings such as inflammatory bowel disease, there are no clinical trials of anti-TNF-α agents in strokes. Further studies are therefore required to clarify the role of TNF-α in strokes.

MCP-1

CC chemokine ligand (CCL2) is known as MCP-1 and is a potent mononuclear cell attractant. MCP-1 is synthesized by several cell types, such as monocytes/macrophages, T-lymphocytes, smooth muscle cells, endothelial cells, and even cerebrovascular endothelial cells. Expression of MCP-1 is upregulated by inflammatory cytokines. Serum levels of MCP-1 are high in patients with ischemic strokes and myocardial infarction (Arkeyalan A 2005), which might be interpreted as a stroke-induced increases in inflammatory events. It is reported that plasma levels of MCP-1 were elevated in patients with essential hypertension in the absence of other diseases (Madej A 2005). The MCP-1-deficient mice model is a unique model to elucidate the role of macrophages in a stroke (Huges PM 2002). Compared with control mice, infarct volume was smaller in MCP-1-deficient mice 24 hours after middle cerebral artery occlusion, and a reduction of phagocytic macrophage accumulation within infarcts and the infarct border in MCP-1 deficient mice 2 weeks after middle cerebral artery occlusion. In addition, MCP-1 deficient mice produced less IL-1β in ischemic tissue. This means that MCP-1 and IL-1β are key factors of macrophages in stroke lesions.

Adipokines

Obesity is also recognized as a risk factor for a stroke, because obesity is associated with hypertension and inflammation via secretion of adipokines, such as adiponectin, leptin, Resistin, adipsin, plasminogen activator inhibitor-1, and inflammatory cytokines (Mathieu P 2009, Yiannikouris A 2010). It is well known that macrophage infiltration into adipose tissue induces inflammation in adipose tissue and influences these adipokine secretions (Bouloumié A 2005). The most commonly studied adipocytokines are leptin and adiponectin. There are a lot of reports about the association of leptin and adiponectin with strokes, and leptin and adiponectin show differential association patterns with ischemic strokes (Kim BJ 2012). It is reported that higher leptin levels and lower adiponectin levels were found in stroke patients (Gerdes S 2012). On the other hand, there is controversial reports that adiponectin, but not leptin, levels are recognized as a predictor of the risk for a stroke (Pruger C 2012), or that leptin, but not adiponectin; levels are recognized as a predictor of the risk for strokes in men, but not women (Söderberg S 2009). It is not clear whether adiponectin and leptin are useful predictors of strokes in obese subjects; however, adiponectin and leptin might directly influence stroke incidence. It is reported that leptin stimulates macrophages and that adiponectin suppresses it. Leptin increases the mRNA and protein levels of IL-1$\beta\beta$, IL-6, IL-12, TNF-α, cyclooxygenase-2, and MCP-1 in macrophages and endothelial cells (Loffreda S 1998). Adiponectin inhibits pro-inflammatory signaling in human macrophages (Folko EJ 2009) and promotes macrophage polarization toward an anti-inflammatory phenotype (Ohashi K 2010). Adiponectin also increases IL-10, an anti-inflammatory cytokine, as well as mRNA expression in human monocyte-derived macrophages (Kumada M 2004). In addition, both adiponectin and leptin receptors are expressed in the brain, suggesting that these adipokines might be directly associated with a stroke (Thundyil J 2012).

Anti-Inflammatory Strategies

There are several reports that treatment with drugs that have anti-inflammatory properties can prevent strokes not only in animal models, but also in humans.

Statins

Rosuvastatin treatment significantly delayed the onset of a stroke and attenuated the transcription of inflammatory biomarkers (Sironi L 2005). Clinical studies using statins already use inflammatory events as endpoints for stroke prevention. In healthy persons without hyperlipidemia but with elevated high-sensitivity CRP levels, rosuvastatin, which lowered high-sensitivity CRP as well as cholesterol levels, reduced the incidence of strokes and myocardial infarction by 50% relative to placebo (Ridker PM 2008). A meta-analysis of statin trials showed that statins might reduce the incidence of all strokes by decreasing LDL-cholesterol without increasing the incidence of hemorrhagic strokes (Amarenco P 2004). In addition to cholesterol dependent effects, cholesterol-independent effects of statins on strokes have also been recognized (Vaughan CJ 2003). However, statin treatment increases the risk of hemorrhagic strokes in patients with a history of cerebrovascular disease, even though it also clearly decreased the risk of an ischemic stroke (Vergouwen MD 2008). Therefore, patients undergoing statin treatment should be carefully monitored to avoid achieving very low levels of cholesterol, which are known risks for hemorrhagic strokes (Puddey IB 1996).

Thiazolizinediones

Thiazolidinediones, including rosiglitazone and pioglitazone, are peroxisome proliferator activated receptor-$\gamma\gamma$ (PPAR-γ) agonists used in the treatment of type 2 diabetes. A systemic review showed that 6 Mediators of Inflammation rosiglitazone and pioglitazone were similarly effective in reducing infarct volume and protecting neurologic function in a rodent model of focal or global cerebral ischemia (White AT 2010). Pioglitazone delayed the onset of a stroke by improving vascular endothelial dysfunction and brain inflammation in SHRSP. Pioglitazone suppressed macrophage infiltration, MCP-1 and TNF-α gene expressions in the brain (Nakamura T 2007). Rosiglitazone induced upregulation of CD36 in macrophages and enhanced the ability of microglia to phagocytose red blood cells, which helped to improve hematoma resolution, and improved functional deficits in an intracerebral hemorrhage mouse model (Xhao H 2009). In humans, the PROspective pioglitAzone Clinical Trial In macroVascular Events (PROACTIVE) (Dormandy JA 2005) showed that pioglitazone significantly reduced the risk of a recurrent stroke in high-risk patients with type 2 diabetes (Wilcox R 2007). On the other hand, one report showed that compared with pioglitazone, rosiglitazone was associated with an increased risk of a stroke, heart failure, and all-cause mortality and an increased risk of the composite of acute myocardial infarction, strokes, heart failure, or all-cause mortality in patients of 65 years or older (Graham DJ 2010).

Other Inflammatory Drugs

Low-dose acetylsalicylic acid (aspirin) also delayed the onset of a stroke in SHRSP via suppression of inflammation. Aspirin reduced salt induced macrophage accumulation and MMP-9 activity at the stroke-negative area in the cerebral cortex of SHRSP (Ishizuka T 2008). Frequent aspirin use might also confer a protective effect for the risk of strokes in humans (Tymianski M 2011). Terutroban, a specific thromboxane/prostaglandin endoperoxide receptor antagonist, decreased cerebral mRNA expressions of IL-1β, transforming growth factor-β, and MCP-1 and increased survival in SHRSP. These effects were similar to rosuvastatin and aspirin (Gelosa P 2010). The Prevention of cerebrovascular and cardiovascular Events of ischemic origin with terutroban in patients with a history of ischemic strokes or transient ischemic attack (PERFORM) study was started in February 2006 (Bousser MG 2009). Recently, it was reported that PERFORM study did not meet the predefined criteria for non-inferiority, but showed similar rates to terutroban and aspirin for the primary endpoint, such as a composite of fatal or nonfatal ischemic strokes, fatal or nonfatal myocardial infarction, or other vascular death (Bousser MG 2011). These reports indicate that antiplatelets agents, which also have anti-inflammatory properties, could suppress inflammation and prevent the onset of a stroke.

Inflammation and Ischemic Tolerance

Inflammatory and immune responses play important roles following an ischemic stroke. Inflammatory responses contribute to damage and also contribute to repair. Injury to tissue triggers an immune response. This is initiated through activation of the innate immune system. There is microglial activation in a stroke. This is followed by an influx of lymphocytes and macrophages into the brain, triggered by the production of proinflammatory cytokines. This inflammatory response contributes to further tissue injury. There is also a systemic immune response to a stroke, and there is a degree of immunosuppression that may contribute to the stroke patient's risk of infection. This immunosuppressive response may also be protective, with regulatory lymphocytes producing cytokines and growth factors that are neuroprotective. The specific targets of the immune response after a stroke are not known, and the details of the immune and inflammatory responses are only partly understood. The role of inflammation and immune responses after a stroke is twofold. The immune system may contribute to the damage after a stroke, but may also contribute to repair processes. The possibility that some of the immune responses after a stroke may be neuroprotective is exciting and suggests that the deliberate enhancement of these responses may be a therapeutic option.

The suppression of inflammation appears to be the means by which ischemic preconditioning protects against a stroke. It is known that a sublethal ischemic event confers protection against subsequent lethal ischemia, in various organs, including the brain (Dhodha VK 2004). In experimental studies, animals that have been subjected to preconditioning have reduced inflammation after a subsequent ischemic challenge and reduced expression of inflammatory molecules (Bowen KK 2006). These changes are thought to be associated with changes in expression of genes such as hypoxia inducible factor 1 (HIF1) (Bernaudin M 2002, Dhodha VK 2004). In summary, it appears that immune suppression after a preconditioning ischemic episode prevents the acute harmful immune response after a subsequent ischemic episode. There is evidence that inflammation participates in tissue damage in strokes, and this is brought about by the activation of the innate immune system. Immunosuppression after a stroke has occurred may be too late to reduce this damage, although further work is required. After the acute injury of a stroke, there appears to be a naturally occurring state of immunosuppression, during which infection can occur. This immunosuppression appears to be due, in part, to circulating T cells. There is evidence that the immune system, possibly through such T cells, but also by other types of T cells, may be able to assist in neural repair. There is some animal work that suggests that tolerization to brain antigens improves outcomes after a stroke. Thus, immune and inflammatory responses after a stroke are both good and bad. Therapeutic possibilities based on this data include the early use of antibiotics to prevent infection (currently undergoing clinical trial), inhibition of the early inflammatory/immune response, although it is perhaps likely, that doing so after the stroke has occurred may be too late, and perhaps enhancing protective immune responses to speed neural repair.

Conclusion

In conclusion, in the presented work, we sought to provide a brief overview of the current understanding of inflammatory mechanisms involved during an acute ischemic stroke and neuroprotective agents that can curtail neuroinflammation and could have utility in the treatment of a stroke (see Table 1). As discussed, evidence suggests that post-ischemic oxidative stress and inflammation contribute to brain injury and to the expansion of the ischemic lesion. On the other hand, an adequate adaptive immune response after acute brain ischemia also plays an important role in response to ischemic injury as shown by the tremendous potential of Treg cells to prevent secondary infarct growth by counteracting the production of proinflammatory cytokines and by modulating the activation of lymphocytes and microglia in the ischemic brain (Liesz A 2009). These results provide new insights into the immunopathogenesis of acute ischemic strokes and could lead to new approaches that involve immune modulation using Treg cells. To date, 1,026 drugs have been tested in various animal models, of which 114 underwent clinical evaluation (De la Ossa NP 2007). The greater part of the agents studied until now have failed. Consequently, rt-PA remains the only agent shown to improve stroke outcomes in clinical trials, despite the many clinical trials conducted. However, its use is limited by its short therapeutic window (three hours), by its complications derived essentially from the risk of hemorrhage, and by the potential damage by R/I injury. Because of these drawbacks the optimum treatment of cerebral focal ischemia remains one of the major challenges in clinical medicine.

References

Allan SM, P.J. Tyrrell, N.J. Rothwell, Interleukin-1 and neuronal injury, *Nat. Rev. Immunol.* 5 (2005) 629–640.

Arakelyan A, J. Petrkova, Z. Hermanova, A. Boyajyan, J. Lukl, and M. Petrek, "Serum levels of the MCP-1 chemokine in patients with ischemic stroke and myocardial infarction," *Mediators of Inflamation*, vol. 2005, no. 3, pp. 175–179, 2005.

Amarenco P, J. Labreuche, P. Lavallée, and P. J. Touboul, "Statins in stroke prevention and carotid atherosclerosis: systematic review and up-to-date meta-analysis," *Stroke*, vol. 35, no. 12, pp. 2902–2909, 2004.

Acalovschi D, Wiest T, Hartmann M, et al. Multiple levels of regulation of the interleukin-6 system in stroke. *Stroke* 2003, 34:1864-1870.

Asahi M, Wang X, Mori T, et al. Effects of matrix metalloproteinase-9 gene knock-out on the proteolysis of blood-brain barrier and white matter components after cerebral ischemia. *J Neurosci* 2001, 21:7724-7732.

Boutin H, LeFeuvre RA, Horai R, et al. Role of IL-1α and IL-1β in ischemic brain damage. J Neurosci 2001, 21:5528-5534.

Barone FC, Feuerstein GZ: Inflammatory mediators and stroke: new opportunities for novel therapeutics. *J Cereb Blood Flow Metab* 1999, 19:819-34.

Bouloumié A, C. A. Curat, C. Sengenès, et al. "Role of macrophage tissue infiltration in metabolic diseases," *Current Opinion in Clinical Nutrition and Metabolic Care*, vol. 8, no. 4, pp. 347–354, 2005.

Bar-Or A, R. K. Nuttall, M. Duddy et al., "Analyses of all matrix metalloproteinase members in leukocytes emphasize monocytes as major in-ammatory mediators in multiple sclerosis," *Brain*, vol. 126, no. 12, pp. 2738–2749, 2003.

Boutin H, R. A. LeFeuvre, R. Horai, et al. Role of IL-1$\alpha\alpha$ and IL-1β in ischemic brain damage," *Journal of Neuroscience*, vol. 21, no. 15, pp. 5528–5534, 2001.

Banwell V, E. S. Sena, and M. R. Macleod, "Systematic review and stratified meta-analysis of the efficacy of interleukin-1 receptor antagonist in animal models of stroke," *Journal of Stroke and Cerebrovascular Diseases*, vol. 18, no. 4, pp. 269–276, 2009.

Barone FC, G.Z. Feuerstein, Inflammatory mediators and stroke: new opportunities for novel therapeutics, *J. Cereb. Blood Flow Metab.* 19 (1999) 819–834.

Becker K, D. Kindrick, J. Relton, J. Harlan, R. Winn, Antibody to the alpha 4 integrin decreases infarct size in transient focal cerebral ischemia in rats, *Stroke* 32 (2001) 206–211.

Blake GJ and P. M. Ridker, "Inflammatory bio-markers and cardiovascular risk prediction," *Journal of Internal Medicine*, vol. 252, no. 4, pp. 283–294, 2002.

Blann AD, W. Tse, S. J. R. Maxwell, and M. A. Waite, "Increased levels of the soluble adhesion molecule E-selectin in essential hypertension," *Journal of Hypertension*, vol. 12, no. 8, pp. 925–928, 1994.

Ban C, L. Sironi, G. De Simoni et al., "Pentoxifylline prevents spontaneous brain ischemia in stroke-prone rats," *Journal of Pharmacology and Experimental therapeutics*, vol. 310, no. 3, pp. 890–895, 2004.

Bousser MG, P. Amarenco, A. Chamorro et al., "Rationale and design of a randomized, double-blind, parallel-group study of terutroban 30 mg/day versus aspirin 100 mg/day in stroke patients: the prevention of cerebrovascular and cardiovascular events of ischemic origin with terutroban in patients with a history of ischemic stroke or transient ischemic attack (PERFORM) study," *Cerebrovascular Diseases*, vol. 27, no. 5, pp. 509–518, 2009.

Bousser MG, P. Amarenco, A. Chamorro et al., "Terutroban versus aspirin in patients with cerebral ischemic events (PERFORM): a randomised, double-blind, parallel-group trial," *the Lancet*, vol. 377, no. 9782, pp. 2013–2022, 2011.

Boutin H, LeFeuvre RA, Horai R, et al. Role of il-1alpha and il-1beta in ischemic brain damage. *J. Neurosci*. 2001;21:5528-5534.

Bradford JR, C.J. Needham, A.J. Bulpitt, D.R. Westhead, Insights into proteinprotein interfaces using a Bayesian network prediction method, *J. Mol. Biol*. 362 (2006) 365–386.

Bruce AJ, Boling W, Kindy MS, et al. Altered neuronal and microglial responses to excitotoxic and ischemic brain injury in mice lacking tnf receptors. *Nat Med*. 1996;2:788-794.

Burge J, T. Lane, H. Link, S. Qiu, V.P. Clark, Discrete dynamic Bayesian network analysis of fMRI data, *Hum. Brain Mapp*. 30 (2009) 122–137.

Bernaudin M, Tang Y, Reilly M, Petit E, Sharp FR: Brain genomic response following hypoxia and re-oxygenation in the neonatal rat. Identification of genes that might contribute to hypoxia-induced ischemic tolerance. *J Biol Chem* 2002; 277:39728–38.

Bowen KK, Naylor M, Vemuganti R: Prevention of inflammation is a mechanism of preconditioning-induced neuroprotection against focal cerebral ischemia. *Neurochem Int* 2006; 49:127–35.

Colobran R, Pujol-Borrell R, Armengol MP, Juan M: The chemokine network. I. How the genomic organization of chemokines contains clues for deciphering their functional complexity. *Clin Exp Immunol* 2007; 148:208–17.

Croce K, Libby P: Intertwining of thrombosis and inflammation in atherosclerosis. *Curr Opin Hematol* 2007; 14:55–61.

Chamorro A. Role of inflammation in stroke and atherothrombosis. *Cerebrovasc Dis*. 2004;17 Suppl 3:1-5.

Ceulemans AG, T. Zgavc, R. Kooijman, et al. The dual role of the neuroinflammatory response after ischemic stroke: modulatory effects of hypothermia, *J. Neuroinflamm*. 7 (2010) 74.

Clausen BH, K.L. Lambertsen, M. Meldgaard, B. Finsen, A quantitative in situ hybridization and polymerase chain reaction study of microglial-macrophage expression of interleukin-1beta mRNA following permanent middle cerebral artery occlusion in mice, *Neuroscience* 132 (2005) 879–892.

Clausen BH, K.L. Lambertsen, A.A. Babcock, et al. Interleukin-1beta and tumor necrosis factor-alpha are expressed by different subsets of microglia and macrophages after ischemic stroke in mice, *J.. Neuroinflamm*. 5 (2008) 46.

Connolly ES, Jr., Winfree CJ, Springer TA, et al. Cerebral protection in homozygous null icam-1 mice after middle cerebral artery occlusion. Role of neutrophil adhesion in the pathogenesis of stroke. *J. Clin. Invest.* 1996;97:209-216.

Clark WM, Rinker LG, Lessov NS, Hazel K, Hill JK, Stenzel-Poore M, Eckenstein F: Lack of interleukin-6 expression is not protective against focal central system ischemia. *Stroke* 2001, 31:1715-1720.

Caso JR, Moro MA, Lorenzo P, Lizasoain I, Leza JC: Involvement of IL-1β in acute stress induced worsening of cerebral ischemia in rats. *Eur Neuropsychopharmacol* 2007, 17:600-607.

Clark WM, Rinker LG, Lessov NS, Hazel K, Eckenstein F: Time course of IL-6 expression in experimental CNS ischemia. *Neurol. Res* 1999, 21:287-292.

Chen WY, Chang MS: IL-20 is regulated by hypoxia-inducible factor and up-regulated after experimental ischemic stroke. *J. Immunol* 2009, 182:5000-5012.

Connolly ES, Jr., Winfree CJ, Prestigiacomo CJ, et al. Exacerbation of cerebral injury in mice that express the p-selectin gene: Identification of p-selectin blockade as a new target for the treatment of stroke. *Circ Res*. 1997;81:304-310.

Clark WM, L. G. Rinker, N. S. Lessov et al., "Lack of interleukin-6 expression is not protective against focal central nervous system ischemia," *Stroke*, vol. 31, no. 7, pp. 1715–1720, 2000.

del Zoppo G, Ginis I, Hallenbeck JM, et al. Inflammation and stroke: Putative role for cytokines, adhesion molecules and inos in brain response to ischemia. *Brain Pathol.* 2000;10:95-112.

Danton GH, W.D. Dietrich, Inflammatory mechanisms after ischemia and stroke, *J. Neuropathol. Exp. Neurol*. 62 (2003) 127–136.

Dhodda VK, Sailor KA, Bowen KK, Vemuganti R: Putative endogenous mediators of preconditioning-induced ischemic tolerance in rat brain identified by genomic and proteomic analysis. *J Neurochem* 2004; 89:73–89.

Denes A, P. Thornton, N.J. Rothwell, S.M. Allan, Inflammation and brain injury: acute cerebral ischaemia peripheral and central inflammation, *Brain Behav. Immun*. 24 (2010) 708–723.

Dormandy JA, B. Charbonnel, D. J. Eckland et al., "Secondary prevention of macrovascular events in patients with type 2 diabetes in the PROactive Study (PROspective pioglitazone Clinical Trial in macroVascular Events): a randomised controlled trial," *the Lancet*, vol. 366, no. 9493, pp. 1279–1289, 2005.

Desouza CA, D. R. Dengel, R. F. Macko, et al. "Elevated levels of circulating cell adhesion molecules in uncomplicated essential hypertension," *American Journal of Hypertension*, vol. 10, no. 12, pp. 1335–1341, 1997.

Dollery CM and P. Libby, "Atherosclerosis and proteinase activation," *Cardiovascular Research*, vol. 69, no. 3, pp. 625–635, 2006.

Dimitrijevic OB, Stamatovic SM, Keep RF, Andjelkovic AV: Absence of the chemokine receptor CCR2 protects against cerebral ischemia/reperfusion injury in mice. *Stroke* 2007, 38:1345-1353.

De la Ossa NP, Davalos A: Neuroprotection in cerebral infarction: the opportunity of new studies. *Cerebrovasc Dis*. 2007, 24:153-156.

Dirnagl U, Iadecola C, Moskowitz MA: Pathobiology of ischemic stroke: an integrated view. *Trends Neurosci* 1999, 22:391-397.

Donnan GA, Fisher M, Macleod M, Davis SM: Stroke. *Lancet* 2008, 371:1612-1623.

Ekdahl CT, Kokaia Z, Lindvall O: Brain inflammation and adult neurogenesis: the dual role of microglia. *Neuroscience* 2009, 158:1021-1029.

Elkind MS, Cheng J, Boden-Albala B, et al. Tumor necrosis factor receptor levels are associated with carotid atherosclerosis. *Stroke*. 2002;33:31-37.

Enlimomab A. Acute Stroke Trial Investigators. Use of antiicam-1 therapy in ischemic stroke: Results of the enlimomab acute stroke trial. *Neurology*. 2001;57:1428-1434.

Elkind MS: Inflammation, atherosclerosis, and stroke. *Neurologist* 2006; 12:140–8.

Emsley HC, P.J. Tyrrell, Inflammation and infection in clinical stroke, *J. Cereb. Blood Flow Metab.* 22 (2002) 1399–1419.

Emsley HCA, C. J. Smith, R. F. Georgiou et al., "A randomised phase II study of interleukin-1 receptor antagonist in acute stroke patients," *Journal of Neurology, Neurosurgery and Psychiatry*, vol. 76, no. 10, pp. 1366–1372, 2005.

Fontaine V, Mohand-Said S, Hanoteau N, et al. Neurodegenerative and neuroprotective effects of tumor necrosis factor (tnf) in retinal ischemia: Opposite roles of tnf receptor 1 and tnf receptor 2. *J Neurosci.* 2002;22:RC216.

Fava M, "Leukocytes and the risk of ischemic diseases," *JAMA*, vol. 258, no. 7, pp. 907–908, 1987.

Fabriek BO, Zwemmer JN, Teunissen CE et al. In vivo detection of myelin proteins in cervical lymph nodes of MS patients using ultrasound-guided fine-needle aspiration cytology. *J. Neuroimmunol* 2005; 161:190–4.

Ferrarese C, Mascarucci P, Zoia C, et al. Increased cytokine release from peripheral blood cells after acute stroke. *J Cereb Blood Flow Metab* 1999, 19:1004-9.

Fassbender K, T. Bertsch, O. Mielke, F. Mühlhauser;, and M. Hennerici, "Adhesion molecules in cerebrovascular diseases: evidence for an in-ammatory endothelial activation in cerebral large- and small-vessel disease," *Stroke*, vol. 30, no. 8, pp. 1647–1650, 1999.

Folco EJ, V. Z. Rocha, M. López-Ilasaca, and P. Libby, "Adiponectin inhibits pro-inflammatory signaling in human macrophages independent of interleukin-10," *the Journal of Biological Chemistry*, vol. 284, no. 38, pp. 25569–25575, 2009.

Furlan AJ, Katzan IL, Caplan LR: Thrombolytic therapy in acute ischemic stroke. *Curr Treat Options Cardiovasc Med* 2003, 5:171-180.

Goussev AV, Zhang Z, Anderson DC, Chopp M: P-selectin antibody reduces hemorrhage and infarct volume resulting from MCA occlusion in the rat. *J Neurosci* 1998, 161:16-22.

Gueorguieva I, Clark SR, McMahon CJ, et al. Pharmacokinetic modeling of interleukin-1 receptor antagonist in plasma and cerebrospinal fluid of patients following subarachnoid hemorrhage. *Br. J. Clin Pharmacol* 2008, 65:317-325.

Gerdes S, S. Osadtschy, M. Rostami-Yazdi, N. et al. "Leptin, adiponectin, visfatin and retinol-binding protein-4—mediators of comorbidities in patients with psoriasis?" *Experimental Dermatology*, vol. 21, no. 1, pp. 43–47, 2012.

Goldstein LB, C. D. Bushnell, R. J. Adams et al., "Guidelines for the primary prevention of stroke: a Guideline for Healthcare Professionals from the American Heart Association/American Stroke Association," *Stroke*, vol. 42, no. 2, pp. 517–584, 2011

Gillum RF, D. D. Ingram, and D. M. Makuc, "White blood cell count and stroke incidence and death: the NHANES I epidemiologic follow-up study," *American Journal of Epidemiology*, vol. 139, no. 9, pp. 894–902, 1994.

Grau AJ, A. W. Boddy, D. A. Dukovic et al., "Leukocyte count as an independent predictor of recurrent ischemic events," *Stroke*, vol. 35, no. 5, pp. 1147–1152, 2004.

Gelosa P, R. Ballerio, C. Ban et al., "Terutroban, a thromboxane/prostaglandin endoperoxide receptor antagonist, increases survival in stroke-prone rats by preventing systemic inflammation and endothelial dysfunction: comparison with aspirin and rosuvastatin," *Journal of Pharmacology and Experimental therapeutics*, vol. 334, no. 1, pp. 199–205, 2010.

Ginsberg MD, Neuroprotection for ischemic stroke: past present and future, Neuropharmacology 55 (2008) 363–389.

Graham DJ, R. Ouellet-Hellstrom, T. E. Macurdy et al., "Risk of acute myocardial infarction, stroke, heart failure, and death in elderly medicare patients treated with rosiglitazone or pioglitazone," *JAMA*, vol. 304, no. 4, pp. 411–418, 2010.

Greenberg AG, M.S. Obin, Obesity and the role of adipose tissue in inflammation and metabolism, *Am. J. Clin. Nutr.* 83 (2006) 461S–465S.

Galkina E, Kadl A, Sanders J, Varughese D, Sarembock IJ, Ley K: Lymphocyte recruitment into the aortic wall before and during development of atherosclerosis is partially L-selectin dependent. *J. Exp. Med* 2006; 203:1273–82.

Galkina E, Harry BL, Ludwig A et al. CXCR6 promotes atherosclerosis by supporting T-cell homing, interferon-gamma production, and macrophage accumulation in the aortic wall. *Circulation* 2007; 116:1801–11.

Heller EA, Liu E, Tager AM et al. Chemokine CXCL10 promotes atherogenesis by modulating the local balance of effector and regulatory T cells. *Circulation* 2006; 113:2301–12.

Hansson GK, Libby P: The immune response in atherosclerosis: a double-edged sword. *Nat Rev Immunol* 2006; 6:508–19.

Hack CE, L.T. Haber, A. Maier, et al. A Bayesian network model for biomarker-based dose response, *Risk Anal.* 30 (2010) 1037–1051.

Hallenbeck JM, Significance of the inflammatory response in brain ischemia, *Acta Neurochir. Suppl.* 66 (1996) 27–31.

Hallenbeck JM, "The many faces of tumor necrosis factor in stroke," *Nature Medicine*, vol. 8, no. 12, pp. 1363–1368, 2002.

Hughes PM, P. R. Allegrini, M. Rudin, V. H. Perry, A. K. Mir, and C. Wiessner, "Monocyte chemoattractant protein-1 deficiency is protective in a murine stroke model," *Journal of Cerebral Blood Flow and Metabolism*, vol. 22, no. 3, pp. 308–317, 2002.

Han HS, M.A. Yenari, Cellular targets of brain inflammation in stroke, *Curr. Opin. Investig. Drugs* 4 (2003) 522–529.

Hughes PM, Allegrini PR, Rudin M, et al. Monocyte chemoattractant protein-1 deficiency is protective in a murine stroke model. *J Cereb Blood Flow Metab* 2002, 22:308-17.

Hill JK, L. Gunion-Rinker, D. Kulhanek, et al. Temporal modulation of cytokine expression following focal cerebral ischemia in mice, *Brain Res.* 820 (1999) 45–54.

Hughes PM, Allegrini PR, Rudin M, et al. Monocyte chemoattractant protein-1 deficiency is protective in a murine stroke model. *J Cereb Blood Flow Metab*. 2002;22:308-317.

Huang J, Kim LJ, Mealey R, et al. Neuronal protection in stroke by an slex-glycosylated complement inhibitory protein. *Science.* 1999;285:595-599.

Iadecola C, Niwa K, Nogawa S, et al. Reduced susceptibility to ischemic brain injury and n-methyl-d-aspartate-mediated neurotoxicity in cyclooxygenase-2-deficient mice. *Proc Natl Acad Sci USA.* 2001;98:1294-1299.

Johnson JL, G. B. Sala-Newby, et al. "Low tissue inhibitor of metalloproteinases 3 and high matrix metallopr teinase 14 levels defenes a subpopulation of highly invasive foam-cell macrophages," *Arteriosclerosis, Thrombosis, and Vascular Biology*, vol. 28, no. 9, pp. 1647–1653, 2008.

Jonasson L, Holm J, Skalli O, Bondjers G, Hansson GK: Regional accumulations of T cells, macrophages, and smooth muscle cells in the human atherosclerotic plaque. *Arteriosclerosis* 1986; 6:131–8.

Kobayashi K, Lopez LR, Shoenfeld Y, Matsuura E: The role of innate and adaptive immunity to oxidized low-density lipoprotein in the development of atherosclerosis. *Ann NYAcad Sci* 2005; 1051:442–54.

Koenig W, Khuseyinova N: Biomarkers of atherosclerotic plaque-instability and rupture. *Arterioscler Thromb Vasc Biol 2007*; 27:15–26.

Kim WK, Alvarez X, Fisher J et al. CD163 identifies perivascular macrophages in normal and viral encephalitic brains and potential precursors to perivascular macrophages in blood. *Am J Pathol* 2006; 168:822–34.

Kumada M, S. Kihara, N. Ouchi et al., “Adiponectin specifically increased tissue inhibitor of metalloproteinase-1 through interleukin-10 expression in human macrophages,” *Circulation*, vol. 109, no. 17, pp. 2046–2049, 2004.

Kim BJ, S.-H. Lee, W.-S. et al. “Adipocytokines and ischemic stroke: differential associations between stroke subtypes,” *Journal of the Neurological Sciences*, vol. 312, no. 1-2, pp. 117–122, 2012.

Kim JS, Gautam SC, Chopp M, et al. Expression of monocyte chemoattractant protein-1 and macrophage inflammatory protein-1 after focal cerebral ischemia in the rat. *J Neuroimmunol* 1995, 56:127-134.

Loffreda S, S. Q. Yang, H. Z. Lin et al., “Leptin regulates proinflammatory immune responses,” *the FASEB Journal*, vol. 12, no. 1, pp. 57–65, 1998.

Lakhan SE, A. Kirchgessner, M. Hofer, Inflammatory mechanisms in ischemic stroke: therapeutic approaches, *J. Transl. Med.* 7 (2009) 97.

Lambertsen KL, K. Biber, B. Finsen, Inflammatory cytokines in experimental and human stroke, *J. Cereb. Blood Flow Metab.* 32 (2012) 1677–1698.

Lambertsen KL, M. Meldgaard, R. Ladeby, B. Finsen, A quantitative study of microglial-macrophage synthesis of tumor necrosis factor during acute and late focal cerebral ischemia in mice, *J. Cereb. Blood Flow Metab.* 25 (2005) 119–135.

Lloyd-Jones D, R. Adams, M. Carnethon, et al. Heart disease and stroke statistics – 2009 update: a report from the American Heart Association Statistics Committee and Stroke Statistics Subcommittee, *Circulation* 119 (2009) e21–e181.

Lucas SM, Rothwell NJ, Gibson RM: The role of inflammation in CNS injury and disease. Br *J Pharmacol* 2006, 147(Suppl 1):S232-40.

Lindsberg PJ, Carpén O, Paetau A, et al. Endothelial ICAM-1 Expression Associated With Inflammatory Cell Response in Human Ischemic Stroke. *Circulation* 1996, 94:939-945.

Liesz A, Suri-Payer E, Veltkamp C, et al. Regulatory T cells are key cerebroprotective Immunomodulators in acute experimental stroke. *Nat Med* 2009, 15:192-199.

Lucas SM, Rothwell NJ, Gibson RM: The role of inflammation in CNS injury and disease. Br *J Pharmacol* 2006; 147(Suppl. 1): S232–40.

Melchior B, Puntambekar SS, Carson MJ: Microglia and the control of auto reactive T cell responses. *Neurochem Int* 2006; 49:145–53.

McColl BW, Rothwell NJ, Allan SM: Systemic inflammatory stimulus potentiates the acute phase and CXC chemokine responses to experimental stroke and exacerbates brain damage via interleukin-1- and neutrophil-dependent mechanisms. *J Neurosci* 2007; 27:4403–12.

Mach F, Schonbeck U, Sukhova GKet al. Functional CD40 ligand is expressed on human vascular endothelial cells, smooth muscle cells, and macrophages: implications for CD40–CD40 ligand signaling in atherosclerosis. *Proc. Natl. Acad. Sci. USA* 1997; 94:1931–6.

Moller F, Andersen CB, Nielsen LB: Adhesion of Tand B lymphocytes to mouse atherosclerotic aortas: association with lesion topology and VCAM-1 expression. *Scand J. Clin Lab Invest* 2005; 65:559–70.

Mor A, Planer D, Luboshits G et al. Role of naturally occurring CD41CD251 regulatory T cells in experimental atherosclerosis. *Arterioscler Thromb. Vasc. Biol.* 2007; 27:893–900.

Montaner J, Alvarez-Sabin J, Molina C, et al. Matrix metalloproteinase expression after human cardioembolic stroke: temporal profile and relation to neurological impairment. *Stroke* 2001, 32:1759-66.

Muir KW, Tyrrell P, Sattar N, Warburton E: Inflammation and ischemic stroke. *Curr. Opin. Neurol.* 2007, 20:334-342.

McCoy MK, M.G. Tansey, TNF signaling inhibition in the CNS: implications for normal brain function and neurodegenerative disease, *J. Neuroinflamm.* 5 (2008) 45.

Morioka T, A.N. Kalehua, W.J. Streit. Characterization of microglial reaction after middle cerebral artery occlusion in rat brain, *J. Comp. Neurol.* 327 (1993) 123–132.

Madej A, B. Okopień, J. Kowalski, M. Haberka, and Z. S. Herman, "Plasma concentrations of adhesion molecules and chemokines in patients with essential hypertension," *Pharmacological Reports*, vol. 57, no. 6, pp. 878–881, 2005.

Mathieu P, P. Poirier, P. Pibarot, I. et al. "Visceral obesity the link among inflammation, hypertension, and cardiovascular disease," *Hypertension*, vol. 53, no. 4, pp. 577–584, 2009.

Newby AC, "Metalloproteinase expression in monocytes and macrophages and its relationship to atherosclerotic plaque instability," *Arteriosclerosis, thrombosis, and Vascular Biology*, vol. 28, no. 12, pp. 2108–2114, 2008.

Newby AC, "Do metalloproteinases destabilize vulnerable atherosclerotic plaques?" *Current Opinion in Lipidology*, vol. 17, no. 5, pp. 556–561, 2006.

Nawashiro H, Tasaki K, Ruetzler CA, et al. Tnfalpha pretreatment induces protective effects against focal cerebral ischemia in mice. *J Cereb Blood Flow Metab.* 1997;17:483-490.

Nawashiro H, D. Martin, and J. M. Hallenbeck, "Inhibition of tumor necrosis factor and amelioration of brain infarction in mice," *Journal of Cerebral Blood Flow and Metabolism*, vol. 17, no. 2, pp. 229–232, 1997a.

Nawashiro H, K. Tasaki, C. A. Ruetzler, and J. M. Hallenbeck, "TNF-α pretreatment induces protective effects against focal cerebral ischemia in mice," *Journal of Cerebral Blood Flow and Metabolism*, vol. 17, no. 5, pp. 483–490, 1997b.

Nimmerjahn A, Kirchhoff F, Helmchen F: Resting microglial cells are highly dynamic surveillants of brain parenchyma in vivo. *Science* 2005; 308:1314–8.

Olsson S, L. Holmegaard, K. Jood et al., "Genetic variation within the interleukin-1 gene cluster and ischemic stroke," *Stroke*, vol. 43, no. 9, pp. 2278–2282, 2012.

Ohashi K, J. L. Parker, N. Ouchi et al., "Adiponectin promotes macrophage polarization toward an anti-inflammatory phenotype," *the Journal of Biological Chemistry*, vol. 285, no. 9, pp. 6153–6160, 2010.

O'Collins VE, Macleod MR, Donnan GA, et al. 1,026 experimental treatments in acute stroke. *Ann Neurol.* 2006, 59:467-477.

Park KP, Rosell A, Foerch C, et al. Plasma and brain matrix metalloproteinase-9 after acute focal cerebral ischemia in rats. *Stroke* 2009, 40:2836-2842.

Pang L, W. Ye, X.M. Che, B.J. et al. Reduction of inflammatory response in the mouse brain with adenoviral-mediated transforming growth factor-ss1 expression, *Stroke* 32 (2001) 544–552.

Planas AM, R. Gorina, A. Chamorro, Signalling pathways mediating inflammatory responses in brain ischaemia, *Biochem. Soc. Trans.* 34 (2006) 1267–1270.

Prentice RL, T. P. Szatrowski, H. Kato, and M. W. Mason, "Leukocyte counts and cerebrovascular disease," *Journal of Chronic Diseases*, vol. 35, no. 9, pp. 703–714, 1982.

Prugger C, G. Luc, B. Haas et al., "Adipocytokines and the risk of ischemic stroke: the PRIME Study," *Annals of Neurology*, vol. 71, no. 4, pp. 478–486, 2012.

Puddey IB, "Low serum cholesterol and the risk of cerebral haemorrhage," *Atherosclerosis*, vol. 119, no. 1, pp. 1–6, 1996.

Ridker PM, Hennekens CH, Buring JE, et al. C-reactive protein and other markers of inflammation in the prediction of cardiovascular disease in women. *N Engl J Med.* 2000;342:836-843.

Ross R, "Atherosclerosis an inflammatory disease," *The New England Journal of Medicine*, vol. 340, no. 2, pp. 115–126, 1999.

Ridker PM, E. Danielson, F. A. H. Fonseca et al., "Rosuvastatin to prevent vascular events in men and women with elevated Creactive protein," *the New England Journal of Medicine*, vol. 359, no. 21, pp. 2195–2207, 2008.

Rallidis LS, Zolindaki MG, Vikelis M, et al. Elevated soluble intercellular adhesion molecule-1 levels are associated with poor short-term prognosis in middle-aged patients with acute ischemic stroke. *Int J Cardiol* 2009, 132:216-220.

Shichita T, Sugiyama Y, Ooboshi H, et al. Pivotal role of cerebral interleukin-17-producing γδT cells in the delayed phase of ischemic brain injury. *Nat Med* 2009, 15:946-950.

Spera PA, Ellison JA, Feuerstein GZ, Barone FC: IL-10 reduces rat brain injury following focal stroke. *Neurosci Lett* 1998, 251:189-92.

Soriano S, Amaravadi L, Wang Y, et al. Mice deficient in fractalkine are less susceptible to cerebral ischemia-reperfusion injury. *J Neuroimmunol* 2002, 125:59-65.

Swanson RA, Ying W, Kauppinen TM: Astrocyte influences on ischemic neuronal death. *Curr Mol Med* 2004, 4:193-205.

Sironi L, E. Gianazza, P. Gelosa et al., "Rosuvastatin, but not simvastatin, provides end-organ protection in stroke-prone rats by antiinflammatory effects," *Arteriosclerosis, Thrombosis, and Vascular Biology*, vol. 25, no. 3, pp. 598–603, 2005.

Söderberg S, D. Colquhoun, A. Keech et al., "Leptin, but not adiponectin, is a predictor of recurrent cardiovascular events in men: results from the LIPID study," *International Journal of Obesity*, vol. 33, no. 1, pp. 123–130, 2009.

Sánchez-Moreno C, J. F. Dashe, T. Scott, et al. "Decreased levels of plasma vitamin C and increased concentrations of in-ammatory and oxidative stress markers a-er stroke," *Stroke*, vol. 35, no. 1, pp. 163–168, 2004.

Scheller A, A. Chalaris, D. Schmidt-Arras, and S. Rose-John, "The pro- and anti-inflammatory properties of the cytokine interleukin-6," *Biochimica et Biophysica Acta*, vol. 1813, no. 5, pp. 878–888, 2011.

Shichita T, Y. Sugiyama, H. Ooboshi, et al. Pivotal role of cerebral interleukin-17-producing gammadeltaT cells in the delayed phase of ischemic brain injury, *Nat. Med.* 15 (2009) 946–950.

Smith CJ, H.C. Emsley, C.M. Gavin, et al. Peak plasma interleukin-6 and other peripheral markers of inflammation in the first week of ischemic stroke correlate with brain infarct volume, stroke severity and long-term outcome, *BMC Neurol.* 4 (2004) 2.

Spalletta G, P. Bossu, A. Ciaramella, et al. The etiology of poststroke depression: a review of the literature and a new hypothesis involving inflammatory cytokines, *Mol. Psychiatry* 11 (2006) 984–991.

Spranger J, A. Kroke, M. Mohlig, et al. Inflammatory cytokines and the risk to develop type 2 diabetes: results of the prospective population-based European Prospective Investigation into Cancer and Nutrition (EPIC)-Potsdam Study, *Diabetes* 52 (2003) 812–817.

Simpson E: A historical perspective on immunological privilege. *Immunol Rev* 2006; 213:12–22.

Tedgui A, Mallat Z: Cytokines in atherosclerosis: pathogenic and regulatory pathways. *Physiol Rev* 2006; 86:515–81.

Tanne D, Benderly M, Goldbourt U et al. C-reactive protein as a predictor of incident ischemic stroke among patients with preexisting cardiovascular disease. *Stroke* 2006; 37:1720–4.

Tanne D, Haim M, Boyko V, et al. Soluble intercellular adhesion molecule-1 and risk of future ischemic stroke: A nested case-control study from the bezafibrate infarction prevention (bip) study cohort. *Stroke.* 2002;33:2182-2186.

Tarkowski E, Rosengren L, Blomstrand C, et al. Intrathecal release of pro- and anti-inflammatory cytokines during stroke. *Clin Exp Immunol* 1997, 110:492-499.

Tuttolomondo A, D. Di Raimondo, R. di Sciacca, et al. Inflammatory cytokines in acute ischemic stroke, *Curr. Pharm. Des.* 14 (2008) 3574–3589.

Tuttolomondo A, D. Di Raimondo, R. Pecoraro, et al. Inflammation in ischemic stroke subtypes, *Curr. Pharm. Des.* 18 (2012) 4289–4310.

Thundyil J, D. Pavlovski, C. G. Sobey, and T. V. Arumugam, "Adiponectin receptor signalling in the brain," *British Journal of Pharmacology*, vol. 165, no. 2, pp. 313–327, 2012.

Tymianski M, "Aspirin as a promising agent for decreasing incidence of cerebral aneurysm rupture," *Stroke*, vol. 42, no. 11, pp. 3003–3004, 2011.

Vakili A, S. Mojarrad, M. M. Akhavan, and A. Rashidy- Pour, "Pentoxifylline attenuates TNF-$\alpha\alpha$ protein levels and brain edema following temporary focal cerebral ischemia in rats," *Brain Research*, vol. 1377, pp. 119–125, 2011.

Vaughan CJ, "Prevention of stroke and dementia with statins: effects beyond lipid lowering," *American Journal of Cardiology*, vol. 91, no. 4, supplement, pp. 23–29, 2003. 10 Mediators of Inflammation.

Vila N, Castillo J, Davalos A, Chammoro A: Proinflammatory cytokines and early neurological worsening in ischemic stroke. *Stroke* 2001, 31:2325-2329.

van Puijvelde GH, Hauer AD, de Vos P et al. Induction of oral tolerance to oxidized low-density lipoprotein ameliorates atherosclerosis. *Circulation* 2006; 114:1968–76.

Vergouwen MD, R. J. De Haan, M. Vermeulen, and Y. hemorrhagic stroke in patients with a history of cerebrovascular disease," *Stroke*, vol. 39, no. 2, pp. 497–502, 2008.

Whiteley C, C. Jackson, S. Lewis et al., "Inflammatory markers and poor outcome a-er stroke: a prospective cohort study and systematic review of interleukin-6," *PLoS Medicine*, vol. 6, no. 9, Article ID e1000145, 2009.

Wang Q, X.N. Tang, M.A. Yenari, The inflammatory response in stroke, *J. Neuroimmunol.* 184 (2007) 53–68.

Wang PY, Kao CH, MuiMY, Wang SJ: Leukocyte infiltration in acute hemispheric ischemic stroke. *Stroke* 1993; 24:236–40.

Whiteley W, C. Jackson, S. Lewis, et al. Inflammatory markers and poor outcome after stroke: a prospective cohort study and systematic review of interleukin-6, *PLoS Med.* 6 (2009)

Wisse BE, The inflammatory syndrome: the role of adipose tissue cytokines in metabolic disorders linked to obesity, *J. Am. Soc. Nephrol.* 15 (2004) 2792–2800.

White AT and A. N. Murphy, "Administration of thiazolidinediones for neuroprotection in ischemic stroke: a pre-clinical systematic review," *Journal of Neurochemistry*, vol. 115, no. 4, pp. 845–853, 2010.

With Noto AT, Bogeberg ME, Amiral J, Vissac AM, Hansen JB: Endothelial dysfunction and systemic inflammation in persons with echolucent carotid plaques. *Thromb Haemost* 2006; 96:53–9.

Xhao H, J. Grotta, N. Gonzales, and J. Aronowski, "Hematoma resolution as a therapeutic target: the role of microglia/ macrophages," *Stroke*, vol. 40, no. 3, pp. S92–S94, 2009.

Xu QB, Oberhuber G, Gruschwitz M, Wick G: Immunology of atherosclerosis: cellular composition and major histocompatibility complex class II antigen expression in aortic intima, fatty streaks, and atherosclerotic plaques in young and aged human specimens. *Clin Immunol Immunopathol* 1990; 56:344–59.

Yang GY, C. Gong, Z. Qin, et al. Tumor necrosis factor alpha expression produces increased blood-brain barrier permeability following temporary focal cerebral ischemia in mice, *Brain Res. Mol. Brain Res.* 69 (1999) 135–143.

Yilmaz G, D.N. Granger, Leukocyte recruitment and ischemic brain injury, *Neuromol. Med.* 12 (2010) 193–204.

Yamasaki Y, Matsuura N, Shozuhara H, et al. Interleukin-1 as a pathogenetic mediator of ischemic brain damage in rats. *Stroke* 1995, 26:676-680.

Yiannikouris A, M. Gupte, K. Putnam, and L. Cassis, "Adipokines and blood pressure control," *Current Opinion in Nephrology and Hypertension*, vol. 19, no. 2, pp. 195–200, 2010.

Zaremba J and J. Losy, "Early TNF-$\alpha\alpha$ levels correlate with ischemic stroke severity," *Acta Neurologica Scandinavica*, vol. 104, no. 5, pp. 288–295, 2001.

Zhang ZG, Zhang L, Jiang Q, et al. Vegf enhances angiogenesis and promotes blood-brain barrier leakage in the ischemic brain. *J Clin Invest.* 2000;106:829-838.

Zhang RL, Chopp M, Li Y, et al.: Anti-ICAM-1 antibody reduces ischemic cell damage after transient middle cerebral artery occlusion in the rat. *Neurology* 1994, 44:1747-1751.

Zhang R, Chopp M, Zhang Z, Jiang N, Powers C: The expression of P- and E-selectins in three models of middle cerebral artery occlusion. *Brain Res* 1998, 785:207-214.

Zhao BQ, Wang S, Kim HY, et al. Role of metalloproteinases in delayed cortical responses after stroke. *Nat. Med.* 2006, 12:441-445.

Zhu Y, Yang GY, Ahlemeyer B, et al. Transforming growth factor-beta 1 increases bad phosphorylation and protects neurons against damage. *J. Neurosci.* 2002, 22:3898-909.

Zhao B, J.C. Mar, S. Maruo, et al. Epstein-Barr virus nuclear antigen 3C regulated genes in lymphoblastoid cell lines, *Proc. Natl. Acad. Sci. USA*. 108 (2011) 337–342.

Zaremba J, J. Ilkowski, and J. Losy, "Serial measurements of levels of the chemokines CCL2, CCL3 and CCL5 in serum of patients with acute ischemic stroke," *Folia Neuropathologica*, vol. 44, no. 4, pp. 282–289, 2006.

Zhu YC, Cui LY, Hua BL, Pan JQ: Correlation between fibrinogen level and cerebral infarction. *Chin Med. Sci. J.* 2006; 21:167–70.

In: Recent Advances in Stroke Therapeutics
Editor: Manzoor Ahmad Mir
ISBN: 978-1-63117-754-5

Chapter IV

Major Advances in the Treatment of Strokes

Abstract

The translation of neuroprotective agents for ischemic stroke from bench-to-bedside has largely failed to produce improved treatments since the development of tissue plasminogen activator (tPA). One possible reason for lack of translation is the failure to acknowledge the greatest risk factor for stroke, age, and other common comorbidities such as hypertension, obesity, and diabetes that are associated with stroke. In this chapter, we highlight both mechanisms of studying these factors and results of those that have been addressed.

We also discuss the potential role of other lifestyle factors associated with an increased stroke risk, such as sleep fragmentation and/or deprivation. Furthermore, many proposed therapeutic agents have targeted molecular mechanisms occurring soon after the onset of ischemia despite data indicating delayed patient presentation following ischemic stroke.

Modulating inflammation has been identified as a promising therapeutic avenue consistent with preliminary success of ongoing clinical trials for anti-inflammatory compounds such as minocycline. In this chapter, we review the role of inflammation in stroke and in particular, the role of inflammatory cell recruitment and macrophage phenotype in the inflammatory process. Emerging evidence indicates an increasing role of neuro-immune crosstalk, which has led to increased interest in identification of peripheral biomarkers indicative of neural injury. It is our hope that identification and investigation of factors influencing stroke pathophysiology may lead to improved therapeutics.

Keywords: Neuroprotective, Plasminogen activator, hypertension, Ischemic, inflammatory, therapeutics, pathophysiology, clinical trials, biomarkers

Introduction

Acute ischemic stroke remains a condition of high morbidity and mortality. Until now, the only established therapy has been intravenous (IV) tissue-type plasminogen activator (tPA). Only 3–10% of patients with acute ischemic stroke receive this treatment. On the basis of data from part 3 of the European Collaborative Acute Stroke Study (ECASS III), the time window for beneficial treatment of ischemic stroke with IV tPA has been extended from 3 to 4.5 h after the onset of stroke symptoms. Beyond that window of opportunity, and additionally to IV treatment, interventional stroke therapy has assumed an important role for the treatment of acute ischemic stroke. Currently, new promising pharmacological and mechanical treatment options are being established as routine procedures to achieve a further improved outcome for stroke patients.

The main challenge in stroke therapy is how to rescue patients who have survived the ischemic insult, considering that by the time they are evaluated, the majority might have passed the 3-h window in which to receive t-PA therapy. Therefore, the prime issues are: i) how to extend the window of treatment; ii) how to minimize the effect of reperfusion injury, considering that the damaging effect due to reperfusion sometimes could be greater than that due to ischemia itself; iii) how to reduce the risks associated with t-PA therapy beyond 3 h; and iv) how to regenerate infarcted brain areas to regain neurological function. New advances that combine the basic understanding of pathobiology of the disease and translational research, including drug delivery approaches and surgical interventions could address the complex issues associated with stroke therapy.

Stroke is a leading cause of death, long-term disability, and socioeconomic costs, highlighting the urgent need for more effective treatments. Intravenous administration of tissue plasminogen activator (t-PA) is the only FDA-approved therapy to re-establish cerebral blood flow. However, because of increased risk of hemorrhage beyond 3 h post stroke, few stroke patients (1–2%) benefit from t-PA; t-PA, which has neurotoxic effects, can also aggravate the extent of reperfusion injury by increasing blood-brain barrier permeability. An alternative strategy is needed to extend the window of intervention, minimize damage from reperfusion injury, and promote brain repair leading to neurological recovery. Reactive oxygen species (ROS), generated soon after ischemia and during reperfusion and thereafter, are considered the main mediators of ischemic injury. Antioxidant enzymes such as catalase, superoxide dismutase, etc. can neutralize ROS-mediated injury but their effective delivery to the brain remains a challenge. In this chapter, we review various therapeutic approaches including surgical interventions, and discuss the potential of nanoparticle-mediated delivery of antioxidants for stroke therapy.

Stroke is a sudden loss of brain function resulting from interference with the blood supply to the central nervous system (CNS). Normal cerebral blood flow (CBF) is approximately 50–60 ml/100g/min. The reduction in CBF below 20 ml/100g/min results in an electrical silence and less than 10 ml/100g/min causes irreversible neuronal injury (Hakim M. 1998, Jones T. H. 1981). Lack of blood circulation to the brain deprives neurons of necessary glucose and oxygen. Neurons are the impulse transmitters; hence they require constant supply of energy. Up to 85% of all strokes are of ischemic origin, with most attributable to blockage of one or more cerebral artery by blood clots, with resulting reduction in cerebral perfusion. The remaining stroke cases are hemorrhagic, involving either intracerebral or subarachnoid hemorrhage.

Mechanisms of Neuronal Injury and the Therapeutic Possibilities

Cerebral ischemia results in a number of hemodynamic, biochemical, and neurophysiological alterations (Ostrowski R. P. 2006). A series of complex acute, subacute and chronic events occur after the incidence of stroke and reperfusion (Jean W. C. 1998). Ischemic injury involves energy failure, loss of cell ion homeostasis, acidosis, increased intracellular calcium excitotoxicity, free radical-mediated toxicity, and pathological permeability of the blood-brain barrier (BBB). Free radicals, specifically reactive oxygen species (ROS) that are generated soon after ischemia, as well as in later stages of ischemic reperfusion (e.g., by inflammatory cells), are the fundamental mediators of reperfusion injury.

The development of hypoxic-ischemic neuronal injury is significantly influenced by the release of excitatory neurotransmitters, primarily glutamate and aspartate in the brain. This process is called excitotoxicity and is activated by depletion of cellular energy stores. Glutamate, normally stored inside the synaptic terminals, is released in the extracellular space in a depleted energy state, which then results in the opening of calcium channels associated with N-methyl- D asapartate (NMDA) and alpha-amino-3-hydroxy-5-methyl-4-isoxanole propionate (AMPA) receptors. This leads to an influx of calcium, sodium and chloride ions and efflux of potassium ions. (Siesjo B. K. 1989, Hademenos G. J. 1997, Garcia J. H. 1994). The influx of calcium is responsible for the activation of a series of destructive enzymes such as proteases, endonucleases and lipases that allow release of cytokines and other inflammatory mediators, resulting in the loss of cellular integrity (Siejo B. K. 1981, Becker K. J. 1998). Inflammatory mechanisms play an important role in tissue injury by inducing the rapid production of many different inflammatory mediators. Within 30 minutes after ischemia and reperfusion, leukocytes recruited to the ischemic area activate mediators of inflammation such as oxygen free radicals, cytokines, and nitric acid.

A vast amount of data implicates oxygen-derived free radicals (especially superoxide and hydroxyl radicals) and high-energy oxidants (such as peroxynitrile) as mediators of inflammation in ischemia/reperfusion injury (Cuzzocrea S. 2001). Free radicals are highly reactive molecules generated predominantly during cellular respiration and normal metabolism. Imbalance between cellular production of free radicals and the ability of cells to defend against them is referred to as oxidative stress (Valko M. 2007).

After brain injury by ischemic stroke, the production of ROS dramatically increases, leading to tissue damage via several different cellular, molecular pathways, and mechanical pressure (Figure 4.1).

ROS can cause damage to cellular components such as lipids, protein, and nucleic acids, leading to subsequent cell death (Janardhan V. 2004). Damage can become more widespread due to weakened cellular antioxidant defense systems in ischemia.

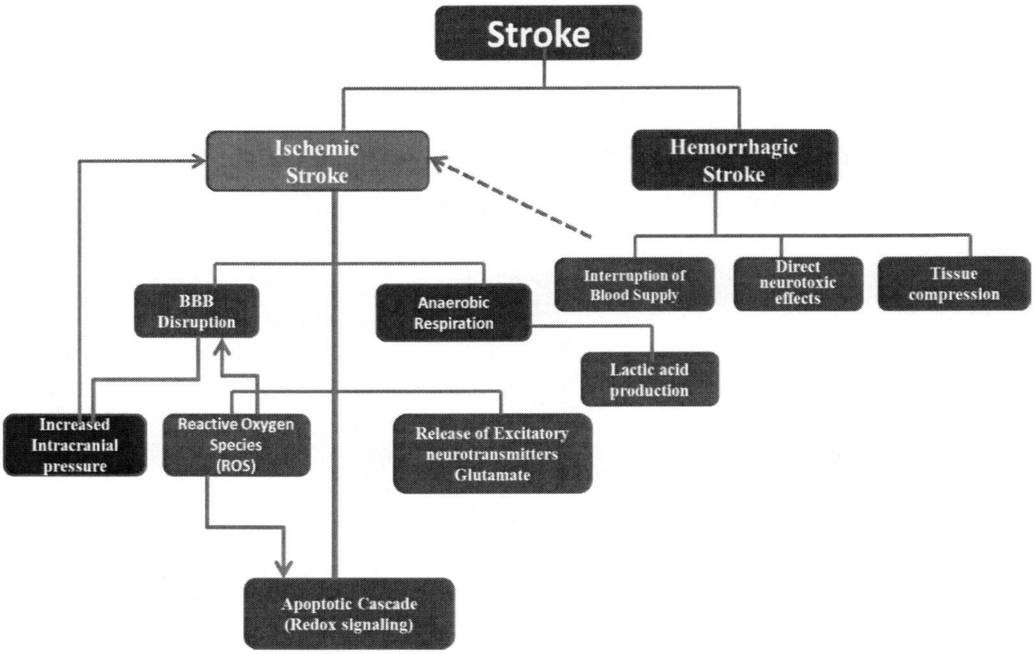

Figure 4.1. Schematic showing different types of stroke and cascade of events following ischemia.

ROS are the major stimulators of inflammatory cytokine production (such as interleukin-1, tumor necrosis factor-α, and interferon-γ) and protease secretion by microglia, leukocytes, and resident cells of the neurovascular unit (Haddad J. J. 2002). As these neuroinflammatory mechanisms become activated, alterations in cytokine profiles, adhesion-molecule expression, and tight-junction components mediate further vascular leakage. Significant evidence exists suggesting that ROS are involved in every fundamental physiological step that leads to neuronal death (Cao W. 1988) and thus are considered an important target in developing an effective stroke therapy (Juurlink B. H. 1997).

Following the onset of ischemic stroke, cerebral blood flow is disrupted throughout the affected region of the brain. Blood flow disruption to the tissue is not uniform due to the presence of collateral circulation resulting in a flow gradient. Consequently, a "core" region of infarct develops in which flow is severely reduced, often approximating upwards of a 90% decrement, and tissue undergoes necrosis within minutes as insufficient adenosine triphosphate (ATP) is present to maintain homeostatic ionic gradients and metabolic functions (Astrup J. 1977). Surrounding this core region in which blood flow is severely reduced is the "penumbra", a tissue distribution in which flow is less severely reduced and remains typically around 35% of baseline flow (Astrup J. 1977). Characterized by normal cellular membrane potential but a disruption in the ability for normal action potential firing, tissue initially residing within the penumbral region progresses to cellular death, ultimately resulting in an expanded core lesion without restoration of cerebral blood flow (Lo E. H. 2008). As such, therapeutic development has focused on achieving reperfusion via tissue plasminogen activator (tPA) and/or restoring homeostasis via administration of 'neuroprotective' pharmacologic agents intended to disrupt the ischemic injury cascade.

Current research in stroke has focused on developing neuroprotective therapies that target many mechanisms involved in stroke pathophysiology.

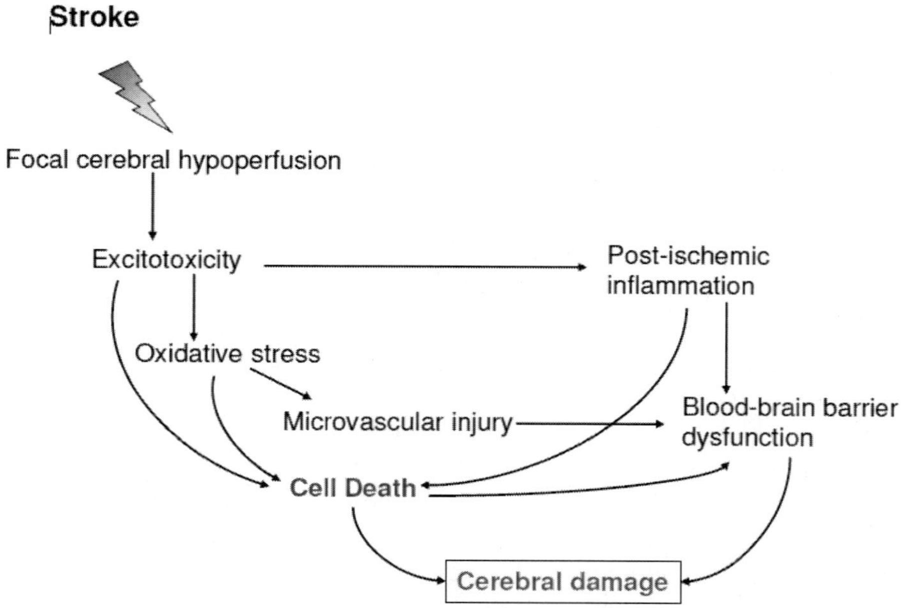

Figure 4.2. Ischemic cascade leading to cerebral damage.Ischemic stroke leads to hypoperfusion of a brain area that initiates a complex series of events. Excitotoxicity, oxidative stress, microvascular injury, blood-brain barrier dysfunction and postischemic inflammation lead ultimately to cell death of neurons, glia and endothelial cells. The degree and duration of ischemia determines the extent of cerebral damage.

Studies from animal and cell models have greatly expanded our knowledge in this field and form the basis of clinical trials of neuroprotective therapies. Results have been variable; it is very likely that no single therapy will be satisfactory, and that multiple agents working through different mechanisms or novel agents that target more than disease mechanism may offer the best hope for a future neuroprotective therapy. In this chapter, we address several disease mechanisms of pathogenesis in stroke, along with some examples of therapies targeting each of these mechanisms.

Current Status of Neuroprotectant Development: Drug Development Shortcomings

Investigation of neuroprotection and the associated concepts have gone through various periods of apparent focus as described by Lo previously (Lo E. H. 2008). Early studies, initiated by Astrup and colleagues, focused on understanding the effect of ischemia produced across a range of cerebral blood flow measurements on neurophysiology and electrical conduction (Astru p J. 2008).

The second phase of investigation sought to identify molecular mechanisms of injury with an emphasis on the acute period of injury. Following molecular biology studies was the discovery and implementation of numerous imaging modalities in both preclinical and clinical studies for assessing both changes in blood flow and the evolution of both the penumbra and infarct core (Lo E. H. 2008). While these various developments have provided much insight and utility in both preclinical and clinical studies, successful translation of a neuroprotectant from bench-to-bedside has yet to occur despite identification of over 1000 "successful" neuroprotectants in preclinical studies and initiation of over 100 clinical trials (O'Collins V. E. 2006).

The reasons for lack of translation and failure are presently unknown but clear discrepancies exist between preclinical models and the clinical population most commonly afflicted by ischemic stroke. These include the age and general health of the population being studied as well as the time point of treatment initiation. Similarly, the endpoints frequently used in preclinical and clinical studies are often different. Furthermore, the vast majority of preclinical work has been conducted in rodents, species that are more distant phylogenetically from the human population in comparison to nonhuman primates. Nonhuman primates more closely resemble humans in vascular anatomy, experience striatal damage following ischemic stroke more comparably to the human, and are gyrencephalic in nature like humans (Fukuda S. 2003). Consequently, nonhuman primates represent perhaps the most ideal preclinical model, but are frequently not utilized due to cost, lack of availability, and expertise required for care and use. For these reasons, nonhuman primate models are not discussed further. The following sections elaborate on these concepts in an attempt to convey the contribution of common comorbidities seen in the clinical population to stroke risk and outcome. Furthermore, the potential impact of other lifestyle factors such as sleep fragmentation and/or deprivation, often related to an altered sleep-wake cycle by something such as shift work, is discussed.

In treating acute ischemic stroke, two primary strategies are followed: 1) limiting the ischemic insult by early reperfusion and 2) interfering with the pathobiochemical cascade leading to ischemic neuronal damage.

In developing an effective therapy, one must also weigh the deleterious consequences of reperfusion injury versus the effects of delay in resuming blood supply to the brain (Wagner K. R. 2004).

Within an hour of ischemia, two layers of cerebrovascular tissue develop: the inner core displaying necrosis of both neuronal as well as supporting glial elements, and the outer layer of less severe ischemia called the ischemic penumbra. The cells within the ischemic penumbra can be recovered if timely therapeutic intervention is administered. The size of the ischemic penumbra (portion of the brain that can be rescued) diminishes with time, as the infarct core progressively becomes hypoperfused tissue that cannot be rescued following reperfusion. Ischemic damage in the penumbra, however, is reversible and is the target of rescue via re-establishing blood flow (Fisher M. 2004).

Drugs Used in Acute Stroke Therapy

Drug therapy is a relatively recent approach to the treatment of stroke, and a large amount of research is focused on finding effective new drugs that can minimize stroke damage. The most relevant drugs evaluated for acute stroke therapy are summarized in Table 4.1.

Table 4.1. Drugs used in endovascular therapy for acute stroke

Group	Drug	Effect
Drugs to improve blood flow	Heparin Abciximab Ancrod	Antithrombotic Antiplatelet Fibrinogen depleting
Thrombolytics	Streptokinase Urokinase Prourokinase Alteplase Reteplase Tenecteplase Tissue plasminogen activator	Plasminogen activators
	Alfimeprase BB10153 Desmoteplase	Direct acting fibrinolytics
New drugs under evaluation	V10153 Microplasmin	

Plasminogen Activators

Plasminogen activators are the primary drugs used as thrombolytic agents in acute stroke therapy. These drugs act by converting plasminogen into plasmin. Plasmin unlocks fibrinogen, fibrin monomers and cross-linked fibrin (as found in a thrombus) into fibrin degradation products (Lisboa R. C. 2002).

Streptokinase a clot buster bind to plasminogen and the streptokinase/plasminogen complex then serves as a plasminogen activator. It is a protein derived from group CS-hemolytic streptococci, which showed significant rates of ICH and systemic hemorrhage (Cornu C. 2000); thus, it is no longer used for acute stroke therapy; rather, Urokinase, a serine protease with a plasma half-life of 14 min, is used (Lisboa R. C. 2002). The randomized trial of intra-arterial infusion of urokinase within 6 h of middle cerebral artery stroke: the middle cerebral artery embolism local fibrinolytic intervention trial (MELT), suggested that intra-arterial fibrinolysis has the potential to increase the likelihood of excellent functional outcome (Ogawa A. 2007). Prourokinase (r-prourokinase) is the proenzyme precursor of urokinase. Despite the favorable results in the PROACT (Prolyse in Acute Cerebral Thromboembolism) I and II trials (de Zoppo D. J. 1998, Furlan A. 1999), the FDA did not approve its use in IA stroke therapy.

Alteplase (recombinant human tissue-type plasminogen activator; rtPA) is a serine protease with a plasma half-life of 3.5 min. This short half-life and the limited penetration of the clot, because of strong binding with surface fibrin, delay recanalization and increase the risk of recurrent occlusion. By the administration of heparin or antiplatelet drugs, reocclusion may be reduced.

Moreover, rtPA seems to have some neurotoxic properties, including activation of metalloproteinases, which may result in increased blood–brain barrier permeability leading to cerebral hemorrhage and edema, as well as amplification of calcium currents through the N-methyl-D-aspartate receptor. This leads to excitotoxicity and neuronal death (Kaur J. 2004). Nevertheless, rtPA represents the first line therapy in the treatment of acute ischemic stroke. More recently licensed plasminogen activators are variants of tPA. These include Reteplase, a truncated tPA variant with a longer half-life and Tenecteplase, a bioengineered tPA variant. Because of their longer half-lives, Reteplase and Tenecteplase can be given as a bolus injection, thereby simplifying administration (Llevadot J. 2001). A case study reported 84% recanalization and no ICH with IA Reteplase in combination with mechanical thrombolysis (Qureshi A. 2002). A pilot clinical trial with Tenecteplase, was terminated owing to symptomatic and asymptomatic ICHs (15% and 23%, respectively) (Haley E. C. 2005). Direct fibrinolytics and new fibrinolytic agents currently under development were built upon advances of tPA derivatives developed to produce less bleeding (Mellot M. J. 1995).

Alfimeprase (ARCA Biopharma Broomfield, CO, USA), a recombinant, truncated form of fibrolase, has been developed to accelerate lysis. It is designed to dissolve clots by directly degrading fibrin when delivered through a catheter directly into the thrombus and is inactivated locally by circulating alpha-2 macroglobulin. Because there is no need for plasmin generation, alfimeprase has the potential to degrade fibrin more rapidly than tPA. This should result in faster recanalization and lower hemorrhagic risk (Deitcher S. R. 2005). Nevertheless, alfimeprase failed to meet the key efficacy end points of revascularization in the phase II trial CARNEROS-1 (Proof-of-Concept Study of the Safety and Efficacy of Alfimeprase to Rapidly Open Arteries and Restore Brain Function Following a Stroke). The full results of this trial have not yet been published.

BB10153 (British Biotech, Oxford, England), a variant form of plasminogen, has the plasminogen activator cleavage site replaced with a thrombin cleavage site. Like plasminogen it binds to fibrin and gets converted to plasmin by fibrin-bound thrombin. In a phase II dose-escalation study 34% of patients achieved complete low in the infarct-related artery. There were no intracranial bleeds (Gibson C. M. 2006) and based on these data, BB10153 is undergoing continued investigation. Desmoteplase (Paion, Aachen, Germany), a recombinant analog of the full-length plasminogen activator isolated from the saliva of the vampire bat, demonstrated safety in the Desmoteplase in Acute Ischemic Stroke (DIAS), Dose Escalation of Desmoteplase for Acute Ischemic Stroke (DEDAS), and DIAS-II trials (Furlan A. J. 2006). A new trial (DIAS-III) was stopped because of lack of efficacy in the desmoteplase-treated patients. The thrust of this study was to determine whether the window for fibrinolytic therapy could be extended beyond 3 h (Hacke W. 2005).

The success of plasminogen activators is, at least in part, highly dependent on the amount of plasminogen in the thrombus. Newer drugs do not depend on the availability of plasminogen.

Ancrod (Viprinex; Neurobiological Technologies, Emeryville, CA, USA) is a defibrinogenating agent derived from the venom of the Malayan pit viper. By defibrinogenating blood an anticoagulant effect is promoted. To study the safety and efficacy of ancrod in patients with acute ischemic stroke administered within 6 h of stroke onset, the Ancrod Stroke Study was performed. No significant difference in overall mean scores on the Scandinavian Stroke Scale could be demonstrated. Those patients with ancrodinduced 6-h fibrinogen levels of 130 mg/dL or less had a marginally significantly better neurological outcome on the Scandinavian Stroke Scale, mortality, and Barthel Index than ancrod-treated patients with higher fibrinogen levels (The Ancord Stroke investigators, 1994).

V10153 (Vernalis, Winnersh, UK) is a novel modified recombinant variant of human plasminogen, which is activated to plasmin by thrombin. Thrombin, as the key enzyme involved in blood clot formation, is utilised to initiate clot destruction (Davson K. M. 1994). V10153 selectively induces lysis of newly formed clots, which should result in a reduced risk of hemorrhage. The V10153 Acute Stroke Thrombolysis Trial (VASTT) was a phase II dose-escalation multicenter study. The trial has been halted because of significant hemorrhagic complications. The trial enrolment is closed and data are currently being analyzed.

Microplasmin (ThromboGenics, Heverlee, Belgium) is a truncated form of plasmin that is more resistant to antiplasmin. In a rabbit stroke model, IV microplasmin infusion resulted in a high rate of clot lysis without increasing the rate of ICH (Lapchak P. A. 2002). These findings were confirmed in the MITI-IV (Microplasmin in Treatment of Ischemic Stroke-IntraVenous) trial, a phase II multicenter, randomized, double-blinded, placebo-controlled ascending-dose clinical trial. Data are yet to be published.

Adjuvant Drugs

Because fibrinolytic agents also have prothrombotic properties, early reocclusion has been demonstrated in 34% of the patients treated with IV rtPA (Alexandrov A. V. 2002). Therefore, the adjuvant use of antithrombotic agents is common practice. IV heparin for systemic anticoagulation during the periprocedural phase of endovascular stoke therapy is controversial. The potential advantages, including augmentation of the thrombolytic effect, prevention of acute reocclusion and reduction in the risk of catheter-related embolism, have to be weighed against the potentially increased risk of ICH when heparin is combined with a thrombolytic agent (delzeppo G. J. 1998). The use of glycoprotein (GP) IIb/IIIa antagonists, such as ReoPro (abciximab – an intravenous platelet aggregation inhibitor, is a monoclonal antibody directed against the platelet glycoprotein GP IIb–IIIa receptor), Integrilin (eptifibatide), or Aggrastat (tirofiban) in ischemic stroke remains investigational. In pilot studies, no major ICH was seen in combination with standard rtPA therapy (Pancioli M. 2008). Conversely, the AbESTT (Abciximab in Emergent Stroke Treatment) Trial-II, a phase III study, evaluating the safety and efficacy of abciximab in acute ischemic stroke, including patients who awoke with stroke symptoms, was permanently stopped owing to a high rate of intracranial hemorrhage in the abciximab-treated patients (Adams H. P. 2008). The data for the use of GP IIb/IIIa inhibitors in conjunction with intraarterial thrombolysis are limited to case reports. The number of cases with symptomatic ICH varied between 0 and 23% (Noguira R. J. 2008)

Endovascular Therapy of Acute Stroke

The relatively high haemorrhage rates, in combination with the low complete recanalization rates, demonstrate the imitations of treatment solely with pharmacological agents. Especially in carotid terminus or basilar artery occlusions with large clot burden, the procedure takes time and may not achieve meaningful recanalization. Platelet-rich clots, old clots and calcified clots or fat emboli cannot be addressed. These factors substantiate the assumption that faster and more complete reperfusion will lead to better long-term outcomes for acute stroke patients. Endovascular therapy promises higher recanalization rates because of the obvious advantages over IV rtPA, which are site specific, reduction of drug amount and potentially longer treatment windows.

Nevertheless, the potential benefit of endovascular therapy must be weighed against the potential risk of the procedure. Intraarterial (IA) stroke therapy has been associated with a 5–7% risk for clinically significant procedural complications (delzeppo G. J. 1998, Furlan A. 1999) and a 6–15% risk for symptomatic ICH (Smith W. S. 2002). Patients with minor strokes, who are treated with IV rtPA, have an 82% chance of a good outcome and the risk of symptomatic hemorrhage and death is 3% and 1%, respectively (The NINDS Stroke study Investigaors, 2005).

Such patients are quite unlikely to benefit from endovascular stroke therapy, as they often show no vessel occlusion on cerebral angiograms (Fisher U. 2005). Most stroke centers offer IA stroke therapy only to patients with major strokes. Different strategies of endovascular therapy are offered to reach reperfusion of occluded vessels in acute stroke. Most techniques focus on removing and dissolving the occlusive thrombus to reestablish antegrade flow, but some use the collateral vessel system of the brain to augment flow retrogradely. The different interventional methods are summarized in Table 4.2.

Table 4.2. Strategies of endovascular stroke therapy

Strategies of endovascular stroke therapy			
Interventional method	Endovascular device used	Reperfusion	
		Ante-grade	Retro-grade
Intraarterial thrombolysis	Microcatheter	X	
Mechanical thrombus disruption	Microguidewire, laser	X	
Percutaneous transluminal angioplasty	Microcatheter with balloon for dilatation	X	
Aspiration of thrombus	Guiding catheter	X	
Endovascular thrombectomy	Clotretriever	X	
Augmented fibrinolysis	Ultrasound	X	
Thrombus entrapment	Stent	X	
Temporary endovascular bypass	Stent		x
Flow augmentation	Balloon catheter		x
Transarterial or transvenous retrograde reperfusion	Balloon catheter		

Intra-Arterial Thrombolysis

The major theoretic advantage of IA thrombolysis over IV thrombolysis is that microcatheter techniques allow direct access to the occluded intracranial vessel and by penetrating the thrombus with the microcatheter the fibrinolytic agent can be infused into the thrombus. This permits a smaller dose of fibrinolytic agent to reach a higher local concentration than reached by systemic infusion and ideally allows more complete recanalization. Additionally, complications from systemic fibrinolytic effects, including ICH, can theoretically be reduced. Thus, the treatment window for endovascular techniques can be extended beyond the typical IV window by 3–6 h, which is important because of the low number of patients who present during the 3-h time window. The first reports about IA administration of thrombolytic agents, mainly in the posterior circulation, were published in the 1980s. An overall recanalization rate of 60% and a mortality rate of 90% in nonrecanalized patients versus 31% in at least partially recanalized patients were found (Zeumer H. 1983, Hacke W. 1988). Multiple non-randomized case series reported successful use of IA thrombolysis. A review of patients treated with urokinase, showed recanalization rates of >75% when additional endovascular techniques (such as mechanical fragmentation of the thrombus, thromboaspiration, percutaneous transluminal angioplasty, and implantation of stents) were used (Noguiera R. J. 2008). Combined IV and IA thrombolysis several studies have evaluated the feasibility, safety and efficacy of combined IV rtPA with IA thrombolysis in patients with acute stroke. This approach has the potential of combining the advantages of IV rtPA (fast and easy to use) with the advantages of IA therapy (directed therapy, titrated dosing, mechanical aids to recanalization and higher rates of recanalization), thus improving the speed and frequency of recanalization. In the Emergency Management of Stroke (EMS) Bridging Trial, no difference in the 7–10-day or 3-month outcomes between the IV rtPA or IV placebo followed by immediate intra-arterial therapy with rtPA group were found, but there were more deaths in the IV/ IA group (Lewandwoski C. A. 1999). The Interventional Management of Stroke (IMS I) Study investigated a combined IV and IA approach to recanalization in patients with ischemic stroke (IMS study Investigators, 2004). The 90-day mortality rate in IMS I subjects (16%) was numerically lower, but not statistically different from the mortality rate of the placebo (24%) or rtPA treated subjects (21%) in the NINDS-rtPA- Stroke-Trial.

Mechanical Thrombectomy

When thrombolysis is ineffective or is not considered as a viable option, mechanical devices are used to recanalize the occluded cerebral vessel to restore the flow (IMS 2007). One such device, the Merci Retriever™ (Concentric Medical, Mountain View, CA), consists of a flexible corkscrew-shaped tapered nitinol wire with 5 helical loops that can be threaded in the thrombus, which is then removed by traction (Smith W. S. 2006). The first prospective study that examined a device-based treatment option for ischemic stroke showed a 43% recanalization rate with the device alone and a 64% recanalization rate with additional intraarterial administration of t-PA (Smith W. S. 2008). The Catch System™ (BALT Extrusion, Montmorency, France) is a tiny wire basket that retrieves the thrombus

(Brekenfeld C. 2008). Another useful new technique has been developed in which the clot is simultaneously aspirated from the vessel as it is being extracted. The Phenox Clot Retriever™ (Phenox, Bochum, Germany) consists of a highly flexible core wire compound resembling a pipe cleaner with perpendicularly oriented polyamide microfilaments that create an attenuated palisade. It is deployed distal to the clot and is slowly pulled back under continuous aspiration via the guiding catheter.

The BONnet™ (Phenox, Bochum, Germany) consists of a self-expanding nitinol braiding with polyamide filaments passing through the interior to enlarge the surface area and enable better fixation of the thrombus mass (Liebig T. 2008). The Penumbra System™ (Penumbra, Alameda, CA) has been FDA-approved as a dual approach to clot extraction using aspiration and debulking of the thrombus to reduce or eliminate the clot burden (Natrajan S. K. 2009, PPST 2009). The system includes reperfusion microcatheters that are connected to an aspiration pump through an aspiration tube. A separator is advanced and retracted within the lumen of the reperfusion catheter to debulk the clot, followed by clot retrieval with a ring device that engages the thrombus by capturing it in clasps with a cylinder that is then withdrawn. The recanalization rate is more than 80% and the device has an excellent safety profile (<3% procedural serious adverse events) (Struffert T. 2009). This system has the potential of reopening a vessel without the use of thrombolytics, thus offering dual options for recanalization via a single access platform, and decreases the need to blindly penetrate into the occluded vascular segment because it operates from the proximal end of the clot (Noguira R. G. 2009). Percutaneous transluminal angioplasty (PTA) is particularly useful in cases of atherothrombotic disease, in which the residual stenosis may reduce flow sufficiently to lead to rethrombosis (Abu Chebl A. 2005). PTA can be used alone or with subsequent thrombolytic therapy for distal embolization. The largest study of angioplasty for acute stroke showed that recanalization was achieved in 63.9% of thrombolytic-only treated patients, versus 91.2% in the combined thrombolytic plus PTA treatment group. Because of the risk of vessel rupture and distal embolization, this technique is generally reserved for patients whose flow cannot be restored by more conservative methods (Abu Chebl A. 2005). Interventional treatment of acute ischemic stroke with self-expanding stents for flow restoration has been shown to be an effective method for achieving re-canalization. In a prospective study, Stent-Assisted Recanalization in Acute Ischemic Stroke, 100% successful recanalization was demonstrated in 20 patients, with only 1 symptomatic hemorrhage. The disadvantage of this approach is the implantation of a permanent prosthesis and the need for continuous antiplatelet therapy (Levy E. I. 2009, Jahan R. 2010).

Several techniques are used for mechanical clot disruption. The most common is probing the thrombus with a microguide wire. This technique appears to be useful in facilitating chemical thrombolysis. Alternatively, a snare (e.g., Amplatz goose-neck microsnare, Microvena) can be used for multiple passes through the occlusion to disrupt the thrombus (Berguie M. 2006). A snare can also be used for clot retrieval, mostly in situations in which the clot has a firm consistency or contains solid material. Two devices that use laser technologies have been used to disrupt intracranial clots. The EPAR (Endovasix, Belmont, CA, USA) is a mechanical clot-fragmentation device based on laser technology. The photonic energy is converted to acoustic energy at the fiberoptic tip through creation of micro cavitation bubbles, causing emulsification of the thrombus which is a mechanical thrombolysis and not a direct laser-induced ablation. In a pilot study with 34 patients, vessel recanalization occurred in 61.1%. There were ICHs in 5.9% and the overall mortality rate was 38.2% (Berlis A. 2004).

The LaTIS laser device (LaTIS, Minneapolis, MN, USA) uses the slow injection of contrast material as a 'light pipe' to carry the energy from the catheter to the embolus. A safety and feasibility trial was stopped because the device could not be deployed to the level of the occlusion in 2 of the first 5 patients.

Intra-arterial (IA) Mechanical Therapies

The limitations to IA lysis are related to clot characteristics. The response to the pharmacological agent may vary according to the source and type of clot. White platelet rich clots are more resistant to lytics than fresh red blood cell rich clots. De novo cardiac clots and paradoxial venous clots respond better than calcified clots from atherosclerotic plaques. The therapeutic approach concerning these limitations changed dramatically in 2004 with the US Food and Drug Administration approval of the first mechanical clot-retriever (Smith W. S. 2005). The mechanical fragmentation of a clot increases the surface area accessible to fibrinolytic agents thus increases the speed of thrombolysis. The use of chemical thrombolytics is lower, or can be avoided, particularly in patients with contraindications to thrombolytic therapy. The treatment window can be exceeded beyond the limit of 6–8 h. Clot-retrieval devices also may be more efficient in catching mature embolic clots and emboli composed of cholesterol, calcium or other debris from atherosclerotic lesions (Smith W. S., 2005 and 2008, Noguiera R. G. 2009).

Surgical Interventions

Surgical reconstruction of the cervical carotid artery may be indicated in patients with transient ischemic attack but who are otherwise in good neurologic condition. Another option, microsurgical embolectomy of intracranial vessels, is an invasive procedure involving craniotomy, opening the occluded artery to remove the clot, and reperfusion of the affected area. However, because the procedure is performed through the subarachnoid space via a small craniotomy with a minimal skin incision, it is relatively safe. This can be a last therapeutic option for those patients who are ineligible to receive intravenous or intraarterial thrombolysis, or in the case of failed mechanical thrombectomy. Again, there is a restrictive time window of less than 6 hours from stroke onset for the intervention to be effective. Another surgical procedure utilized in ischemic stroke patients is brain decompression. In the case of major vessel occlusion, large cerebral infarcts is developed, commonly associated with rapidly progressing malignant cerebral edema (Hofmeijer J. 2004). This leads to compromised neuronal metabolism, decreased cerebral perfusion, and impaired oxygenation. In addition, shifting of intracranial contents and transtentorial herniation, is the leading cause of death in these patients (Hacke W. 1996). Because this kind of cerebral edema is refractory, i.e., not amenable to other forms of treatment, brain decompression is considered a therapy of last resort. Decompressive hemicraniectomy with duraplasty is a complex procedure in which a part of the skull vault is removed and the dura is opened to give more room for the expanding brain. Then, a Silastic sheet, watertight Lyodura, or pericranial grafts are placed over the craniectomy for brain protection. This procedure has been shown to result in increased cerebral perfusion, better survival, improved neurological outcomes, and a reduction in the volume of the infarction (Adams H. P. 2007, Schwab S. 2007). Another, more invasive craniotomy involves resection of infarcted tissue and/or uncal resection. Resection of dead tissue makes room for reperfusion of live tissue in the affected area. Both types of procedures appear to yield satisfactory outcome results.

The disadvantages of the mechanical approaches include the difficulty of navigating devices into the intracranial circulation, excessive trauma to the vasculature (potentially leading to vasospasms, vessel dissection, perforation or rupture) and fragmented thrombus causing distal embolization into previously unaffected territories.

Percutaneous Transluminal Angioplasty

The feasibility and high efficacy of percutaneous transluminal angioplasty (PTA) in acute stroke has been shown (Ueda T. 1997). Partial or complete recanalization could be achieved in 91% of patients treated with direct PTA versus 64% treated with thrombolytic therapy alone. ICH was seen in 3% versus 19%, and good outcome occurred in 73% versus 50% of the patients, respectively (Nakano S. 2002). 92% recanalization was achieved with the use of balloon angioplasty and adjuvant low-dose eptifibatide and/or thrombolytics with 42% good outcomes (Noguire R. G. 2008). PTA may also be particularly useful in the cases of atherothrombotic disease, in which the residual stenosis may reduce flow sufficiently to lead to rethrombosis (Quereshi A. I. 2002).

Endovascular Thromboaspiration

The use of large 7 to 8-F guide catheter with syringe suction is a simple approach that has been used to remove occlusive thrombus and restore flow in symptomatic acute internal carotid artery occlusion. The guide catheter is slowly withdrawn to facilitate more complete removal of the thrombus (Brekenfield C. 2005). Suction thrombectomy or thromboaspiration through either a microcatheter or a guiding catheter may be an option for a fresh clot. Aspiration devices cause fewer embolic events and vasospasm, but can be difficult to navigate into the intracranial circulation.

The Penumbra System (Penumbra, Alameda, CA, USA) uses a microcatheter and a separator, which is advanced and retracted through the catheter to dislodge the clot and a suction device removes it. This system was initially tested in a pilot trial, where 23 subjects were enrolled. Recanalization before IA lysis was achieved in all treated cases (48%). Good outcome at 30 days was demonstrated in 45% of patients. The mortality rate was 45%. The use of adjunctive IA thrombolytic therapy was associated with a higher incidence of hemorrhage (Bose A. 2008).

The Angiojet (Possis Medical, Minneapolis, MN, USA) is an endovascular rheolytic thrombectomy device that combines local vortex suction, created by high-pressure saline jets, with mechanical disruption. The generated clot fragments are then sucked into the 4- or 5-F access catheter, which is not flexible enough to allow its navigation into the intracranial arteries. The NeuroJet (Possis Medical) has been designed specifically for intracranial navigation. Unfortunately, vessel dissections and the inability to navigate through the carotid siphon were noted in a pilot study, and the trial was discontinued (Molina C. A. 2005).

Endovascular Thrombectomy

Endovascular thrombectomy means the extraction of the thrombus with the help of an endovascular tool through a catheter, and should provide rapid recanalization and flow restoration with a reduced risk of distal embolic complications. It is used alone or in conjunction with thrombolytic drugs. The limitations of these devices are intracranial navigation and capture of thrombus within the tortuous cerebral vasculature, and the risk of vessel wall damage or perforation. Some of the devices grasp the thrombus and apply force proximally; others are basket like devices and use a distal approach to the clot.

The Merci Retrieval System (Concentric Medical, Mountain View, CA, USA) is a nitinol wire with an imprinted shape memory effect covered with a platinum coil to improve the visibility under fluoroscopy. It is inserted through a braided microcatheter to a position distal to the thrombus. After release from the microcatheter, it assumes a shape similar to a cork screw and has to be slowly pulled back under continuous aspiration via a balloon guiding catheter.More than 10,000 patients have been treated with this device. Currently the third-generation devices (V series) are used. With a 4.3F distal access catheter (DAC) an additional coaxial support can be added to the system, resulting in improved deliverability with the potential for simultaneous thrombo aspiration or IA thrombolysis. The Merci embolectomy system has been studied in the MERCI and Multi MERCI trials, where a recanalization up to 55% of treatable vessels was reported, and in 68% after adjunctive therapy (IA rtPA, mechanical). Clinically significant procedural complications occurred in 5.5% and ICH in 9.8% of patients (Bose A. 2008, Smith W. S. 2008). As an example how clot-retrievers are supposed to work the Merci retriever is shown in Figure 4.3.

The Phenox Clot Retriever (Phenox, Bochum, Germany) has been CE marked for the treatment of acute stroke in Europe since. It consists of a highly flexible nitinol/platinum-alloy compound core wire surrounded by a palisade of perpendicularly oriented stiff polyamide microfilaments trimmed in a conical shape. It is introduced into the target vessel through a microcatheter deployed distal to the thrombus and slowly pulled back under continuous aspiration via the guiding catheter. The smallest version of the device is used to recanalize distal MCA branches. Recently the second generation of the device (Phenox Clot Retriever CAGE), which incorporates a nitinol cage into the previous design, was constructed for the treatment of thrombi with firmer consistency. Recanalization was achieved in 56.3% of 45 patients with stroke with no device-related morbidity and mortality (Henkes H. 2006). The Neuronet device (Abbot Vascular, Temecula, CA, USA) has also been used successfully to retrieve intracranial clots.

It is a microguidewire-based laser-cut nitinol basket open proximally with the crisscrossing basket portion tapering to a shapable platinum-tipped wire (Mayer T. E. 2002).Very similar is the Catch (Balt Extrusion, Montmorency, France) device, a derivative of a self-expanding braided nitinol stent.

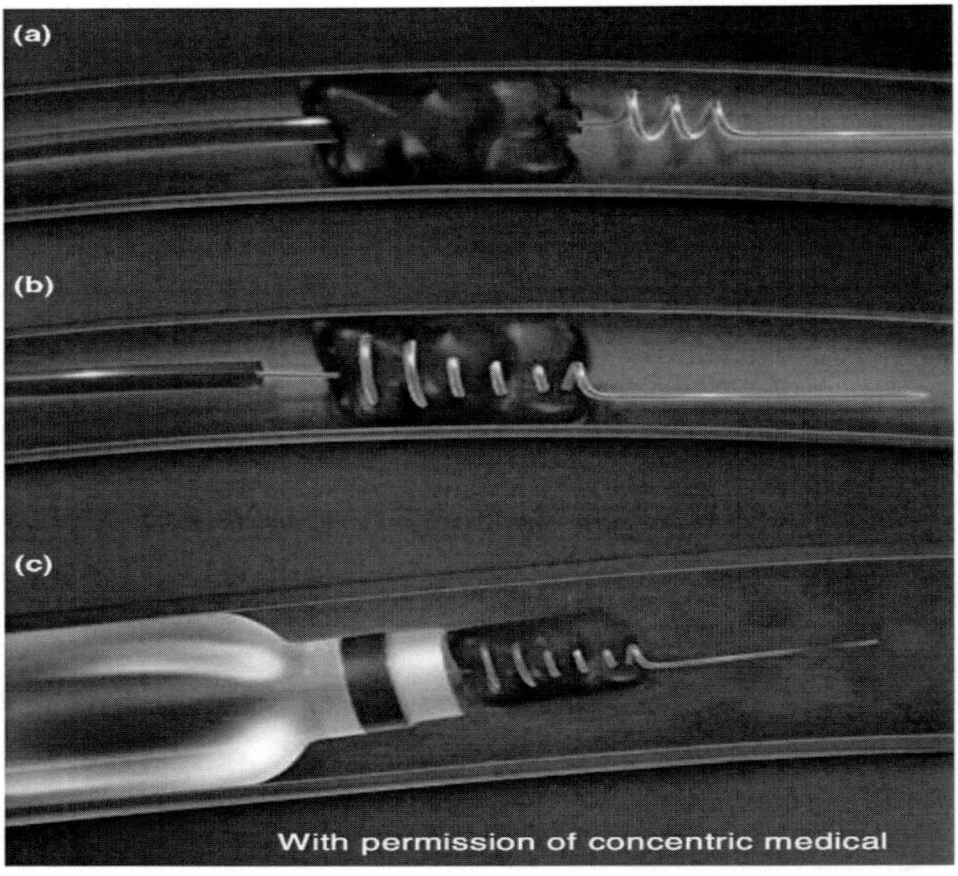

Figure 4.3. *Endovascular Therapy for acute stroke:* The principle of clot retrieving. The Merci System. Endovascular therapy for acute stroke is always performed under general nesthesia. First the MerciBalloon Guide Catheter is placed in the common or internal carotid artery for anterior circulation occlusion. Using standard cerebral catheterization techniques, a microcatheter is guided then through the guide catheter into the occluded vessel and passed beyond the thrombus (a). The Merci Retriever is now advanced through the microcatheter, and several of the helical loops are deployed distal to the thrombus. The Merci Retriever is then retracted to the face of the thrombus, and the proximal loops are deployed within the thrombus (b). The balloon of the Merci Balloon Guide Catheter has to be inflated now to arrest orthograde blood flow during removal of the thrombus. At least the Merci Retriever with the ensnared thrombus and the microcatheter are withdrawn together into the balloon guide catheter lumen. Continuous aspiration is applied to the guide catheter to promote complete evacuation of the thrombus (c). Once a retrieval attempt is completed, the balloon of the balloon guide catheter is deflated to re-establish flow. If the clot could not be removed with the retriever, the procedure can be repeated up to 5 times.

It is a nitinol basket, closed at its distal end and anchored with a pair of nitinol wires for insertion and withdrawal at the proximal end (Chapot R. 2005).

A comparison between the Merci and the Catch devices in an animal model has demonstrated superiority of the Merci retriever, which resulted in higher rates of overall recanalization (90% versus 70%), higher chances of recanalization at the first attempt, and a lower rate of thrombus fragmentation/distal embolization (Brekenfield C. 2008).

The Alligator Retrieval Device (Chestnut Medical Technologies, Menlo Park, CA, USA) is a retriever with 4 small grasping jaws attached to the tip of a flexible wire. This device has been used to treat 6 patients with intracranial clots (predominantly MCA), resulting in rapid clot removal and clinical improvement in all patients. In limited experience it provided a rapid, safe, and effective means for achieving revascularization (Kerber C. W. 2007). The In-Time Retriever (Boston Scientific, Natick, MA, USA) has 4–6 wire loops and tends to bow when opened but has no specific opening to capture the embolus. This device has been successfully used in case studies (Bergui M. 2006). The performance of 5 different embolectomy systems was recently evaluated using an in vitro pulsatile flow model. The Merci, Catch, and Phenox retrievers were equally able to mobilize and remove most thrombi, whereas the In-Time and Attractor devices achieved only partial thrombus removal at best, and with considerable difficulty during initial thrombus penetration and placement of the device (Liebig T 2008).

Augmented Fibrinolysis

The MicroLysUS infusion catheter (EKOS, Bothell, WA, USA) is a microcatheter with a piezoelectric element at its distal tip, which creates a microenvironment of ultrasonic vibration to facilitate thrombolysis. This is achieved by a combination of a noncavitating sonography, which reversibly separates fibrin strands, and acoustic streaming, which increases fluid permeation, resulting in increased drug-thrombus surface interaction. In a pilot study 14 patients were treated with IA rtPA or reteplase infusion through the EKOS microcatheter and simultaneous sonography transmission for 60 min. Recanalization was achieved in 57% of patients and good clinical outcome in 43%. The mortality rate was 36%. A comparison of angiographic outcomes between subjects treated in the IMS-II trial with the EKOS catheter and IMS-I subjects treated with the standard microcatheter demonstrated recanalization in 73% versus 56% respectively. This device is being investigated further in the IMS-III trial (Noguiera R. G. 2008).

Thrombus Entrapment

Stent placement of an acutely occluded intracranial vessel may provide fast recanalization by entrapping the thrombus between the stent and the vessel wall. This may be followed by thrombus dissolution via either endogenous or pharmacologic thrombolysis (Noguiera R. G. 2008). Treatment with balloon-expandable stents showed a recanalization rate of 79% and no symptomatic ICHs (Levi E. I. 2006). Multiple intracranial self-expandable stents are used in acute stroke therapy, although primarily designed for the treatment of wide neck aneurysms: the Neuroform (Boston Scientific), the Enterprise (Cordis, Miami Lakes, FL, USA), the LEO (Balt Extrusion, Montmorency, France) and the Solitaire/Solo stent (ev3 Endovascular, Plymouth, MN, USA). The Wingspan stent (Boston Scientific) is approved for the treatment of intracranial artherosclerotic lesions. Using these stents during stroke treatment, Gp IIb/IIIa inhibitors are administered intra- or immediately post procedurally to avoid acute in-stent thrombosis. Isolated case reports of successful intracranial recanalization with these stents have been reported (Fitzesimmonis B. F. 2006). The Pharos Vitesse stent (Micrus Endovascular), the only balloon-expandable stent approved for intracranial use, was used successfully in 4 patients with acute strokes (Killer M. et al. unpublished). The prospective ‘First Food and Drug Administration-Approved Prospective Trial of Primary Intracranial Stenting for Acute Stroke’ trial, called SARIS (Stent-Assisted Recanalization in Acute Ischemic Stroke) suggested primary intracranial stenting for acute stroke may be a valuable addition to the stroke treatment armamentarium (Levi E. I. 2009).

Temporary Endovascular Bypass

The need for an aggressive antithrombotic therapy after stent implantation remains one of the major limitations to its use in acute stroke. However, the advent of closed-cell stents has allowed resheathing and removal of the stent after recanalization. The need for post-treatment dual antiplatelet therapy, which could potentially increase the risk of hemorrhagic conversion of the infarct, is not necessary. Recently the preliminary data about the use of the Solitaire/SOLO device as a temporary endovascular bypass and clot retriever were presented (Liebig T. et al. unpublished). A clinical case in which partial deployment of an Enterprise stent resulted in immediate recanalization of an occluded MCA that was refractory to IV and IA rtPA, IA abciximab, and mechanical manipulation, confirmed this therapeutic concept (Hussain M. S. 2010). The currently newest available device is the TrevoTM System (Concentric Medical, Mountain View, CA, USA), an innovative, easy-to-use thrombus retrieval system. The main component of the Trevo System is a stentrieverTM, a new generation of retrieval devices which is able to restore flow in the occluded brain territory and remove the clot under aspiration with the guiding catheter. The first 24 cases, recently been performed in Europe, showed promising results (Liebig T. et al. unpublished). The alternative reperfusion strategies use the collateral vasculature of the brain as well as retrograde and reversed flow. Retrograde reperfusion and flow reversal are experimental treatment techniques that cause total reversal of the cerebral circulation and perfusion of the venous system with arterial blood into the capillary bed, which is then physiologically proximal to the occluded artery.

Flow Augmentation

Global reperfusion or flow augmentation tries to increase cerebral blood flow (CBF) to perfuse the brain tissue distal to the occlusive thrombus via leptomeningeal collaterals. This retrograde reperfusion strategy may potentially lead to better recanalization rates when used as an adjunct to antegrade reperfusion treatments. The increase in CBF should result in the better delivery of thrombolytic drugs to the occlusion site, theoretically leading to better recanalization with systemic thrombolysis. Flow augmentation can be achieved mechanically with the NeuroFlo device (CoAxia, Maple Grove, MN, USA). The NeuroFlo device is a dual balloon catheter designed for partial occlusion of the aorta above and below the origin of the renal arteries. It is intended to increase blood flow to the brain and thus potentially reduce the damage caused by stroke. The recently completed SENTIS Phase III trial (Safety and

Efficacy of NeuroFlo Technology in Ischemic Stroke) assesses the safety and efficacy of the NeuroFloTM catheter for use in patients with ischemic stroke. The results are not yet published. Another ongoing 'Study to Evaluate the Effects of the Neuroflo Device in People Who Have Had a Stroke' investigates the feasibility and safety of the NeuroFloTM in patients with persistent arterial occlusion after attempted thrombectomy with the Merci1 Retriever System. Delayed symptomatic reocclusion after initial endovascular stroke therapy can lead to sudden clinical deterioration and has been linked to poor clinical outcomes (Hussain M. S. 2010). The rate of reocclusion after endovascular treatments is 18% (Janjua N. 2008). This may be underestimated as many patients present with large clinical deficits at time of presentation and explain the low rate of good clinical outcome despite of a high rate of revascularization.

Reperfusion Therapies

The advantages of pharmacological thrombolysis over mechanical means are: The drugs are easier to administer and – 'Time is Brain': they can be started faster. Future newer generation lytics and platelet inhibitors may be even faster, effective and specific. The disadvantages are that often no success can be achieved, and although the therapy can be initiated quickly, the effect occurs slowly and the risk of local and systemic hemorrhagic complications is evident. The major disadvantages of an invasive procedure are additional risks and high costs compared with IV rtPA that are weighted against achieving higher reperfusion rates. The current approach to acute endovascular stroke therapy is the use of mechanical clot-retrievers in combination with pharmacological agents. Future trials will address that and explore combined treatment strategies with neuroprotectants, antithrombotics, and supplementary mechanical strategies.

Thrombolytic Agents

The critical time period during which this volume of brain tissue is at risk is referred to as the "window of opportunity". At present, intravenous administration of tissue plasminogen activator (t-PA) within 3 h of symptom onset is the only US FDA-approved treatment available to re-establish cerebral blood flow. Early reperfusion with t-PA increases recovery from stroke symptoms by ~30%, with a low rate of serious complications. This will not only rescue neuronal and glial cells within the penumbra, but also glial cells from the central ischemic core zone, thereby limiting the size of infarcted tissue (Turner R. 2007). However, despite the beneficial outcome of early reperfusion, only 3%–8.5% of eligible stroke patients receive t-PA because of the possibility of intracranial hemorrhage (Bambeur K. Z. 2006). The American Heart Association recently suggested that selected patients may benefit from t-PA up to 4.5 h after stroke, but some counter that the risk of hemorrhagic complications beyond 3 h following ischemia is significantly greater due to breakdown of the BBB (Sue E. J. 2008). In addition, the increase in cerebrovascular permeability results in diffusion of t-PA to the brain parenchyma (Yepes M. 2003), causing neurotoxicity (Gotto H. 2007). To extend treatment availability to patients with stroke and to reduce the potential for intracranial hemorrhage, intraarterial thrombolysis is a viable option for those who present for medical treatment in the 3–6 hour time window (Zaidat O. O. 2002). The strategy behind intraarterial administration is rapid local delivery of a thrombolytic agent through a microcatheter placed near the site of occlusion. This leads to improved recanalization and reduced hemorrhagic complications due to lower doses of thrombolytic agent required to resume blood flow (Rha J. H. 2007). The disadvantages include the relative complexity of the procedure, delays in initiation of treatment, required technical expertise, and the invasiveness of the procedure (Nougueira R. G. 2009). To address the above issues, particularly to compensate for the delay in receiving the treatment, a combination therapy of intravenous and intraarterial thrombolysis has been tested. The initial partial recanalization with intravenous injection of t-PA is followed by complete recanalization via direct intraarterial delivery (Lawendowski C. A. 1997).

Promising Directions and Potential Targets in Neuroprotectant Development

Despite past shortcomings in neuroprotectant development, multiple pharmacologic agents are currently under investigation in advanced phases of clinical trial development and appear promising based on early phase results. This includes Arundic Acid (ONO-2506), an astrocyte modulator, and minocycline, an inhibitor of microglia.

Modulating Astrocyte Activity

While neuroprotection research has been largely neurocentric in nature and failed to emphasize the prominent role of glia in both homeostasis and injury response, the suggestion has been made that preservation of neuronal survival and function may not be possible without significant regulation of the microenvironment by astrocytes. Astrocytes, frequently described as "housekeeping cells of the nervous system", are involved in regulating blood-brain barrier (BBB) integrity, removal of metabolic waste products, release of neural growth factors, and uptake of excess neurotransmitter release during synaptic activity. As such, astrocyte modulation represents a promising strategy for future therapeutic development for ischemic stroke (Takano T. 2009). The effect of ischemia on astrocytes is widespread in that signaling amongst astrocytes, as well as between astrocytes and neurons or microglial cells, is likely altered in addition to the potential for necrotic or apoptotic cellular death. This disrupted signaling likely has significant consequences on the control of basic physiologic functions including cerebral blood flow, glutamate uptake by astrocytes, and the ability of astrocytes to serve as an energy reserve during ischemia (Bambrick L. 2004, Carmignoto G. 2010, Rosi D. J. 2007, Zonta M. 2003). Perhaps the hallmark event involving astrocytes following neural injury, and specifically ischemia, is the development of reactive gliosis and associated morphologic changes and altered gene expression. One of the challenges in modulating astrocyte activity, and associated gliosis, for therapeutic benefit is the emerging evidence that astrocytes have both protective and detrimental roles, potentially a result of multiple astrocyte subtypes (Zamanian J. L. 2012). Recent work by Zamanian, et al. haveillustrated this concept in that ischemia appears to promote a protective astrocytic response whereas neuroinflammation induced by lipopolysaccharide (LPS) produces a potentially detrimental phenotype.

Notably, these two different stimuli each induced significantly altered gene expression yet the expression shared between stimuli was less than 50%, furthering the notion of a stimulus-specific astrocyte response or multiple astrocyte subtypes (Zamanian J. L. 2012). The influence of astrocytes on outcome following neurologic injury, and the potential for conflicting roles (beneficial or detrimental), has been seen clearly in a variety of preclinical models including ischemia, experimental autoimmune encephalitis (EAE), and spinal cord injury to name a few. In a preclinical model of ischemia, Li and colleagues demonstrated a protective role of astrocytes by knocking out glial fibrillary acidic protein (GFAP) and vimentin.

Deletion of this combination of intermediate filaments, characteristic of astrocytes, resulted in infarct volumes two to three times larger than in wild-type animals (Li L. 2008). In spinal cord injury, a dual role of astrocyte reactivity has been observed in which initially, astrocytes appear to modulate inflammation and contain inflammatory cells to the damaged region.

On the other hand, astrocytes are the primary component of the glial scar that prevents axonal re-growth in the chronic period post-injury (Okada S. 2006). In a model of demyelinating disease, experimental autoimmune encephalitis (EAE), targeted genetic removal of reactive astrocytes resulted in diminished perivascular scar formation and increased leukocyte infiltration into brain parenchyma. The exacerbated inflammatory response was associated with a detrimental outcome (Voskuhl R. R. 2009).

Despite the expanded understanding of astrocyte roles in homeostasis and disease, clear knowledge gaps remain. This includes more clear elucidation of the timing of beneficial versus detrimental responses to injury, how these responses can be pharmacologically manipulated, and how the astrocyte response is altered in association with disease comorbidities and the aging process. Our laboratory and others have begun to explore these factors with the hope of improving the understanding of neural injury in order to develop future therapeutics (Cotrina M. L. 2002, Dinapoli V. A. 2010). One potentially promising therapeutic that alters astrocyte activation, and synthesis of S-100B, that has advanced to clinical trials is (*R*)-(−)-2-propyloctanoic acid (ONO-2506). S-100B is expressed by reactive astrocytes throughout the penumbral region following ischemia and leads to nitric oxide release from the astrocyte, potentiating neuronal cell death (Teteshi N. 2002). In an early phase clinical trial, ONO-2506, also known as arundic acid, proved safe and produced a trend towards functional improvement based on the National Institutes of Health Stroke Scale (NIHSS) (Pettigrew L. C.2006).

Inhibiting Effects of Microglia

Much like astrocytes, microglial modulation may represent a promising therapeutic target for ischemic stroke based on the progression of compounds such as minocycline in clinical trials.

Microglial activation, a hallmark of the inflammatory response within the central nervous system post-stroke, has been described as both beneficial and detrimental in nature (Yenari M. A. 2010). Ablation of Mac-2 positive microglia, a marker of activated microglia, resulted in enhanced infarct volume and altered temporality of pro-inflammatory cytokine release. These changes were associated with a nearly three-fold increase in apoptotic cells and a nearly two-fold decrease in IGF-1, a neurotrophic factor, levels (Lalancetti-Hebert M. 2007). In contrast, numerous other studies have shown an improvement in outcome following ischemia by reducing microglial activation (Hayakawa K. 2008, Sakata H. 2012). This is achieved by administration of minocycline, traditionally used as an antibiotic, which has been associated with diminished Iba-1 expression, an activation marker, by microglia (Hayakawa K. 2008). Importantly, the microglial response post-stroke begins rapidly but takes hours to days to develop fully, potentially resulting in an extended window of therapeutic opportunity (Yenari M. A. 2010). The idea of an extended window, at least in comparison to that used for thrombolytic therapy, is consistent with preclinical findings in which a clinically relevant dosage of minocycline decreased infarct volume at both 4 and 5 h post-stroke while reducing functional deficits with 4 h administration (Xu L. 2004). In addition to the effects on microglia, minocycline has been shown to alter the function of other immune cells previously implicated in ischemic damage such as macrophages (Camphbel J. H. 2011). While not previously investigated specifically with regards to ischemia, the effect of minocycline on macrophages may be related to alterations in macrophage recruitment and/or macrophage polarization, a topic that is discussed at greater length in subsequent sections. The effect of minocycline on subsequent inflammatory processes is logical in that microgliosis following injury is associated with not only the acute and rapid activation of microglial cells but also the recruitment of marrow-derived inflammatory cells that migrate to the brain and penetrate the parenchyma (Lalancette-Hebert, M. 2007). The precise mechanism via which minocycline mediates protection through microglial-mediated effects remains unclear but has been shown to decrease expression of high-mobility group protein B1 (HMGB1) and *in vitro*, reduces oxidative stress via diminished superoxide release (Hayakawa K. 2008, Yenari M. A. 2006). Minocycline may also prove beneficial in other reparative therapies post-stroke, such as stem-cell delivery. Sakata and colleagues demonstrated that minocycline pre-conditioning of neural stem cells prior to transplantation resulted in production of beneficial paracrine factors and diminished graft cell death via upregulation of antioxidant genes associated with Nrf2 (Sakata H. 2012). In early phase clinical trials, minocycline has exhibited similar promise in that it has been proven safe when administered alone or in combination with thrombolytics and also exhibited potential efficacy in these small studies. Namely, NIHSS and modified Rankin Scale (mRS) scores were lower, and Barthel Index (BI) scores higher, in the group given minocycline. This improvement was seen as soon as 7 days post-stroke and persisted at day 30 of follow-up (Lampl Y. 2007). While a large efficacy trial is needed to confirm preliminary findings, minocycline appears promising for the treatment of ischemic stroke (Fagan S. C. 2011). Notably, clinical studies have also shown that minocycline administration results in diminished levels of matrix metalloproteinase-9 (MMP-9) (Switzer J. A. 2011). Preclinical studies have shown a reduction in blood-brain barrier (BBB) permeability following minocycline administration and due to previous associations between BBB permeability and MMP-9 activity, it would appear that these clinical findings indicate a potential effect of minocycline on restoration or maintenance of BBB integrity (Yenari MA 2006, Switzer JA 2011).

Neuroprotective Therapies

Thrombolysis is likely an effective therapeutic modality because it helps restore blood flow and improve cellular metabolism in ischemic regions not yet irreversibly injured. However, thrombolysis is not targeted at the cellular consequences of ischemia. Therefore, it is essential to add a component that would act as a neuroprotective or prevent the damage caused by reperfusion injury. In fact, the Stroke Progress Review Group, which is charged with assisting the National Institute of Neurological Disorders and Stroke (NINDS) in addressing the Institute's Stroke Research Program, has recommended research on combinations of neuroprotectants or neuroprotectants plus reperfusion therapy. Addition of neuroprotectants would protect neurons, which are susceptible to apoptosis, and could minimize the damage due to reperfusion injury.

Modulating the Blood-Brain Barrier (BBB)

As focus has gradually shifted from solely the neuron to include glial cells and the associated neurovascular unit, the role of the blood-brain barrier in ischemic injury has received renewed interest. Much of the work involving BBB permeability has focused on potential mechanisms of degradation, such as matrix metalloproteinases, creating a natural target for pharmacologic agents (Lee S. R. 2004a, Lee S. R. 2004b, Lo E. H. 2002, Rossel A. 2008, Zhao B. Q. 2006). In work by Pfefferkorn and colleagues, the authors showed the ability to reduce BBB disruption and improve survival following delayed tPA administration by using BB-94, a matrix metalloproteinase inhibitor (Pfefferkorn, T. 2003). In more recent work using a model of traumatic brain injury, a similar phenomenon was shown using Kollidon VA64, a pharmacological agent described as resealing membranes. Improving membrane integrity resulted in diminished neural injury and improved functional outcome (Mbye L. H. 2012). It is clear that more investigation is required to understand not only the role of BBB permeability in disease but also how to target BBB permeability therapeutically, but studies such as those described herein provide a potential proof-of-concept and perhaps most importantly, further indicate the need for a comprehensive approach to ischemic stroke therapeutic development.

Targeting Inflammation

As demonstrated by the early phase success of agents currently under investigation, such as minocycline and arundic acid, targeting inflammation may offer promise in the quest for identification of neuroprotective compounds. Inflammation offers many opportunities and targets for modulation, many of which persist for hours to days, sometimes even longer, following injury. Consequently, these targeted therapeutics are more likely to be administered within the window of opportunity for a given pathologic process compared to some of the previously tested agents that target events occurring almost immediately post-stroke. Inflammation, while generally thought of in a negative connotation, is an essential component of recovery and repair-associated processes as well, further complicating experimental investigations. In this work, we focus on the dual responses associated with inflammation, particularly with regards to macrophage polarization, an emerging topic in both the inflammation and neuroscience literature.

Inflammation: A Deleterious Event or a Beneficial Response?

The inflammatory process is further complicated due to the fact that various elements can serve a deleterious or a beneficial role in the injury and recovery process, as highlighted earlier in this work with discussion of astrocytes and microglia. Another prime example of this potentially dual response to neural injury is that of macrophages. Macrophages and microglia may contribute to secondary injury processes via production of inflammatory cytokines and reactive oxygen species while also potentially reducing injury through maintenance of the cellular microenvironment by phagocytic clearance of cellular debris and apoptotic cells (David S. 2011, Popovich P. G. 2008). Emerging evidence indicates that many of these inflammatory cell types may never truly exist in a resting state and rather may almost constantly be undergoing changes in state through intermediary forms, evident by both morphologic and functional changes, in response to the cellular environment and signals from the surrounding regions (Pollazi E. 2010). This is perhaps most adequately described, and potentially targeted therapeutically, by macrophages. In the following section, we attempt to highlight some of the recent developments in the macrophage literature, particularly those related to various macrophage subsets and neural injury.

Inflammation

Several inflammatory mediators such as leukocytes, adhesion molecules, acute phase reactants, cytokines and proteases increase in the plasma of patients with cerebral ischemia. The early central inflammatory events include the production of reactive oxygen species (nitric oxide, superoxide) expression of proteolytic enzymes (MMP-9, MMP-2), vasoactive substances (prostaglandins and cyclooxygenases) and vascular adhesion molecules (ICAM-1, P-selectin, L-selectin). Neutrophils and macrophages are considered early contributors to the production of ROS and cytokines, while activation of microglia and proliferation of astrocytes in the ischemic area further promotes the inflammatory response in later stages (Dennis A. 2009). Inflammatory mediators, (such as IL-1β, IL-6, TNFα, IL-10, transforming growth factor beta (TGFβ) and chemokines including MCP-1, macrophage inflammatory protein-1 (MIP-1), keratinocyte-derived chemokine/chemokine (CXC motif) ligand 1/(KC/CXCL1) and fractalkine (CX3CL1)), are also found in increased levels in brain tissue in animal models of stroke.

The expression of IL-1β mRNA is increased in the ischemic rat brain within hours after the induction of stroke (Liu T. 1993), elevated levels of IL-6 are seen in the plasma and cerebrospinal fluid (CSF) 3–6 h after experimental stroke in mice (Clark W. M. 1999), and levels of pro-inflammatory cytokines such as IL-6, IFNγ, MCP-1 become elevated in the plasma within 6 hours in rodents (Offner H. 2006).

The intercellular adhesion molecule-1 (ICAM-1) antibody, Enlimomab, can reduce the size of stroke when given within 1 hr reperfusion after transient, but not permanent ischemia, in a rat stroke model.

However, its use was associated with significant worsening in the modified Rankin scale and higher mortality at 90 days compared to placebo in a large clinical trial (Enlimomab Group 2001). Blocking neutrophil activiation by a recombinant protein inhibitor of the CD11b/CD18 receptor, UK 279,276 (Rovelizumab), within 6 hrs of stroke also failed to show any benefits in one clinical trial which was stopped prematurely. Despite promising results for interleukin (IL)-1 receptor antagonist (RA) in several animal studies, this drug has not been investigated in humans (Banwell V. 2009). FK506 also demonstrates benefits, particularly after transient ischemia, in animal studies and remains a potential target for studies in humans (Mecleod M. R. 2005).

Systemic administration of minocycline is protective in experimental models of focal (Yrjanheikki J. 1998) or global (Yrjanheikki J. 1999) cerebral ischemia. Inhibition of IL-1β converting enzyme (Harra H. 2007) or deletion of IL-1β and IL-1α results in markedly reduced ischemic damage and neuronal death in animal studies (Boutin H. 2001). Deficiency of inflammatory chemokines such as MCP-1 (Huges P. M. 2002) or fractalkine (Soriano S. G. 2002) is associated with less vulnerability to ischemic injury.

Cerebral ischemia activates an inflammatory reaction within hours of the injury. The suppression of inflammation using a variety of drugs has been shown to reduce infarct area in animal studies. Commonly used anti-inflammatory agents are aspirin and the lipid lowering statins.

A combination of aspirin and extended release dipyridamole was found to be more efficacious than aspirin alone for nonfatal stroke by the second European Stroke Prevention Study (ESPS-2) and the European/Australian Stoke Prevention in Reversible Ischemia Trial (ESPRIT) (Deb P. 2007).

In an investigation of the anti-inflammatory and neuroprotective properties of statins, the Stoke Prevention by Aggressive Reduction in Cholesterol Level study showed that treatment with high-dose atovastatin reduces the risk of stroke in patients with the first attack of stroke and no known coronary artery disease (Gedikli O. 2008). In addition to aspirin and statins, two leukocyte adhesion inhibitors, Enlimomab and LeukArrest, were studied in patients with ischemic stroke. Although Enlimomab was shown to reduce the damage in stroke models, patients who received it experienced significantly more negative effects relative to placebo controls (Cheng Y. D. 2004).

Another neuroprotective approach was explored in the "Intravenous Thrombolysis Plus Hypothermia for Acute Treatment of Ischemic Stroke (ICTuS-L)" study of the effects of induced hypothermia and thrombolysis after acute ischemic stroke. Hypothermia is thought to serve a neuroprotective role in stroke via inhibition of the MIP-3α-CCR6 inflammatory pathway (Shintani Y. 2011).

Although hypothermia has been shown to confer some protection against damage in cardiac arrest and neonatal hypoxic-ischemic encephalopathy patients (Lundby J. B. 2011, Jacobs S. E. 2011), its effectiveness in acute ischemic stroke has not been definitively demonstrated. Negative consequences, including pneumonia, were seen more frequently in patients who had undergone hypothermia treatment, compared to controls in this study.

Disappointingly, there was no significant benefit in mRS between the two trial groups (Hemmen T. M. 2010).

Excitotoxicity and NMDA Glutamate Receptors

Excessive NMDA (N-methyl D-aspartate) receptor activation has been implicated in the pathophysiology of several neurodegenerative diseases and in stroke. Excitotoxicity has been a widely investigated area in stroke. Ischemic neuronal injury in vitro is dependent on synaptic release of excitatory amino acids and resultant elevation of intracellular free calcium. Even transient exposure to excess excitatory amino acids (EAAs) is toxic to cultured neurons, and alterations in neuronal energy balance increases the vulnerability of neurons to excitotoxic damage even in the presence of physiological concentrations of EAAs (Muir K. W. 1995). Evidence that this process progresses over several hours after the ischemic insult highlights a potential role for neuroprotective strategies administered during the critical window prior to irreversible loss, although the exact duration of this window in humans remains unknown. The action of glutamate on NMDA receptors seems to play an important role in glutamate-mediated toxicity. Compounds that decrease glutamate levels or interfere with its binding to this receptor have been the focus of many studies in this area (Nagai Y. 2008). NMDA antagonists, which have been investigated in stroke include Aptiganel hydrochloride (CNS 1102, Cerestat), dextrorphan and dextromethorphan. Their use was associated with side effects and no clear clinical benefit in clinical trials (Muir K. W. 1995). Phase 2 trials of both oral and IV forms of remacemide hydrochloride in stroke are currently underway. Magnesium ion, which electrophysiologically behaves as a noncompetitive NMDA antagonist, has demonstrated efficacy as a neuroprotective agent in focal and global models of cerebral ischemia. Two preliminary trials of IV magnesium show no evidence of adverse effects (Muir K. W. 1994, Wester P. 1985), and phase 3 trials are currently underway. A phase 2 trial of Selfotel (CGS 19755) in acute stroke patients, reported evidence of a dose-dependent toxicity (Clark W. 1994). Selective NMDA antagnosits such as ifenprodil and eliprodil (SL82.0715) have demonstrated preclinical neuroprotective efficacy, and eliprodil is currently being investigated in early phase 3 trials in stroke patients. Other compounds under investigation are 3-(2-carboxypiperazin-4-yl)propyl-1-phosphonic acid (CPP), its derivative d-CPPene, and CGS 19755 (Taylor C. P. 1994). Neuroprotection is evident for the presynaptic glutamate release inhibitors 619C89 and ubeluzole when administered within 6 hours of induced ischemia. Both drugs are currently in phase 2 trials in stroke. Partial glycine agonists, such as HA 966, L687414, and 1-aminocyclopropanecarboxylic acid (ACPC), or full antagonists, such as 7-chlorokynurenic acid and its derivatives or ACEA 1021, are effective in stroke models. Glutamate antagonists at other receptor subtypes, such as the AMPA receptors, are under evaluation (Muir K. W. 1995).

Mitochondrial Dysfunction

The release of multiple apoptogenic proteins from mitochondria has been identified in ischemic and post-ischemic neurons. Results from animal models strongly implicate caspase-dependent and caspase-independent apoptosis and the mitochondrial permeability transition as important contributors to tissue damage, particularly when induced by short periods of temporary focal ischemia (Sims N. R. 2009). Prophylactic administration of oral creatine reduces the size of ischemic brain infarctions in mice. The anti-oxidant Szeto-Schiller peptide (SS-31) plays an important role in modulating ROS-induced mitochondrial permeability transition and cell death, and has been found to be protective in several in vitro and in vivo models of ischemia and reperfusion injury. Synthetic triterpenoids (TP) are analogues of oleanolic acid, which exert anti- oxidative effects through stimulation of the antioxidant response element (ARE)–Nrf2–Keap1 signaling pathway, and have been shown to be protective in a rat model of cerebral ischemia (Chatturvedi R. K. 2008).

Anti-apoptotic Agents

Caspase is a group of cysteine proteases that induce apoptotic cascade when activated. Inhibition of caspase activity has been shown to reduce the size of infarction in rodent stoke models (Cheng Y. 1998, Endres M. 1998). However, none of the caspase inhibitors have yet been tested in clinical trials. A 2009 study on the efficacy of erythropoietin as a neuroprotectant yielded negative effects and safety concerns after it was shown that not only did erythropoietin not confer a neuroprotective benefit, but erythropoietin in combination with the current standard of care, rt-PA, increased the risk of death, intracerebral hemorrhage, brain edema, and thromboembolic events (Ehrenreich H. 2009). Thus, future studies should evaluate the effect of putative therapeutic agents in conjunction with the use of rt-PA where appropriate. These studies demonstrate some of the challenges faced in seeking neuroprotective agents to reduce the initial damage wrought by ischemic stroke.

In general, anti-apoptotic mechanisms being evaluated in neuroprotection include strategies to prevent caspase-dependent apoptosis (e.g., caspase inhibitors) or strategies to prevent caspase-independent apoptosis (e.g., PARP inhibitors). Both caspase-dependent and caspase-independent mechanisms of cell death are implicated in focal cerebral ischemia. Increased expression of Fas and of mediators of the extrinsic caspase-dependent pathway have been shown following focal ischemia. Increased expression of caspase-1, -3, -8, and -9, and of cleaved caspase-8, has been observed in the penumbra. The role for apoptosis in ischemia is further supported by reports that the inhibition of caspase-3 reduces infarct size after transient focal ischemia (Ferrer I. 2003).

Intranuclear MMP activity facilitates oxidative injury in neurons during early ischemia through the cleavage of PARP-1 and XRCC1, and resultant disturbance of DNA repair mechanisms. Inhibition of MMP with the broad-spectrum inhibitor, BB1101, significantly attenuated ischemia-induced PARP-1 cleavage, and resultant cell death in rat model of focal cerebral ischemia (Yang Y. 2009). The p53-dependent receptor pathway also seems to be involved in stroke induced apoptosis. Injection of netrin-1, a ligand of the receptor uncoordinated gene 5H2 (UNC5H2), was associated with significantly reduced infarct volume at 3 days after focal ischemia in an animal model of stroke, through its inhibition of p53-mediated apoptosis (Wu T. W. 2008). Estrogen has also been shown to prevent Fas-mediated apoptosis in experimental models of stroke (Jia J. 2009).

Antioxidant Therapy

Excessive production of reactive oxygen species (ROS) after cerebral ischemia and reperfusion is implicated in brain damage through different cellular and molecular mechanisms, and it is further aggravated by impaired cellular antioxidant defense systems under ischemic conditions. Upon reperfusion, cells are often in a state of oxidative stress, which results in further tissue injury, known as reperfusion injury (Adibhatla 2008a and 2008b). ROS are usually scavenged by antioxidant enzymes, primarily superoxide dismutase (SOD), by catalyzing the dismutation reaction of the superoxide anion to hydrogen peroxide (H2O2).

Catalase and glutathione peroxidase, on the other hand, protect cells from the toxic effects of H2O2 by catalyzing its decomposition into water (Margail I. 2005). However, two pharmacodynamic factors impede the straightforward use of native forms of antioxidant enzymes in cerebral ischemia. First, their molecular weight is well below the renal glomerular filtration cutoff, resulting in their rapid clearance from systemic circulation (e.g., t1/2 of SOD in rats = 4–8 min, catalase = 8–10 min). Second, they are negatively charged at physiologic pH and therefore do not readily cross cell membranes (Francis J. W. 1997). Transient disruption of BBB permeability might permit some access of exogenous enzymes to ischemic neuronal tissue, but they do not permeate cells; neurons and astrocytes do not appear to take up the native enzyme under normal conditions, and hence cannot neutralize ROS formed intracellularly (Schaller B. 2004). Because of these challenges, animal studies have shown no improvement in cerebral blood flow or neurological recovery with SOD or SOD with catalase (Forsmann M. 1998, Schurer L. 1990).

Different alternatives have been investigated to address these issues: for instance, PEGylation and lecithinization to improve the circulation half-life (Tsubokawa T. 2007) and fusion of enzymes, e.g., SOD, with cell membrane-penetrating peptides like transactivator of transcription (TAT) of human immunodeficiency virus or tetanus toxin fragment to increase its ability to cross the BBB (Kim D. W. 2005). However, there are limitations to these modifications. For example, PEGylated SOD (PEG-SOD) increases the enzyme's stability in circulation from 6 min to 36 h, but it limits the permeability of SOD across cerebral cell membranes and its ability to be taken up by neuronal cells (Veronesse F. M. 2002). Similarly, fusion of different cell-penetrating or cell-specific peptides to target proteins requires a crosslinker via a chemical process that could cause denaturation and loss of activity of the target protein (Morris M. C. 2001).

There is also a concern regarding the possible immune-mediated anaphylactic responses to hybrid proteins given to patients (Francis J. W. 1997). Intravenous delivery of SOD loaded into liposomes has shown partial inhibition of infarct volume, but the instability of liposomes *in vivo* (half-life ~4.2 h) limits the duration of SOD activity and efficacy (Imazumi S. 1990, Sinha J. 2008). Our approach uses biocompatible, biodegradable nanoparticles (NPs) loaded with superoxide dismutase (SOD-NPs) with the aim to reduce the damaging effect of ROS. These NPs are formulated using poly dl-lactide *co*-glycolide (PLGA) with antioxidant enzymes encapsulated. The enzyme encapsulated in NPs is released in active form. Our initial studies demonstrated the neuroprotective effect of SOD-NPs in oxidative stress-challenged human neural cells, whereas SOD in solution and PEG-SOD were ineffective. The mechanism of protective efficacy of SOD- NPs appears to be due to sustained bioavailability of antioxidants and intracellular delivery of antioxidant enzymes (Reddy M. K. 2008). In our first *in vivo* ischemic middle cerebral arterial occlusion rat stroke model (Reddy M. K. 2009), we determined that the most efficient method of delivery of NPs is via intracarotid artery injection. The study with dye-loaded NPs demonstrated NP localization primarily to the cortex and striatal regions of the ischemic hemisphere, but not to the nonischemic hemisphere.

Our results demonstrated that over 75% of SOD-NP-treated animals showed increased survival and neurological recovery over a time period of 28 days. In addition, a reduction in breakdown of the blood-brain barrier in treatment animals was evidenced by significantly decreased Evans blue leakage in the brain. These results have driven further research into the neuroprotective effects of SOD-NPs, as well as investigation into how we can further abrogate the negative effects of ROS production in ischemic stroke.

The protective effect of SOD-NPs could be due to the direct antioxidant effect of the active enzyme released from the NPs localized in the brain. It is possible that SOD-NPs prevented the cascade of events or acted on several stages in the pathophysiology of reperfusion injury. Breakdown of the BBB is an early event arising from free-radical damage, especially from superoxide radicals generated in endothelial cells during ischemia and reperfusion (Rosenberg G. A. 2007). SOD-NPs localized in the lining of the cerebral vasculature protected the BBB from free-radical injury, which then could have prevented the leukocyte adhesion that otherwise is a common event following reperfusion as well as prevented edema formation (Kuroda S. 1997).

We are investigating further to understand the mechanism of recovery of animals with time. It is quite possible that the conducive conditions created in the brain as a result of the sustained free-radical scavenging effect of SOD released from NPs localized in the brain (Yasui K. 2006) could have played a role in facilitating the process of angiogenesis and neurogenesis in the infarcted brain. Recently, we began working on developing a thromboembolic rat stoke model to mimic the clinical scenario (Zhang Z. 1997). We are now testing how SOD-NPs and catalase-loaded NPs, or combination of these formulations, would perform in the presence of t-PA and whether we can extend the window of t-PA treatment with effective antioxidant delivery.

Therapeutic strategies based on exogenous delivery of the native form of superoxide dismutase (SOD), a free radical scavenger, are limited because of its short half-life (~6 min) *in vivo* and poor permeability across the blood-brain-barrier (BBB). We encapsulated SOD in biodegradable poly(D,L-lactide *co*-glycolide) nanoparticles (SOD-NPs) and tested their efficacy in a rat focal cerebral ischemia-reperfusion injury model. We hypothesized that localized brain delivery of SOD-NPs would sustain the protective effect of SOD by neutralizing the deleterious effects of ROS formed following ischemia-reperfusion. SOD-NPs were administered at the time of reperfusion *via* the intracarotid route to maximize their localization in the brain. Animals receiving SOD-NPs (10,000 U of SOD/kg) demonstrated a 65% reduction in infarct volume, whereas an equivalent dose of SOD in solution (SOD-Sol) increased it by 25% over saline control ($P<0.001$; data at 6 h following reperfusion). Control NPs alone or mixed with SOD-Sol were ineffective in reducing infract volume, with results similar to saline control, indicating the protective effect of the encapsulated enzyme. SOD-NPs maintained BBB integrity, thereby preventing edema, reduced the level of ROS formed following reperfusion, and protected neurons from undergoing apoptosis. Animals treated with SOD-NPs demonstrated greater survival than those with saline control (75% *vs.* 0% at

28 days) and later regained most vital neurological functions. SOD-NPs may be an effective treatment option in conjunction with a thrombolytic agent for stroke patients.—Reddy, M. K., Labhasetwar, V. Nanoparticle-mediated delivery of superoxide dismutase to the brain: an effective strategy to reduce ischemia-reperfusion injury.

Glutamate antagonists

Radical scavengers (such as vitamin E, sulfhydryl compounds and nitrone spin traps), agents that promote detoxification of ROS (superoxide dismutase, catalase or peroxidase conjugates), and agents that prevent radical generation (e.g., the xanthine oxidase inhibitor allopurinol, nitric oxide synthase inhibitors, or nonsteroidal anti-inflammatory agents and cyclooxygenase-inhibitors) have been studied in stroke. The use of NXY-059 has been associated with clinical benefits in animal models of stroke, and was associated with a significant improvement in the modified Rankin functional scale in the Stroke-Acute Ischemic NXY Treatment-I (SAINT-I) (Lees K. R. 2006). However, these results were not reproduced in the expanded SAINT-II trial (Feuerstein G. Z. 2008, Shuaib A. 2007). Ebselen and the radical scavenger edaravone (MCI- 186, Radicut) were associated with clinical improvement in a small trials (Green A. R. 2005).

Glutamate antagonists are the most studied neuroprotective agents. As mentioned earlier, glutamate is one of the excitatory CNS neurotransmitters and is released excessively during ischemia (Guyot L. L. 2001). Several receptors relevant to neuroprotection, such as NMDA, AMPA, KA, and metabotropic receptors, are activated by glutamate. Since the activation of most of these receptors is associated with calcium influx leading to cell damage, both glutamate receptor antagonism and calcium channel blockers might serve a neuroprotective role. Although glutamate receptor antagonists have shown excellent neuroprotective effects in animal studies, these effects have not been validated in clinical studies. As a result, studies of several NMDA antagonists- Selfotel (CGS19755) (Boast C. A. 1988), Eliprodil (Gotti B. 1988) and Aptiganel (Cerestat, CNS 1102) (Aranowski J. 1994)- have been halted. Calcium channel blockers such as Nimodipine (Horn J. 2000) and Flunarizine also showed no significant benefit versus placebo in clinical trials. Despite these failures and various side effects at both the psychiatric and cardiovascular levels, the possibility of a role for glutamate receptor antagonists in neuroprotection still exists. A phase III trial with YM872, an AMPA receptor antagonist, is ongoing, and seeks to determine its potential efficacy in combination with *t*-PA thrombolysis. No clinical trials with metabotropic glutamate receptor antagonists have been conducted. It was recently reported that SP-8203, an NMDA antagonist, has dual effects that protect cells against excitotoxicity and improve memory in brain ischemic injuries (Noh S. J. 2011), suggesting a potential therapeutic role of SP-8203 in cerebral ischemic injuries. The main cause of failure of many approaches in clinical studies is inadequate dosing and timing of therapeutics, particularly an unrealistic time window derived from animal models that cannot be duplicated in humans (Leker R. R. 2002). The reasons for the failure of the most promising drug in a clinical study (NXY-059 in the SAINT II trial) are that the drug was not given to most patients within a 4- to 6-h time window as was used in animal studies and its inadequate drug levels in the brain (Feur Stein G. Z. 2008). One phase III trial, the FAST-MAG study, which aims to determine the safety of magnesium sulfate when administered acutely in the first minutes after stroke onset, addresses these issues by arming paramedics with tools to obtain consent and administer the experimental therapy within a hyperacute therapeutic window (Saver J. L. 2004). A pilot study for this trial found significantly improved modified Rankin scores (mRS) at day 90 for trial patients, and the study design has contributed a novel experimental strategy that could benefit other researchers in translating pre-clinical study results to field applications. Recognizing the benefits of pre-hospital neuroprotective agent administration, the Stroke Treatment Academic Industry Roundtable (STAIR) meeting sets recommendations for priorities in stroke research, noting that the hyperacute treatment window could potentiate other interventions and increase the time window for other time-sensitive interventions (Albers G. W. 2011).

Ion Channel Modulators

As previously discussed, the influx of calcium, sodium and of potassium during the ischemic cascade leads to brain tissue damage (Ohta K. 2001). Therefore, ion channel modulators might have a neuroprotective role. Nimodipine, a calcium channel blocker that dilates intracranial blood vessels and improves the regional blood flow in the margins of the brain infarct, did not show any benefit in clinical trials. Similarly, Fosphenytoin, the sodium channel blocker, was shown to decrease the amplitude of sodium-dependent action potentials and to block voltage- dependent calcium entry into synaptosomes. Again, phase III clinical trials were terminated due to the lack of demonstrated benefit. The potassium channel activator Maxipost also failed at phase III clinical trials, even though it was expected to protect neurons by inducing neuronal hyperpolarization and decreasing the release of excitatory amino acids (Gribkoff V. K. 2001).

Repair and Recovery Strategies of Stroke: Trophic Factors and Cell-Based Therapies

No matter how successful acute neuroprotective strategies become, many stroke patients may still fall outside of clinical time windows for effective treatment. Hence, approaches that promote repair and recovery will be essential for an integrated stroke armamentarium. Logically, these approaches can be divided into two categories—pharmacologic or trophic factor treatments that seek to amplify and augment endogenous processes of neurovascular plasticity and recovery and cell based therapies that seek to replace damaged or lost brain cells.

Many approaches that augment endogenous recovery have been explored. Growth factors such as NGF, FGF, GDNF, and BDNF have all met with variable degrees of success in animal models (Semkova and Krieglstein, 1999). But a limiting factor in many of these studies is their relatively large molecular weight, making transport into brain difficult. Some alternatives may yet exist, such as smaller peptides, transnasal delivery of growth factors to bypass the blood-brain barrier (Fletcher et al., 2009), peptidomimetics and compounds that can upregulate endogenous trophic factor production but do not require direct infusion into brain (Zhang and Chopp, 2009).

Additionally, one may also target inhibitory molecules that accumulate in the area surrounding the injury and block neuronal repair, such as chondroitin sulfate proteoglycans, myelin associated proteins, NOGO, and semaphorins (Silver and Miller, 2004). Although stroke-damaged brain usually exhibits varying degrees of spontaneous recovery, there will always be significant areas where endogenous repair is insufficient. In this regard, cell-based therapies may represent a new frontier.

To date, a variety of cell sources have been tested, including neural stem cells, bone-marrow-derived mesenchymal cells, as well endothelial progenitor cells (Koch et al., 2009). Treatments have typically involved direct transplantations into brain parenchyma, catheter infusions into cerebral ventricles, as well as systemic injections into circulating blood. The latter approach is especially intriguing, as complex mechanisms of cell targeting seem to be operational in brain. Infarcted brain tissue upregulates and releases various chemokines, such as SDF-1, to establish gradients that broadly serve to attract stem and precursor cell populations (Madri, 2009).

Induced pluripotent stem cells may also provide an alternative cell source to embryonic stem cells (Takahashi and Yamanaka, 2006). One advantage is the theoretical possibility that cell repair can be custom designed to suit specific diseases or individual needs, as described in a flurry of recent studies showing that neurons can be successfully derived from pluripotent cells taken from patients with Huntington's disease, ALS, and spinal muscular atrophy (Dimos et al., 2008; Ebert et al., 2009; Park et al., 2008). Whether similar methods can be applied to stroke victims remains to be tested.

Overall, cell-based therapies in models of experimental stroke suggest that delayed repair is a viable treatment approach. But more work is needed to translate these promising results into effective stroke therapies. Many questions remain, and the precise mechanisms of cell-induced repair are still unclear. For example, do the reported benefits occur because cells are being explicitly replaced or because transplanted cells serve as a source of trophic factor production? How well do transplanted cells survive? Will adjunctive therapies to decrease apoptotic dropout be necessary? If cells survive, how well do they integrate into existing neural or vascular networks? What is the optimum timing for such therapy? What types of cells should be used?

And finally, what subtypes of stroke patients should be selected for robust clinical trial results? As the basic mechanisms of trophic and cell-based repair continue to be defined, an interesting underlying theme has emerged that links the survival of newborn or transplanted cells to the host environment. As discussed in the previous sections, activated vascular cells and microglia may be detrimental to cell survival in the early stages of cerebral ischemia, due to production of cytokines, ROS, and toxic amount of NO. In the recovery phase, however, chronically activated microglia may now secrete beneficial factors such as BDNF and GDNF. Hence, prolonged inflammation can serve biphasic roles—dampening cellular recovery acutely but then enhancing tissue repair later on.

In fact, this principle of biphasic mediators may be broadly applicable in stroke pathophysiology. There are many examples. Overactivation of NMDA receptors induces acute excitotoxicity (Besancon et al., 2008), but without NMDA signaling, chronic neuronal remodeling cannot take place (Young et al., 1999). Matrix metalloproteinases degrade and damage neurovascular substrates in the acute phase (Rosenberg, 2009), but the same proteases are critically important for neurovascular remodeling during the recovery phase (Zhao et al., 2006; Lee et al., 2006).

The intracellular mediator HMGB1 promotes necrosis and expands the core infarct during acute cerebral ischemia (Qiu et al., 2008), but during the repair phase, HMGB1 release from reactive astrocytes promotes angiogenesis and synaptic plasticity (Hayakawa et al., 2010a, 2010b) Altogether, the boundaries between cell death and cell repair may be blurred (Lo, 2008b). Future studies that dissect these biphasic mechanisms should prove fruitful if we are to develop clinically meaningful strategies for both neurovascular protection as well as repair.

Macrophage Polarization as Therapeutic Tool

Macrophages have long been recognized as a key element in the inflammatory response, particularly in reference to the invasion of the body by foreign material such as bacteria. Besides their role as immune effector cells, macrophages are perhaps most important for normal homeostatic processes such as cellular turnover and clearance of cellular debris, hence the description of macrophages as the "janitorial" cell of the body. For example, macrophages are intimately involved in the clearance of over 200 billion erythrocytes each day as well as clearance of apoptotic cells. Consequently, macrophages respond to both endogenous stimuli produced through injury as well as to foreign cell types (Mosser D. M. 2008). As such, work in both the nervous system as well as other body systems indicates that macrophages can be shifted to either a pro-inflammatory or anti-inflammatory state depending on disease states and environmental cues.

Gaining a better understanding of the processes mediating this phenotypic shift may lead to therapeutic advances (David S. 2011). Perhaps the greatest challenge in this process is the complexity of elucidating these mechanisms *in vivo*. *In vitro* studies allow for rapid stimulation of inflammatory cells with antigens or cytokines but this response often does not translate to *in vivo* work, or is at the very least, often modified in a significant way (Morray P. J. 2011).

M1 versus M2: Classical Versus Alternative Activation

Literature focusing on macrophage polarization and subtypes has followed a similar path to that of T-cell literature and, consequently, macrophages have largely been classified as M1 or M2, a description that persists despite evidence showing greater complexity, particularly amongst the M2 population (Figure 1) (Mosser D. M. 2011). In spite of the potential for additional subtypes, we use the conventional M1 and M2 descriptions for organizational purpose but do explore the potential for various M2 subtypes within this work.

Classically Activated Macrophages (M1)

Classical macrophage activation refers to those designated as effector cells as part of cell-mediated immune responses. In the past, classical activation occurred in response to two primary signals—interferon gamma (IFNγ) and tumor necrosis factor (TNF) (Mosser D. M. 2008). This results in increased secretion of pro-inflammatory cytokines and mediators such as IL-12, IL-23, IL-1β, TNF-α, reactive oxygen species (ROS), and nitrosylated species (NS), ultimately producing increased microbicidal or tumoricidal capability (David S. 2011). While emerging evidence indicates that other signals may also induce an M1 response, such as certain toll-like receptor (TLR) agonists, the idea remains the same in that M1 macrophages, while vital for host defense, must be carefully regulated due to the possibility of host-tissue damage with unchecked activation. Persistent inflammation and the associated host-tissue damage is a hallmark of numerous autoimmune diseases such as rheumatoid arthritis and inflammatory bowel disease, demonstrating the need for regulation and strict control of activation processes (Mosser D. M. 2007).

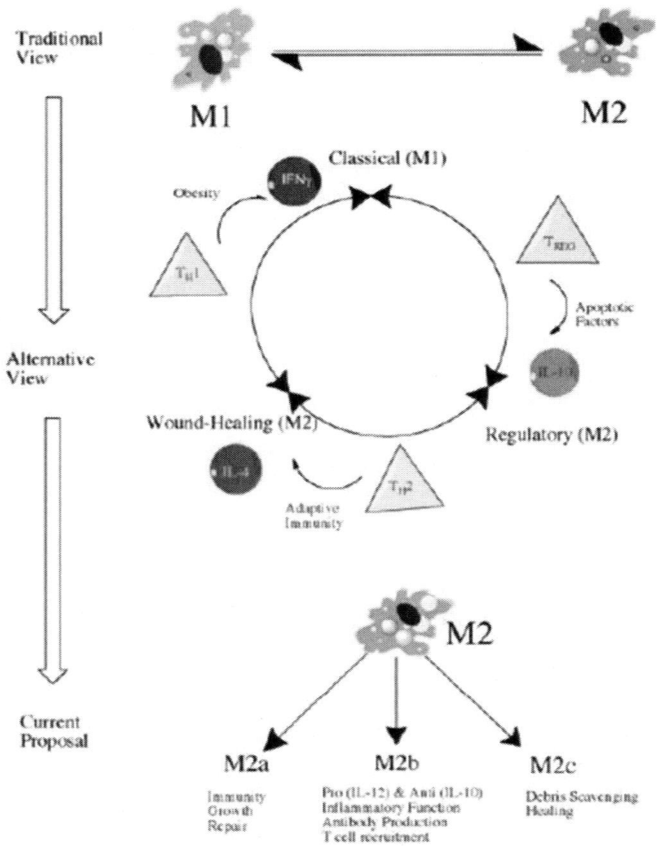

Figure 4.4. *Macrophage polarization*: Classical M1 vs Alternative M2: Evolution of views of macrophage polarization from the more simplistic M1 or M2 characterization without subtypes to the alternative or developing view with the M2 population divided into "wound-healing" and "regulatory" subtypes. Even more current proposals identify three populations of M2-related macrophages involved in a range of functions.

Alternatively Activated Macrophages (M2)

Alternative macrophage activation, similar to classical macrophage activation, can occur in response to both innate and adaptive signals (Mosser D. M. 2007). The primary signaling molecule responsible for activation is interleukin-4 (IL-4), a cytokine released upon initial tissue injury as well as upon initiation of the adaptive immune response.

Alternatively activated macrophages are largely described as beneficial, particularly when it comes to wound healing. Specifically, alternative macrophage activation is responsible for production of extracellular matrix, a property essential in the reparative response. Alternatively activated macrophages are also associated with a reduced expression of pro-inflammatory cytokines, namely TNFa, IL-1b, IL-2, IL-8, IL-12, and CXCL10 (David S. 2011). The response of IL-4 stimulated alternatively activated macrophages is much more characteristic of a TH2-mediated response in comparison to the classical macrophage activation which more closely parallels that of a TH1 response. Despite the previous characterization of alternatively activated macrophages as a distinct cellular population, emerging evidence indicates the presence of further subtypes under the M2 umbrella and that they are involved in a variety of functions ranging from wound-healing to regulatory functions. In fact, some have described M2 macrophages as actually three distinct subtypes—M2a, M2b, and M2c, each of which is generated through a unique polarization process and performs distinct functions (Figure 4.4) (David S. 2011). M2a and M2c have been attributed clear anti-inflammatory and reparative roles, whereas M2b are somewhat unique in that they produce high amounts of IL-10, an anti-inflammatory cytokine, but low-levels of IL-12, a pro-inflammatory cytokine. Similarly, M2b macrophages may produce TNF□, IL-1β, and IL-6, indicating a more complex role in the inflammatory response than previously recognized (David S. 2011).

Neuronal Rescue

Another critical issue in stroke therapy is how to recover areas of infarcted brain that appear irreversibly damaged due to ischemia. To address this issue, research is now focused on understanding neurogenesis, particularly endogenous repair mechanisms such as the involvement of neuronal progenitor cells and their proliferation and differentiation into neural cells (Wiltrout C. 2007). However, use of a small population of endogenous neuronal progenitor cells and their limited capacity to regenerate under inflammatory conditions may not be enough to achieve significant neurological recovery. Therefore, several growth factors (e.g., epidermal, fibroblast, and vascular endothelial growth factors, erythropoietin) have been tested to increase proliferation and migration of progenitor cells. The major challenge seems to be inducing sufficient proliferation to repair the devastating neuronal damage following ischemia, promoting survival of the newly formed cells in the hostile environment, and more importantly, inducing proper connectivity of the newly formed cells with the existing circuitry (Wiltrout C. 2007). An alternative approach is the transplantation of stem cells, but a number of factors could influence the success of this approach, the main one being the survival of the transplanted cells and the likelihood of their proper differentiation into neuronal cells (Kennea N. L. 2002, Roitberg B. 2004).

Future Directions: Therapeutic Targeting of Macrophage Subsets

Therapeutically, it is clear that shifting from the pro-inflammatory macrophage phenotype, M1, to the anti-inflammatory phenotype, M2, may confer an advantage in both initial injury and long-term recovery. How precisely to alter the phenotype and at what time post-injury is not clear but the idea is promising, particularly considering that recent studies have demonstrated that macrophage subsets may not be truly distinct entities and rather may undergo switching. This idea has been demonstrated *in vitro* in which activating macrophages with LPS resulted in diminished reactivity to subsequent pro-inflammatory stimuli (Lawerence 2011). In contrast, these macrophages maintained the ability to express other genes associated with anti-inflammatory activities such as IL-10. The ability to diminish responsiveness to pro-inflammatory stimuli while maintaining the anti-inflammatory capabilities is referred to as endotoxic tolerance and is generally associated with a switch from the M1 to M2 phenotype (Lawerence 2011). While inflammation is clearly a promising therapeutic target, our understanding of inflammatory processes and when precisely each event occurs remains somewhat unclear and likely varies across individuals. As such, a need exists for not only improved measurement and insight into inflammatory processes but also a personalized approach, a common theme discussed throughout medical research in recent years. One method for potentially achieving both these goals is the use of blood-based or CSF-based biomarkers.

Moving Forward: Charting a Course toward New Stroke Therapies

Tremendous progress has been made in the understanding of fundamental mechanisms of neuronal cell death. However, the translation of these powerful molecular and cellular principles into clinically effective neuroprotective therapies in stroke has been challenging. More recently, emerging data from both experimental and clinical studies now suggest that all cell types in the brain participate in the complex pathophysiology of brain injury following stroke. Consequently, therapeutic approaches should target multiple cell types in an attempt to protect their structural and functional integrity and their reciprocal interactions. Protecting the Neurovascular Unit The so-called ''neurovascular unit'' provides a conceptual framework that integrates responses in all cell types, including neuronal, glial, and vascular elements (del Zoppo, 2009; Iadecola, 2004; Zacchigna et al., 2008) (Figure 4.5). Cell-cell interactions in the neurovascular unit form the basis of brain function. Dysfunctional signaling in the neurovascular unit underlies the basis for disease. Whereas the intricate molecular pathways of cell death in the neuron have been dissected in detail, the mechanisms of how the entire neurovascular unit responds to stroke are not completely understood. As discussed in the previous sections, cerebral ischemia can rapidly induce perturbations in cell-cell signaling and function within the neurovascular unit. How each cell type succumbs or adapts to injury is dependent on responses in other cells. For example, genomic and proteomic responses in neurons subjected to metabolic stress have been fairly well described. But how each cell type might alter its response to vascular risk factors and ischemia in the context of other elements in the neurovascular unit remains to be elucidated. As the nexus of cell-cell interactions grows, a systems biology approach may eventually be required to rigorously define mechanisms as well as targets for complete neurovascular protection. The importance of cell-cell signaling in the neurovascular unit has been underscored by many studies (Arai and Lo, 2009a, 2009b; Dugas et al., 2008; Eroglu et al., 2009; Guo et al., 2008). Hence, under normal conditions, trophic coupling within the neurovascular unit helps maintain homeostasis. In contrast, under diseased conditions, it is likely that loss of coupling would lead to the pathophysiology (Grammas et al., 1999; Nagai et al., 2007). Loss of trophic coupling is also likely to play a role in the way vascular risk factors render neurons and glia more vulnerable, such as in the link between leukoaraiosis and brain dysfunction underlying cognitive impairment. Recently, BDNF has been implicated as a candidate factor that mediates trophic coupling between vascular and neuronal compartments (Arai and Lo, 2009b; Guo et al., 2008). So far as BDNF polymorphisms have been implicated in modulating synaptic plasticity (Kleim et al., 2006), these neurovascular trophic signals may also influence the mechanisms of recovery after stroke.

The concept of the neurovascular unit may provide an integrated framework for investigating mechanisms and therapies. Salvaging neurons alone may not be sufficient. One has to protect glial and vascular elements as well. Future investigations might be better served by pursuing targets that are expressed on multiple cell types in brain. Furthermore, prevention of cell death alone may also not be sufficient. In order for therapies to be clinically meaningful, cellular function must be preserved and/or restored.

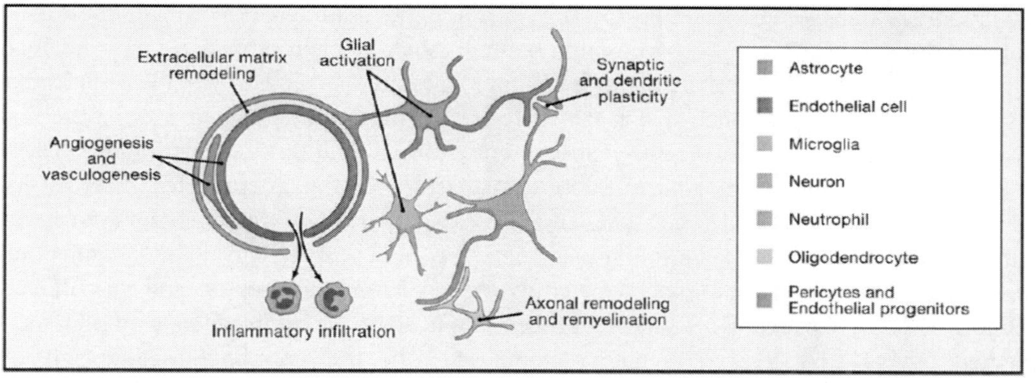

Figure 4.5. *Remodeling the Neurovascular Unit*: This schematic depicts a cerebral blood vessel and surrounding brain parenchyma that comprise the neurovascular unit. The neurovascular unit encompasses cell-cell and cell-matrix interactions between component vascular, glial, and neuronal cells. Homeostatic signaling in the neurovascular unit sustains normal brain function. Dysfunctional neurovascular signaling mediates injury after stroke. During the recovery phase after stroke, neurovascular signalingmay also be critically important with repair mechanisms that may involve angiogenesis, vasculogenesis, and endothelial precursor mechanisms. As the blood-brain barrier heals, inflammation may convert from a deleterious to beneficial role. Reactive glia (astrocytes, microglia, pericytes) may secrete trophic factors. Synaptic and dendritic plasticity as well as axonal remyelination may provide parenchymal substrates for functional recovery. Emerging data now suggest that these phenomenon do not occur in isolation. All components of the neurovascular unit are likely to remodel coordinately (Arai et al., 2009; Murphy and Corbett, 2009; Zhang and Chopp, 2009).

Neurons that are alive but lack proper connectivity or do not express the correct array of transmitter release-reuptake and synaptic activity may not be functional.

Astrocytes that survive, but cannot provide hemodynamic coupling would be unable to link neuronal activation with the required vascular responses. Oligodendrocytes that are respiring but metabolically impaired might not provide the necessary myelination for axonal conduction. Endothelial cells that survive but do not maintain blood-brain barrier properties would facilitate damage to adjacent parenchyma. Ultimately, any stroke therapy must include both prevention of cell death as well as rescue of integrated neurovascular function. Ischemic tolerance and postischemic hypothermia are some of the most potent protective strategies for ischemic brain injury and represent examples of multimodal therapies targeting the neurovascular unit as a whole. These are described in the next sections.

How Does the Brain Protect Itself? Lessons from Ischemic Tolerance

Some of the very same mechanisms implicated in the tissue damaging responses after stroke can also be engaged to protect the brain after threatened injury and to induce ischemic tolerance (IT). IT is a concerted organ response to protect itself against tissue injury and has been widely studied over the past three decades in an effort to identify endogenous mechanisms of protection and to exploit them for therapeutic purposes (Obrenovitch, 2008). In its delayed form, it is induced after challenge by a subthreshold noxious stimulus, developing within 1–3 days and lasting for several additional days. Experimentally it can be induced by exposure to preconditioning stimuli such as neurotoxins (e.g., glutamate), substrate deprivation (e.g., ischemia, hypoxia), or inflammation (e.g., cytokines and immune responses) and engages mechanisms that detect, transduce, and promote a complex tissue reaction that reflects a fundamental genomic reprogramming after threatened injury (Dirnagl et al., 2009; Gidday, 2006; Stenzel-Poore et al., 2004). In this altered physiological state, tissue damage is mitigated when challenged by exposure to a wide range of deleterious stimuli, even if unrelated to the initial challenge. It is mediated by highly redundant cellular, molecular, and physiological mechanisms involving neurons, astrocytes, and vascular cells (Gidday, 2006). Upstream sensors have been implicated, including adenosine and its A1 receptor, the NR2A NMDA receptor subunit, and the transcriptional regulator hypoxia inducible factor (HIF). HIF is an attractive candidate because it regulates a constellation of genes, including those whose protein products facilitate oxygen transport (erythropoietin), regulate glycolytic metabolism (e.g., glucose transporters), and promote angiogenesis (e.g., VEGF), by way of example.

Unexpectedly, genetic deletion of HIF1a improves infarct volume after middle cerebral artery occlusion, implicating as yet unknown pathogenic mechanisms activated by ischemia (Helton et al., 2005). Erythropoietin, one of the gene products of HIF1a, promotes PI3 kinase/AKT activity and the expression of NFkB-dependent protective genes (Digicaylioglu and Lipton, 2001).

Erythropoietin also downregulates hypoxia-induced proapoptotic mechanisms (Noguchi et al., 2007; Prass et al., 2003; Ruscher et al., 2002), and erythropoietin-based therapies have been investigated in the clinical arena (Ehrenreich et al., 2009). Heat shock protein family members are upregulated in ischemic tolerance and, based on their multiple cytoprotective actions, may promote survival. Preconditioning stimuli preserve connexin hemichannels in astrocytes facilitating ATP released from these cells and increasing the extracellular concentration of the beneficial nucleoside adenosine (Lin et al., 2008).

At the same time, preconditioning safeguards the function of cerebral blood vessels from the deleterious effects of cerebral ischemia, resulting in improved penumbral flow and reduced brain damage (Kunz et al., 2007b). These astrocytic and vascular changes are coupled with mechanisms that reduce energy demands, lessen inflammatory responses and ion channel activity, and decrease cascades promoting blood clotting and apoptotic cell death (Dirnagl et al., 2009; Obrenovitch, 2008; Gidday, 2006). Factors involving mitochondria as well as its uncoupling proteins have also been suggested and include improved efficiency of ATP synthesis, preservation of the mitochondrial membrane potential, and delayed opening of mitochondrial transition pore formation, as well as opening of mitochondrial ATP-dependent K+ channels (Dirnagl and Meisel, 2008). One of the key questions defying explanation at the moment is how and why diverse preconditioning stimuli targeting single genes or key steps in seemingly unrelated cascades all impact infarct injury in genetically engineered and wild-type mice. It may be telling us that the mechanisms through which the brain protects itself involve a highly integrated network response that emphasizes multiple cells within the neurovascular unit. If true, comparable multicellular approaches are needed that capitalize on this integrated response in the design of successful treatments.

Therapeutic Hypothermia: Engaging Pleiotropic Mechanisms in Multiple Cell Types

The therapeutic hypothermia field has advanced significantly during the past decade, inspired by positive outcomes from clinical trials in cardiac arrest victims (Bernard et al., 2002). Satisfactory neurological recovery was achieved in about half of the treated patients when treatment was begun within 2 hr of cardiac arrest. Promising results were reported in small feasibility studies in neonatal ischemia (Shankaran et al., 2005). Current efforts are directed toward translating these successes in cardiac arrest and neonatal ischemia to patients with ischemic stroke, but there remain unresolved technical issues surrounding the timing and method for inducing hypothermia, and the deleterious effect of rewarming (Wagner and Zuccarello, 2005). It is now well accepted that hypothermia reduces ischemia in animal models of stroke, and so far, preclinical results have helped guide the design of clinical trials in human subjects. Combining hypothermia with thrombolysis is one example. Experimental evidence suggests that hypothermia protects the brain through pleiotropic effects, acting on multiple cell types within the neurovascular unit. Hypothermia reduces brain metabolism, thereby significantly decreasing oxygen consumption and the workload of the entire organ (Sakoh and Gjedde, 2003). Hypothermia also reduces glutamate release, ROS production, and peri-infarct depolarizations. Inflammatory markers decrease, as well as microglial activation, leucocyte infiltration, MMP activation, and BBB disruption. In addition, hypothermia suppresses apoptotic cell death, decreases mitochondrial release of cytochrome C and apoptosis inducing factor (see for review Tang and Yenari, 2010). Cell survival pathways are upregulated and appear to contribute to the multiplicity of neuroprotective mechanisms. To what extent each of these promotes tissue protection or interacts synergistically to enhance tissue survival is not known and remains for further investigation. Nevertheless, therapeutic hypothermia does illustrate the potential power of approaching stroke therapy using combinations of modalities that engage multiple cell types to enhance protection and recovery.

Gaining Insight from the Bedside: Utility of Biomarkers

Biomarkers for Diagnosis and Prognosis

With the recent advances in technology and research, many look for biomarkers as a new avenue to further understand, diagnose, and treat diseases. A biomarker is a biological component that can be tangibly quantified to understand normal or pathological functioning in the body (Figure 2) (Bettermann K. 2011, Mayeux R. 2004). The roles of biomarkers in the laboratory and clinical setting are vast. They can be used in diagnosing pathologies, monitoring progress of disease or injury, identifying targets for intervention, and assessing risk of pathology. The measurement of biomarkers translated successfully from bench-to-bedside with troponin-1, a well-known example of a biomarker used to aid in diagnosis of myocardial infarction (Than M. 2012). Within the neuroscience community, biomarker research has become an area of increased interest and investigation for a variety of pathologies ranging from stroke to traumatic brain injury (TBI) to Alzheimer's disease (AD).

The remainder of our discussion of biomarkers will focus on ischemic stroke, but it is important to recognize the similarities of many disease states, particularly stroke and TBI. Timing of an accurate diagnosis is essential for patients with stroke. The only FDA-approved treatment, tissue plasminogen activator (tPA), has traditionally had a 3-h window for administration after onset of stroke (Weant K. A. 2012).

While recent guidelines suggest up to a 4.5 h window (Lansberg M. G. 2012), tPA administration has the potential to result in numerous well-documented adverse effects, such as hemorrhagic transformation (HT) or even death (Montaner J. 2011). Consequently, numerous contraindications for tPA administration exist and many patients go untreated. The identification of biomarkers for stroke therefore may not to be limited to traditional diagnostic or prognostic avenues but also more appropriate identification of patients at risk for tPA-associated morbidities.

Likewise, biomarkers may also be useful in determining patients in which tPA administration may be beneficial despite the presence of a comorbidity or risk-factor that would normally result in exclusion from tPA-based treatment. Previous studies have demonstrated differences in numerous markers that may one day potentially play a role in detection of ischemic stroke, stroke-mimic, and transient attack, as well as predict patient outcome (Navaro Sobrino M. 2011, Quin L. 2012), determine stroke severity, predict the risk of recurrent stroke (Tsai T. H. 2012) or hemorrhagic transformation (HT) (Ramos-Fernadez M. 2011) increase understanding of pathophysiology behind cerebral ischemia (Vangilder R. L. 2012), and provide possible targets for therapeutic intervention (Denes A. 2011).

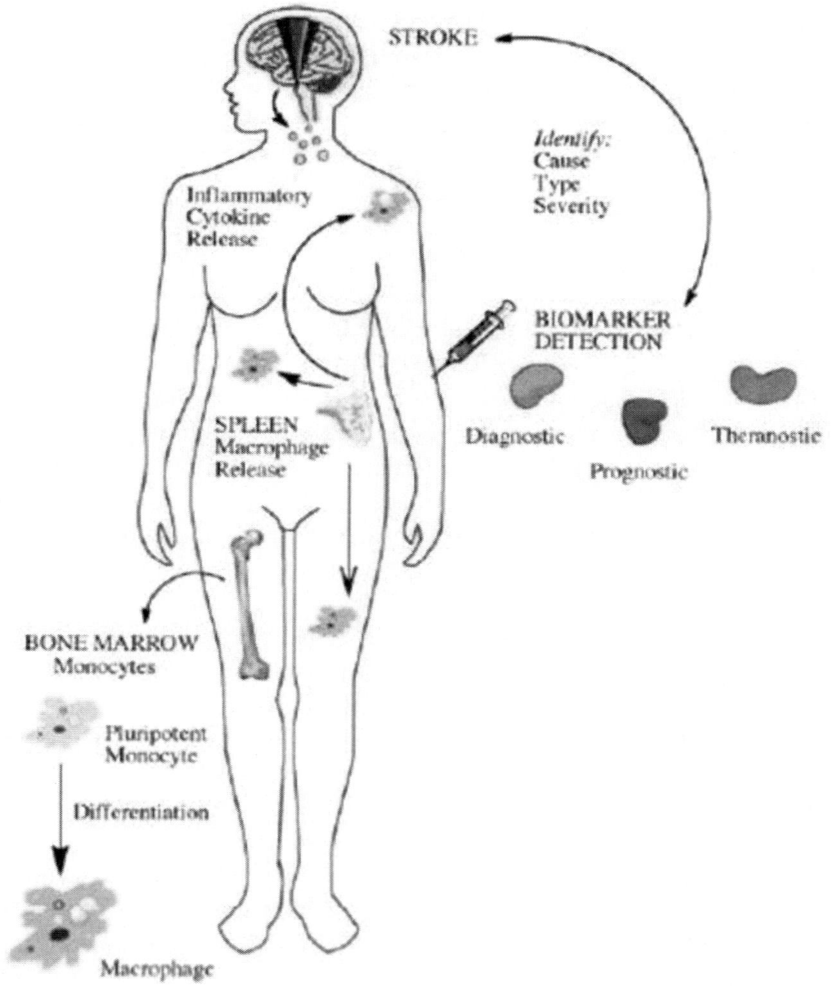

Figure 4.6. *Potential uses of biomarker in Stroke:* Potential uses of biomarkers include identification of stroke cause, type, and severity allowing for potential diagnosis, prognostication, and therapeutic selection or monitoring (theranosis). Biomarkers may also play a role in understanding disease pathophysiology, particularly in regards to inflammation and macrophage release and/or polarization.

While additional studies are certainly required to elucidate the most appropriate use of the markers discussed in the cited studies, each of these studies has provided valuable insight and potential examples of biomarker utilization at various time-points in the therapeutic or prognostic decision-making process, particularly as related to patient suitability for tPA administration.

Historically, biomarker-based studies sought the identification of a single marker for diagnostic/prognostic purposes. However, the investigated biomarkers have proven to be not specific or sensitive enough across multiple populations for clinical usage. Thus, researchers have transitioned largely towards identification of a panel of biomarkers rather than a single marker. The discovery of a group of biomarkers, instead of a sole marker, may improve the specificity, sensitivity, and prediction values across time (Ramos-Fernadez M. 2011, Bettermann K. 2011). A panel could therefore additionally provide the healthcare provider with more information than a single biomarker could reliably do alone (Ramos-Fernadez M. 2011). Due to biomarker discovery and investigation being a relatively new field, our discussion below is limited primarily to single marker studies.

Multiple biomarkers of stroke have been identified in the literature. A popular biomarker of note is matrix metalloproteinase 9 (MMP-9). High levels are correlated with current neurological deterioration, stroke severity, and infarct size (Montaner J. 2001). Interestingly, before administration of tPA, high levels also have been shown to accurately predict HT (Castellanos M. 2003, Montaner J. 2003). Despite MMP-9 playing a clear role in stroke pathology, a major pitfall of its use in the clinical setting is that it is not specific to the brain. It is involved with inflammation and matrix remodeling throughout the body and in different pathologies such as diabetes, hypertension (Tayebjee M. H. 2004), atherosclerosis (Sundstrom J. 2006), and many others. Therefore, MMP-9 likely cannot be used as a stand-alone biomarker for stroke; however it may be a helpful addition to a biomarker panel. Another biomarker of note is glial fibrillary acidic protein (GFAP). High levels of GFAP have been found to be indicative of hemorrhagic stroke in the acute stage, and therefore, GFAP may be an important biomarker to consider when deciding the appropriateness of thrombolytic administration (Hasan N. 2012). Importantly unlike MMP-9, GFAP is released strictly by astrocytes in the brain (Marginean I. C. 2011).

Outside of stroke, GFAP possesses prognostic value for outcome in cases of mild and severe traumatic brain injuries, though it is suggested that it is not an independent factor (Metting Z. 2012, Wiesmann M. 2010). A high concentration of S100 calcium binding protein (S100B) also has the ability to distinguish between hemorrhagic and ischemic stroke (Montaner J. 2012) and positively correlates with infarct volume (Jonsson H. 2001). When measured along with MMP-9, Glickman and colleagues revealed that S100B levels can differentiate between ischemic stroke and stroke mimic (Glickman S. W. 2011). Yet also like MMP-9, evidence indicates that S100B is expressed outside of the brain, such as in cancer, and therefore suffers from the same lack of specificity associated with other markers previously mentioned (Peric B. 2011, Strobel K. 2007). D-dimer concentration shows promise as a biomarker of stroke. As a component of a blood clot, d-dimer is useful for diagnosing the subtype (Hirano K. 2012), specifically cardioembolic stroke (Alvarez-Perez F. J. 2011), and distinguishing between ischemic stroke and stroke-mimic (Montaner J. 2011). As a thrombotic biomarker, d-dimer has many uses in regards to stroke, but it too is found throughout the body and, therefore, is not reflective solely of central nervous system events. Regardless, d-dimer has proven useful in the diagnosis of post-stroke cardiovascular complications such as pulmonary embolism, deep vein thrombosis and others (Glickman S. W. 2011).

The idea of individualized therapy, particularly when it concerns the selection of patients for thrombolytic therapy, has been further explored in recent years by Ning and colleagues. They showed significant prolonged effects on cellular signaling following tPA as evident by prolonged patterns of degradomic protein expression up to 5 days post-treatment, a finding in distinct contrast to that of non-tPA treated stroke patients in which a hyperacute response was evident but ceased by 24 h (Ning M. 2010). Besides demonstrating widespread effects of tPA on the extracellular matrix and brain parenchyma, far outside of the acute therapeutic window, their work could potentially demonstrate the utility of biomarkers in identification of patients at risk for adverse effects following therapeutic administration.

Biomarkers for Elucidating Disease Pathophysiology

While biomarkers are often thought of primarily for diagnostic and prognostic purposes, emerging work indicates a potentially greater role for biomarkers in elucidation of disease pathophysiology, especially communication between the brain and systemic responses. For example, Hayakawa and colleagues showed that by disrupting either the release of high-mobility-group-box-1 (HMGB1) from reactive astrocytes, or the HMGB1 receptor on endothelial progenitor cells, neurovascular remodeling is altered, and worsened deficits result (Hayakawa K. 2012). This work demonstrates the ability to isolate cell-specific events by taking in vitro based findings, such as the release of HMGB1 into astrocyte-conditioned media, and applying them to in vivo studies to determine the effect of HMGB1 systemically on post-ischemic injury. Other studies have used in vitro models in a similar fashion to demonstrate complex signaling relationships amongst neurons and glia. Specifically, Chu et al. showed the protective role of factors released by ischemic microglia, astrocytes, and neurons on astrocytes subjected to ischemia (Chu L. F. 2008). While space constraints prevent the mention of all applicable works, studies such as those described illustrate the potential for an expanded role of biomarkers in elucidation of disease pathophysiology and crosstalk between various cells within the brain and systemically.

Key Advances in Stroke

- ST-3 reinforces the need for further efforts to increase the proportion of ischaemic strokes treated within 3 h, but provides reassurance that thrombolysis in elderly patients or within 6 h from stroke onset does not increase mortality (Sandercock, P. 2012)
- Under the conditions of the ICTUS trial, citicoline is not effective in the treatment of moderate to severe acute ischaemic stroke (Dávalos, A. 2012)
- Atrial tachyarrhythmia must be considered as a new source of embolism in patients with cryptogenic stroke (Healey, J. S 2012)
- Patent foramen ovale closure with a device did not offer a greater benefit than medical therapy alone for the prevention of recurrent stroke or TIA (Takahashi, K. 2006)
- An animal study provides the first evidence that transplantation of cells derived from human induced pluripotent stem cells is a safe and efficient approach to promote recovery after stroke (Oki, K. 2012)

Several clinical trials and experimental studies that could have a major impact on the treatment of patients with ischaemic stroke were published in 2012. The studies cover all therapeutic options, including stroke prevention, recanalization and thrombolysis, neuroprotection, and promising new therapeutic approaches focused on neurorepair. Despite improvements in its management in recent years, cerebrovascular disease remains a major cause of mortality and morbidity. The current framework of therapeutic options to prevent or treat stroke comprises a spectrum of five fields of treatment—primary prevention, recanalization and thrombolysis, neuroprotection, secondary prevention, and neurorepair

(Figure 5.6). In 2012, we witnessed developments in all five areas, with important implications for stroke treatment. When primary prevention fails, an effective protocol for acute stroke treatment is imperative, early reperfusion of ischemic tissue being the primary goal. Currently, thrombolytic therapy with recombinant tissue plasminogen activator (rtPA) is the most effective approach. However, the extensive exclusion criteria, together with the short therapeutic window and narrow age range, severely restrict its use. The Third International Stroke Trial (IST-3) (Sandercock, P. 2012) was conducted to establish the balance between benefits and harms of rtPA treatment in patients who did not accomplish the licence criteria and, hence, to determine whether a wider range of patients might benefit up from rtPA up to 6 h from stroke onset. IST-3 enrolled 3,035 patients (1,515 in the rtPA group and 1,520 controls), 53% of whom were aged >80 years. No differences were found between groups with respect to the primary end point (37% in the rtPA group versus 35% of controls survived and achieved independence).

The global benefits of rtPA treatment seemed to be greatest within the first 3 h from stroke onset, but the analyses had insufficient power to define the benefit in a therapeutic window beyond 3 h. Interestingly, treatment efficacy was similar between patients older and younger than 80 years.

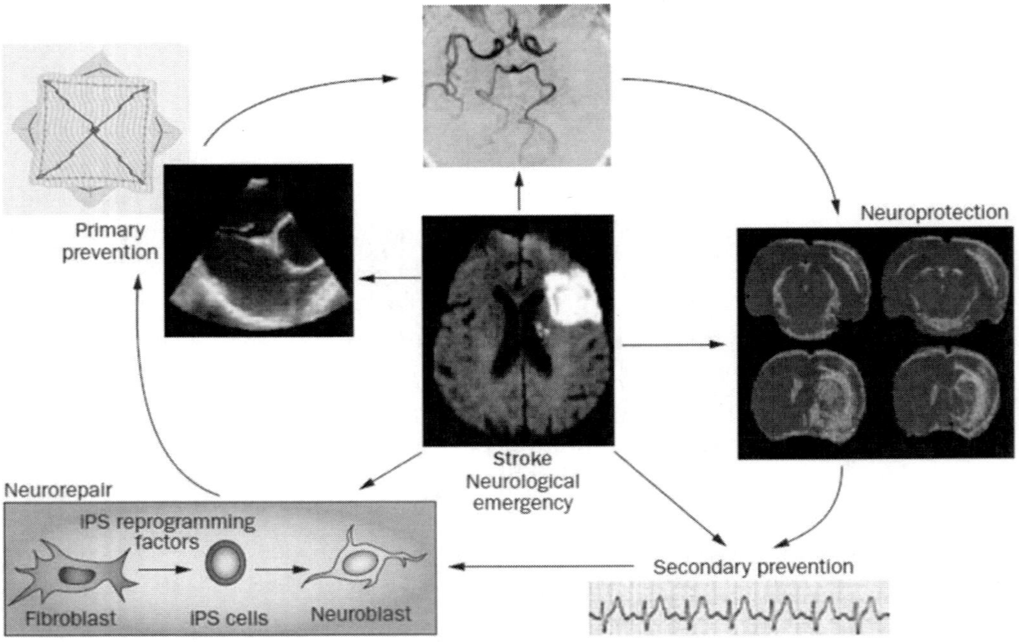

Figure 5.6. *Recent advances in stroke:* Spectrum of therapeutic options to prevent or treat stroke. In 2012, key advances were made in stroke prevention (primary and secondary), recanalization and thrombolysis, neuroprotection, and neurorepair strategies. Abbreviation: iPS, induced pluripotent stem.

The IST-3 data reinforce the need for further efforts to increase the proportion of ischemic strokes treated within 3 h, but they provide reassurance that rtPA treatment in elderly patients and within 6 h from stroke onset does not increase mortality. Although clinical trials with neuroprotective agents have systematically failed, neuroprotection remains a treatment option for acute ischemic stroke. In 2012, the results of ICTUS (International

Citicoline Trial on acUte Stroke) were published (Dávalos, A. 2012). In this trial, patients with moderate to severe acute ischemic stroke were treated with either citicoline or placebo within 24 h after symptom onset. The primary outcome was recovery at 90 days measured by a global test combining three measures—NIH Stroke Scale score ≤1, Modified Rankin Scale score ≤1, and Barthel Index score ≥95—in accordance with a pooled meta-analysis of previous randomized trials with citicoline.

(Dávalos, A. 2002) 2,298 patients (1,148 assigned to citicoline and 1,150 to placebo) were enrolled in ICTUS.2 Global recovery was similar in both groups, and no significant differences were reported in the safety variables or the rate of adverse events. Although ICTUS followed a protocol nearly identical to that of the pooled meta-analysis, (Dávalos, A. 2002) with minimal differences in statistical analysis, none of the benefits for citicoline were confirmed. However, the previous clinical trials with citicoline were conducted 10 years ago, and the standard of stroke care has substantially improved in the meantime. Also, the patients in ICTUS were, on average, 4 years older, and were over three times more likely to have received rtPA treatment, than those in previous trials. Comparison with the older studies suggests that the benefits of citicoline have become diluted in parallel with improvements in the standard of care for acute ischaemic stroke—a fact that should be taken into account for future trials of neuroprotective drugs.

To initiate appropriate secondary prevention, it is essential to know the cause of stroke, yet at least one-quarter of strokes are still classified as cryptogenic. The ASSERT investigators recruited 2,580 individuals >60 years without a history of atrial fibrillation (AF) in whom a pacemaker or defibrillator had been implanted. (Healey, J. S 2012) Patients were monitored for 3 months to detect subclinical atrial tachyarrhythmias (ATs; episodes of atrial rate >190 bpm for >6 min), and were followed up for a mean of 2.5 years for the primary outcome of ischemic stroke or systemic embolism. At least one AT was detected in 10.1% of patients. During the follow-up period, 4.2% of patients in whom subclinical AT had been detected had an ischemic stroke or systemic embolism, compared with 1.7% in whom subclinical AT was not detected. The attributable risk of ischemic stroke or systemic embolism associated with subclinical AT was 13%, which is similar to the stroke risk associated with AF (Wolf, P. A. 1991) On the basis of these results, AT must be considered as a new source of embolism in patients with cryptogenic stroke.

The prevalence of patent foramen ovale (PFO) ranges from 20–26% in the general population, but may be as high as 56% in patients under 55 years who have experienced a cryptogenic stroke. (Lamy, C. 2002) The CLOSURE I investigators evaluated the potential benefits of percutaneous device closure versus medical therapy for secondary stroke prevention in patients with PFO (Furlan, A. 2012) This multicentre, randomized, open-label trial compared PFO closure (using the STARFlex device) with medical therapy (warfarin, aspirin or both) in patients 18–60 years of age with PFO who had presented with cryptogenic stroke or TIA within the previous 6 months.

The primary end point was a composite of stroke or TIA during 2 years of follow-up, death from any cause during the first 30 days, or death from neurological causes between 31 days and 2 years. 909 patients—447 percutaneous device and 462 medical therapies—were enrolled. At 2 years, effective closure was maintained at 86.7% of cases. The incidence of the primary end point was 5.5% in the percutaneous device group and 6.8% in the medical group. Stroke incidence was 2.9% in the percutaneous device group and 3.1% in the medical group. No deaths occurred by 30 days in either group, and there were no deaths from neurological causes during the 2-year follow-up period. AF was significantly more frequent in the closure group (5.7% versus 0.7%). In conclusion, closure did not offer greater benefits than medical therapy alone for the prevention of recurrent stroke or TIA. Over the past two decades, stem cell based neurorepair has emerged as a promising therapeutic option for ischemic stroke.

Animal experimental data with embryonic stem (ES) cells, neural progenitor cells or bone marrow-derived progenitor cells are encouraging; however, no proven stem cell-based therapy is currently available for stroke. Despite the supposed immune-privileged status of the CNS, allogeneic grafts of stem cell-derived neurons and glia remain susceptible to rejection.

A novel alternative strategy to avoid graft rejection and immunosuppression is to generate induced pluripotent stem cells (iPSCs) from somatic cells. In 2006, it was reported that skin fibroblasts from adult mice could be reprogrammed to a pluripotent state by retroviral expression of four transcription factors (Takahashi, K. 2006). The resulting iPSCs are indistinguishable from ES cells in morphology, proliferative capacities, surface antigens, gene expression, epigenetic status, and telomerase activity. The Nobel Prize in Physiology or Medicine 2012 was awarded to Sir John B. Gurdon and Shinya Yamanaka for this breakthrough. The Laboratory of Neural Stem Cell Biology and Therapy, Lund, Sweden transplanted long-term self-renewing neuroepithelial-like stem cells, generated from adult human fibroblast-derived iPSCs, into stroke-damaged mouse and rat striatum or cortex. (Oki, K. 2012).

The transplanted cells stopped proliferating, could survive without forming tumors for at least 4 months, and differentiated into morphologically mature neurons. Grafted cells exhibited electrophysiological properties of mature neurons and received synaptic input from host neurons. Most importantly, the recovery of forepaw movements was observed by 1 week after transplantation. This study provides the first evidence that transplantation of human iPSC-derived cells is a safe and efficient approach to promote repair and recovery after stroke.

Current Devices Used for Mechanical Embolus Removal in Cerebral Ischemia

The mechanical embolus removal in cerebral ischemia (MERCI) trial evaluated the efficacy and safety of a mechanical endovascular device (which consists of a Nitinol core wire with shaped loops at the distal end designed to engage the thrombus) in the revascularization of an occluded large cerebral vessel within 8 hours of stroke onset (Figure 5.7) (Smith W. 2005 and 2008). The original study was subsequently updated with the Multi-MERCI trial incorporating a newer generation of the device (Smith W. 2008) The population of patients included in both studies were those ineligible to receive IV tPA (either arriving too late or having a contraindication for its use). The MERCI trial was a multicenter, prospective, single-arm trial that referred to the control arm of the PROACT II trial as historical control. Although the therapeutic window was 8 hours, the median time from onset to treatment was 4.3 hours in both studies. The recanalization rate was significantly higher than that in the control arm of PROACT II (48% vs 18%, respectively), but lower than that in the IA tPA group (66%). The proportion of patients achieving mRS2 at 90 days was comparable to that in the control arm of PROACT II (22.6% vs 25%, respectively). In contrast, the mortality rate of 43.5% was significantly higher than that reported in most prospective studies of the treatment of acute stroke. The investigators attributed this elevated mortality to a higher baseline NIHSS score (median 18) and higher proportion of basilar artery and internal carotid artery terminus occlusions. The introduction of a new generation of the device in the Multi-MERCI trial resulted in a significantly higher recanalization rate (55%) and an improvement in the mortality or neurological outcome at 90 days, although statistically insignificant.

Penumbra Device

The Penumbra device was introduced in the United States in 2008 after results from a European safety trial were published (Figure 5.8) (Penumbra Pivotal Stroke Group 2009). The system consists of a thrombus debulking and aspiration component as well as a direct thrombus extraction component.

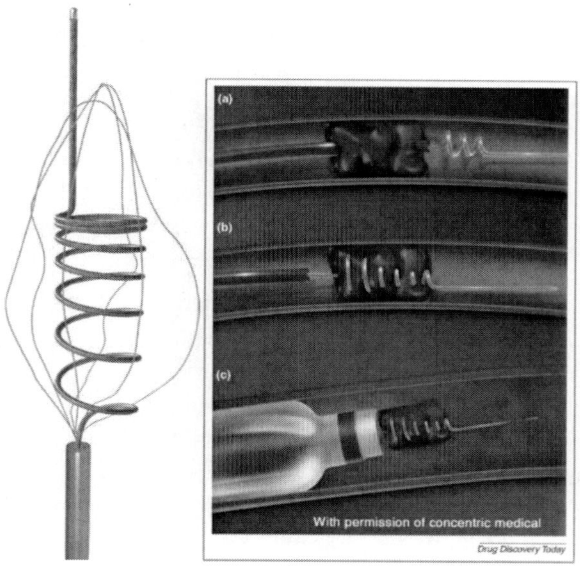

Figure 5.7. *(A) Merci Retriever device* which is a corkscrew-shaped product designed to remove blood clots from large vessels in patients experiencing acute ischemic stroke. (B) *Endovascular Therapy for acute stroke:* The principle of clot retrieving. The Merci System. Endovascular therapy for acute stroke is always performed under general nesthesia. First the MerciBalloon Guide Catheter is placed in the common or internal carotid artery for anterior circulation occlusion. Using standard cerebral catheterization techniques, a microcatheter is guided then through the guide catheter into the occluded vessel and passed beyond the thrombus (a). The Merci Retriever is now advanced through the microcatheter, and several of the helical loops are deployed distal to the thrombus. The Merci Retriever is then retracted to the face of the thrombus, and the proximal loops are deployed within the thrombus (b). The balloon of the Merci Balloon Guide Catheter has to be inflated now to arrest orthograde blood flow during removal of the thrombus. At least the Merci Retriever with the ensnared thrombus and the microcatheter are withdrawn together into the balloon guide catheter lumen. Continuous aspiration is applied to the guide catheter to promote complete evacuation of the thrombus (c). Once a retrieval attempt is completed, the balloon of the balloon guide catheter is deflated to re-establish flow. If the clot could not be removed with the retriever, the procedure can be repeated up to 5 times.

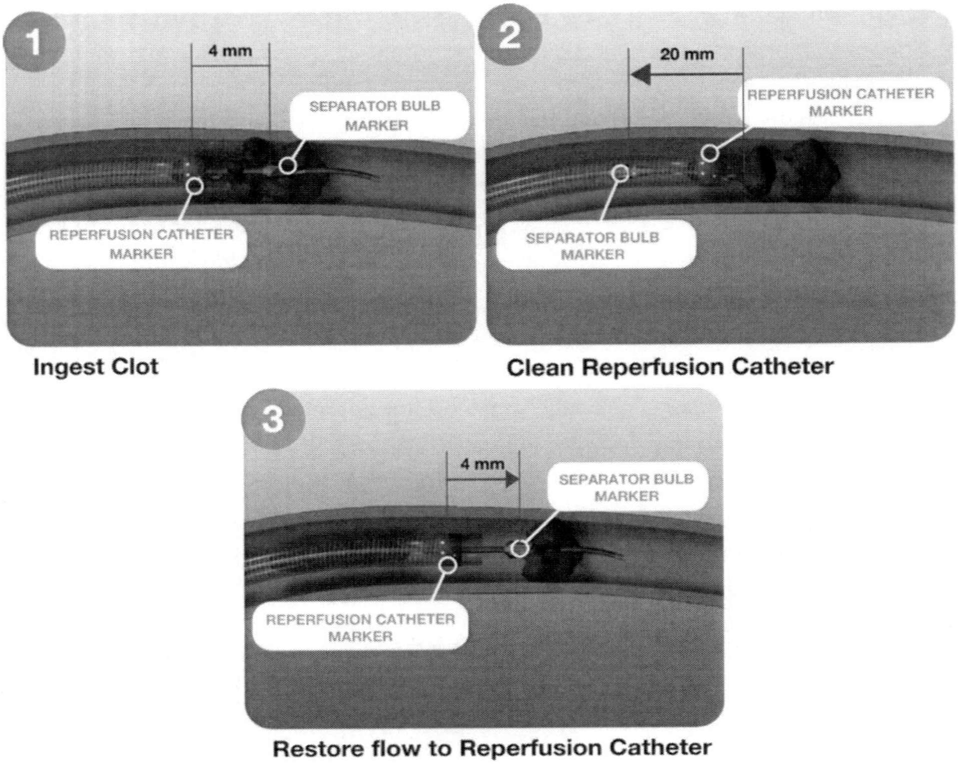

Figure 5.8. Penumbra Device.

The safety and efficacy of the device were reported in a multicenter, prospective, single-arm trial with the goal of establishing substantial equivalence to its predicate device—the Merci clot retrieval system.

Although the revascularization rate using the Penumbra device was the highest of the prospective trials at 81.6% (compared with 55% in the Multi-MERCI trial and 66% in the PROACT II trial), the neurological outcome was comparable or lower (25% with mRS 2, vs 36% in the Multi- MERCI trial and 40% in the PROACT II trial).

The investigators attribute this disparity to the lack of sufficient power and higher baseline NIHSS score.

Stent-Assisted Recanalization in Acute Ischemic

Stroke The use of endovascular stents has been recently advocated in the setting of acute stroke (Levy E. 2009). Based on retrospective data regarding the use of intracranial stents as a salvage technique in acute stroke, the SARIS trial (stent-assisted recanalization in acute ischemic stroke) aimed to evaluate the safety of stent deployment as a primary therapeutic intervention for acute stroke using a prospective, single-arm study design.

The investigators used the Wingspan (Boston Scientific, Natick, MA) and the Enterprise (Cordis, Bridgewater, NJ) intracranial self-expanding stents.

All 20 cases included in the trial were successfully revascularized, although 60% of patients required the use of an adjuvant intraprocedural pharmacological infusion (eptifibatide or tPA) or angioplasty. The risk of subsequent asymptomatic and symptomatic hemorrhage was 10% and 5%, respectively, and no procedure-related complications were reported. With regard to neurological outcomes, 45% of patients achieved an mRS score of 1 or less at 1 month follow-up. The results of the SARIS trial are difficult to directly compare with the large randomized prospective trials because it included a small number of patients with a relatively low median NIHSS score (13% vs 19% in IMS II and 17% in PROACT II), was nonrandomized, and included only short follow-up; nonetheless, the results represent an encouraging foundation for further investigation into the role of stenting for stroke treatment

Future Directions in Stroke Therapy: Logistics of Care

Improved stroke care begins at the pre-hospital stage; The California Acute Stroke Prototype Registry investigators estimate >10-fold increase in the number of patients receiving appropriate treatment if the hospital arrival time is within 1 hour of symptom onset, (California Acute stroke Pilot Registry (CASPR 2005)) highlighting the importance of public education and emergency medical services response time.

Future first responders to the scene of a suspected stroke may be able to perform real-time neuroimaging rapidly with subsequent transmission of images to the receiving medical center such that the time to diagnosis, triage, and catheterization (if deemed necessary) is optimized. Real-time neuroimaging using transcranial ultrasonography, especially with the concurrent use of ultrasonography contrast agents, may prove beneficial in providing such rapid assessment of occluded cerebral vessels in the field (Seidel G. 2009) Color-coded duplex ultrasonography has been shown to correctly differentiate hemorrhagic stroke from ischemic stroke in 95% of cases when compared with computed tomography scanning (Maurer M. 1998).

Furthermore, the use of cerebroprotective agents, again possibly administered in the field or early in the provision of stroke care, may further contribute to improved outcomes. With our current knowledge, patients arriving at a stroke treatment center outside of the defined windows for thrombolysis have few options outside of future stroke prevention and rehabilitation; therefore, extension of the therapeutic window is critical for allowing more patients to benefit from acute stroke treatment. The replacement of the traditional "stopwatch" approach to stroke with a more dynamic and functional time window is likely to take place, with growing evidence in clinical trials with the usefulness of magnetic resonance imaging-based patient selection for thrombolysis (desmoteplase in acute ischemic stroke (DIAS), diffusion and perfusion imaging evaluation for understanding stroke evolution (DEFUSE), and dose escalation of desmoteplase in acute stroke (DEDAS) trials) (Goldberg M. 2012).

The ongoing Third International Stroke Trial and Mechanical Retrieval and Recanalization of Stroke Clots Using Embolectomy (MR RESCUE) trial will also likely impact whether future patients are offered thrombolysis outside the conventional window.

Technological Advances

The incorporation of interventional approaches as an adjunct or alternative to intravenous thrombolysis in the setting of acute stroke is a rapidly growing field with a recent explosion in the number of devices available to the interventionalist. The PROACT trial was one of the first large multicenter trials to investigate the use of intravenous thrombolytic agents for the treatment of acute stroke; the study was followed by several other randomized trials, including the IMS study, which described the use of IV tPA as a bridge toward catheter-directed arterial infusion of the thrombolytic. IMS II introduced data regarding the use of low-energy sonography in addition to local thrombolysis. Subsequent studies have evaluated mechanical clot retrieval devices, including the MERCI and Penumbra trials (Goldberg M. 2012). Investigations and breakthroughs are likely to continue in both pharmacological and mechanical thrombolysis, with the future generation of devices likely to include a combination of the 2 modalities to achieve increased recanalization rates (Hopkins L. 2008, Sugrue P. A. 2009). Future devices are also likely to address the issue of distal emboli during clot manipulation (Leibig T. 2008). In addition to clot removal and microinfusion devices, the use of retrievable stents for the acute revascularization of thromboembolic stroke is a topic of great interest that is currently being evaluated (Wakhloo A. 2008, Zaidaat O. O. 2008). Stenting may prove useful as an adjunct to thrombolysis for immediate reperfusion with subsequent retrieval, or alternatively left in place for permanent deployment.

Pharmacological Advances

Promising pharmacological options for the treatment of acute ischemic stroke can be organized in 1 of 3 categories:

1. Novel thromboembolic agents and adjuvants (including antiplatelet and anticoagulation agents). Microplasmin, a recombinant form of human plasmin, may have a reduced propensity to cause bleeding compared with tPA and has been shown to be tolerable in human volunteers and efficacious in animal models of stroke. Microplasmin is currently under investigation to determine the clinical efficacy in human acute ischemic stroke patients (Thijis V. 2009).
2. Neuroprotective agents that have been an attractive but so far elusive target. At the time of this writing, more than 160 trials for ischemic stroke neuroprotective agents have been initiated (Internet Stroke Centre W. U. 2010). Unfortunately, few have produced positive results. However, notable recent exceptions include high-dose human albumin therapy, which showed promising results in the original Albumin in Acute Stroke trial (Palesch Y. Y. 2006).A larger randomized multicenter placebo-controlled efficacy trial is now underway (Goldberg M. 2012). Additionally, magnesium, which has been shown so far to be a rather weak neuroprotectant, (Muir K. W. 2004) continues to be under investigation because it is a safe and relatively inexpensive agent that may be administered in the hyperacute pre-hospital setting or during interventional procedures (Goldberg M. 2012).

3. Agents that contribute to the recovery of lost or dormant neuronal function. Although currently at its infancy stages, future interventional approaches may include local administration of neurorestorative agents, such as stem cells of both exogenous and endogenous origins, or neurotrophic molecules that promote and direct endogenous neurogenesis (Burns T. C. 2009, Chen J. 2001).

Conclusion

The lack of successful therapeutic translation from bench-to-bedside for a devastating disease such as stroke, despite the progression of over 100 proposed therapeutics to clinical trials, necessitates a closer review of both how stroke research is conducted as well as the therapeutic targets selected. While preclinical studies have improved in rigor, particularly with the advent of the Stroke Therapy Academic and Industry Roundtable (STAIR), clear deficiencies remain. Perhaps most notably, the lack of emphasis on the aging process and commonly associated comorbidities found in stroke patients, is persistent throughout the literature. As aging is the greatest risk factor for stroke, and numerous works have identified a role of aging in response to injury, inclusion of more preclinical models utilizing aged animals may lead to the development of promising therapeutics. Other promising avenues of investigation into stroke research include the role of glia, particularly with regards to the inflammatory response.

Stroke remains a major public health issue, and thrombolysis have been proven effective as therapy for cerebral ischemia, either administered intravenously within 3 hours or intra-arterially within 3 to 6 hours. Whereas the development of new thrombolytic agents and regimens as well as the rapid evolvement of endovascular therapies are an exciting component of the future of stroke treatments, one of the main challenges remains the wide availability and use of treatment for acute stroke patients. Even in its most basic version, intravenous thrombolysis has been demonstrated to be effective and safe when used in small medical centers. The advent of telemedicine and the use of robotics play an important role in making the therapy available to all stroke patients, as does community education, training of primary care providers, allied health professionals, and emergency medical services.

A number of promising thrombolytic strategies are currently being investigated, which may push the field further forward, including the following: The pilot nonrandomized safety and feasibility study, Interventional Management of Stroke, analyzed a combination of intravenous and intra-arterial thrombolysis, bringing together the speed of initiation of intravenous therapy and the higher recanalization rates of intraarterial thrombolysis. Endovascular therapies are rapidly evolving and continue to offer patients in whom intravenous thrombolysis fails a real chance at recanalization. These developments are of great importance to the endovascular neurosurgeon, and it is expected that as a result, endovascular neurosurgeons will be intimately involved in the treatment of stroke patients in the futures. And finally, ultrasound enhanced thrombolysis, developed by Alexandrov et al., using high-frequency ultrasonography to accelerate enzymatic fibrinolysis by increasing penetration of drug molecules into the clot, may offer an enhanced noninvasive option of effective thrombolysis.

Promising preclinical studies and early phase clinical studies, such as the work with minocycline, indicate a potential protective effect associated with microglial inhibition. Similarly, astrocytic modulation via administration of arundic acid may result in improved outcome. Other areas of investigation with regards to inflammation, such as understanding how to manipulate macrophage polarization for therapeutic benefit may lead to breakthroughs in drug development. Lastly, biomarker discovery, while often thought of in a diagnostic or prognostic sense, may in fact serve a much broader role in understanding disease pathophysiology and therapeutic selection. By improving preclinical models to more accurately emulate the clinical scenario and targeting disease pathophysiology beyond the nearly immediate events, the likelihood of successful translation from laboratory to clinic may be improved.

Neurointerventional surgery for the treatment of ischemic stroke is a rapidly expanding field with constantly improving tools and ever evolving indications. Recanalization rates appear to be on the rise in more recent studies compared to early studies. As data continues to accumulate regarding new treatment modalities and technologies, neurosurgeons, radiologists and neurologists should come together to design new treatment paradigms. Much work remains to streamline the care of stroke patients so that appropriate patients can be treated in a timely manner. The advances described above reflect progress across the spectrum of therapeutic options in stroke, from primary prevention to neurorepair. Every step takes us towards the ultimate aim of better outcomes and quality of life for patients with stroke.

References

Abou-Chebl A., Bajzer C. T., et al. Multimodal therapy for the treatment of severe ischemic stroke combining GPIIb/IIIa antagonists and angioplasty after failure of thrombolysis. *Stroke,* 2005; 36(10):2286–8.

Adams, H. P., Jr. et al. (2008) Emergency administration of abciximab for treatment of patients with acute ischemic stroke: results of an international phase III trial–Abciximab in Emergency Treatment of Stroke Trial (AbESTT-II). *Stroke,* 39, 87–99.

Adams H. P. Jr., del Zoppo G., et al. Guidelines for the early management of adults with ischemic stroke: a guideline from the American Heart Association/American Stroke Association Stroke Council, Clinical Cardiology Council, Cardiovascular Radiology and Intervention Council, and the Atherosclerotic Peripheral Vascular Disease and Quality of Care Outcomes in Research Interdisciplinary Working Groups: the American Academy of Neurology affirms the value of this guideline as an educational tool for neurologists. *Stroke,* 2007; 38(5):1655–711.

Adams, H. P., Jr. et al. (1996) Guidelines for thrombolytic therapy for acute stroke: a supplement to the guidelines for the management of patients with acute ischemic stroke – a statement for healthcare professionals from a Special Writing Group of the Stroke Council. American Heart Association. *Circulation,* 94, 167–174.

Adibhatla R. M., Hatcher J. F. Altered lipid metabolism in brain injury and disorders. *Subcell Biochem.,* 2008; 49:241–68.

Adibhatla R. M., Hatcher J. F. Tissue plasminogen activator (tPA) and matrix metalloproteinases in the pathogenesis of stroke: therapeutic strategies. *CNS Neurol. Disord. Drug Targets,* 2008; 7(3): 243–53.

Albers G. W., Goldstein L. B., et al. Stroke Treatment Academic Industry Roundtable (STAIR) recommendations for maximizing the use of intravenous thrombolytics and expanding treatment options with intra-arterial and neuroprotective therapies. *Stroke,* 2011; 42(9):2645–50.

Alexandrov, A. V. and Grotta, J. C. (2002) Arterial reocclusion in stroke patients treated with intravenous tissue plasminogen activator. *Neurology,* 59, 862–867.

Alvarez-Perez, F. J. et al. Usefulness of measurement of fibrinogen, D-dimer, D-dimer/fibrinogen ratio, C reactive protein and erythrocyte sedimentation rate to assess the pathophysiology and mechanism of ischaemic stroke. *J. Neurol. Neurosurg. Psychiatry,* 2011, 82, 986–992.

Astrup, J.; Symon, L.; Branston, N. M.; Lassen, N. A. Cortical evoked potential and extracellular K+ and H+ at critical levels of brain ischemia. *Stroke,* 1977, 8, 51–57.

Aronowski J., Ostrow P., et al. Graded bioassay for demonstration of brain rescue from experimental acute ischemia in rats. *Stroke,* 1994; 25(11): 2235–40.

Brekenfeld C., Schroth G., et al.et al. Mechanical thromboembolectomy for acute ischemic stroke: comparison of the catch thrombectomy device and the Merci Retriever in vivo. *Stroke,* 2008; 39(4):1213–9.

Boast C. A., Gerhardt S. C., et al. The N-methyl-Daspartate antagonists CGS 19755 and CPP reduce ischemic brain damage in gerbils. *Brain Res.,* 1988; 442(2):345–8.

Bambauer K. Z., Johnston S. C., Bambauer D. E., Zivin J. A. Reasons why few patients with acute stroke receive tissue plasminogen activator. *Arch. Neurol.,* 2006; 63(5):661–4.

Bergui, M. et al. (2006) Mechanical thrombolysis in ischemic stroke attributable to basilar artery occlusion as first-line treatment. *Stroke*, 37, 145–150.

Berlis, A. et al. (2004) Mechanical thrombolysis in acute ischemic stroke with endovascular photoacoustic recanalization. *Stroke,* 35, 1112–1116.

Becker K. J. Inflammation and acute stroke. *Curr. Opin. Neurol.,* 1998; 11(1):45–9.

Bambrick, L.; Kristian, T.; Fiskum, G. Astrocyte mitochondrial mechanisms of ischemic brain injury and neuroprotection. *Neurochem. Res.,* 2004, 29, 601–608.

Banwell V., Sena E. S., Macleod M. R. Systematic review and stratified meta-analysis of the efficacy of interleukin-1 receptor antagonist in animal models of stroke. *J. Stroke Cerebrovasc. Dis.,* 2009;18:269.

Bonafe, M.; Storci, G.; Franceschi, C. Inflamm-aging of the stem cell niche: Breast cancer as a paradigmatic example: Breakdown of the multi-shell cytokine network fuels cancer in aged people. *Bioessays,* 2012, 34, 40–49.

Bose, A. et al. (2008) The Penumbra System: a mechanical device for the treatment of acute stroke due to thromboembolism. *Am. J. Neuroradiol.,* 29, 1409–1413.

Brekenfeld, C. et al. (2005) Endovascular neuroradiological treatment of acute ischemic stroke: techniques and results in 350 patients. *Neurol. Res.,* 27, 29–35.

Brekenfeld, C. et al. (2008) Mechanical thromboembolectomy for acute ischemic stroke: comparison of the catch thrombectomy device and the Merci Retriever in vivo. *Stroke,* 39, 1213–1219.

Bettermann, K. Biomarkers for stroke: In search of fingerprints. *J. Stroke Cerebrovasc. Dis.,* 2011, 20, 173–176.

Boutin H., LeFeuvre R. A., Horai R., et al. Role of IL-1alpha and IL-1beta in ischemic brain damage. *J. Neurosci.*, 2001;21:5528.

Burns T. C., Verfaillie C. M., Low W. C.: Stem cells for ischemic brain injury: A critical review. *J. Comp. Neurol.,* 515:125-144, 2009.

Chen J., Sanberg P. R., Li Y., et al: Intravenous administration of human umbilical cord blood reduces behavioral deficits after stroke in rats. *Stroke,* 32:2682, 2001.

Carmignoto, G.; Gomez-Gonzalo, M. The contribution of astrocyte signalling to neurovascular coupling. *Brain Res. Rev.,* 2010, 63, 138–148.

Cao W., Carney J. M., Duchon A., Floyd R. A., Chevion M. Oxygen free radical involvement in ischemia and reperfusion injury to brain. *Neurosci. Lett.,* 1988; 88(2):233–8.

California Acute Stroke Pilot Registry (CASPR) Investigators: Prioritizing interventions to improve rates of thrombolysis for ischemic stroke. *Neurology,* 64:654-659, 2005.

Campbell, J. H.; Burdo, T. H.; Autissier, P. et al. Minocycline inhibition of monocyte activation correlates with neuronal protection in SIV neuroAIDS. *PLoS One,* 2011, 6, e18688.

Castellanos, M.; Leira, R.;et al. A. Plasma metalloproteinase-9 concentration predicts hemorrhagic transformation in acute ischemic stroke. *Stroke*, 2003, 34, 40–46.

Chapot, R. (2005) First experience with the Catch, a new device for cerebral thrombectomy. *Intervent. Neuroradiol.,* 11, 58.

Chaturvedi R. K., Beal M. F. Mitochondrial approaches for neuroprotection. *Ann. N Y Acad. Sci.,* 2008;1147:395.

Cheng Y. D., Al-Khoury L., Zivin J. A. Neuroprotection for ischemic stroke: two decades of success and failure. *NeuroRx.,* 2004; 1(1):36–45.

Cheng Y., Deshmukh M., et al. Caspase inhibitor affords neuroprotection with delayed administration in a rat model of neonatal hypoxic-ischemic brain injury. *J. Clin. Invest.,* 1998; 101(9):1992–9.

Chu, L. F.; Wang, W. T.; et al. Ischemic brain cell-derived conditioned medium protects astrocytes against ischemia through GDNF/ERK/NF-kB signaling pathway. *Brain Res.,* 2008, 1239, 24–35.

Clark W. M. C. B. Randomised trial of CGS19755, a glutamate antagonist, in acute ischemic stroke treatment. *Neurology,* 1994;44(suppl 2):A270.

Clark W. M., Rinker L. G., Lessov N. S., et al. Time course of IL-6 expression in experimental CNS ischemia. *Neurol. Res.,* 1999;21:287.

Cotrina, M. L.; Nedergaard, M. Astrocytes in the aging brain. *J. Neurosci. Res.,* 2002, 67, 1–10.

Cornu, C. et al. (2000) Streptokinase in acute ischemic stroke: an individual patient data meta-analysis – the Thrombolysis in Acute Stroke Pooling Project. *Stroke,* 31, 1555–1560.

Cuzzocrea S., Riley D. P., Caputi A. P., Salvemini D. Antioxidant therapy: a new pharmacological approach in shock, inflammation, and ischemia/reperfusion injury. *Pharmacol. Rev.,* 2001; 53(1): 135–59.

Deitcher, S. R. et al. (2005) Non-clinical and clinical characterization of a novel acting thrombolytic: alfimeprase. *Pathophysiol. Haemost. Thromb.,* 34, 215–220.

David, S.; Kroner, A. Repertoire of microglial and macrophage responses after spinal cord injury. *Nat. Rev. Neurosci.*, 2011, 12, 388–399.

Deb P., Sharma S., Hassan K. M. Pathophysiologic mechanisms of acute ischemic stroke: An overview with emphasis on therapeutic significance beyond thrombolysis. *Pathophysiology,* 2007, 17(3): 197–218.

Denes, A.; Pinteaux, E.; Rothwell, N. J.; Allan, S. M. Interleukin-1 and stroke: Biomarker, harbinger of damage, and therapeutic target. *Cerebrovasc. Dis.,* 2011, 32, 517–527.

Dinapoli, V. A.; Benkovic, S. A.; et al. Age exaggerates proinflammatory cytokine signaling and truncates signal transducers and activators of transcription 3 signaling following ischemic stroke in the rat. *Neuroscience,* 2010, 170, 633–644.

Dávalos, A. et al. Citicoline in the treatment of acute ischaemic stroke: an international, randomised, multicentre, placebo-controlled study (ICTUS trial). *Lancet,* 380, 349–357 (2012).

Dávalos, A. et al. Oral citicoline in acute ischemic stroke: an individual patient data pooling analysis of clinical trials. *Stroke,* 33, 2850–2857 (2002).

Dawson, K. M. et al. (1994) Plasminogen mutants activated by thrombin. Potential thrombus-selective thrombolytic agents. *J. Biol. Chem.,* 269, 15989–15992.

Denes A., Thornton P., Rothwell N. J., et al. Inflammation and brain injury: Acute cerebral ischaemia, peripheral and central inflammation. *Brain Behav. Immun.,* 2009.

Enlimomab Study Group Use of anti-ICAM-1 therapy in ischemic stroke: results of the Enlimomab Acute Stroke Trial. *Neurology,* 2001;57:1428.

Emergency Management of Stroke (EMS) Bridging Trial. *Stroke,* 1999; 30(12):2598–605.

Endres M., Namura S., et al. Attenuation of delayed neuronal death after mild focal ischemia in mice by inhibition of the caspase family. *J. Cereb. Blood Flow Metab.,* 1998; 18(3): 238–47.

Ehrenreich H., Weissenborn K. et al. Recombinant human erythropoietin in the treatment of acute ischemic stroke. *Stroke,* 2009; 40(12):e647–56.

Feuerstein G. Z., Zaleska M. M., et al. Missing steps in the STAIR case: a Translational Medicine perspective on the development of NXY-059 for treatment of acute ischemic stroke. *J. Cereb. Blood Flow Metab.,* 2008; 28(1):217–9.

Fagan, S. C.; Cronic, L. E.; Hess, D. C. Minocycline development for acute ischemic stroke. *Transl. Stroke Res.,* 2011, 2, 202–208.

Fisher M. The ischemic penumbra: identification, evolution and treatment concepts. *Cerebrovasc. Dis.,* 2004; 17 (Suppl 1):1–6.

Fischer, U. et al. (2005) NIHSS score and arteriographic findings in acute ischemic stroke. *Stroke,* 36, 2121–2125.

Fitzsimmons, B. F. et al. (2006) Rapid stent-supported revascularization in acute ischemic stroke. *Am. J. Neuroradiol.,* 27, 1132–1134.

Flint, A. C. et al. (2007) Mechanical thrombectomy of intracranial internal carotid occlusion: pooled results of the MERCI and Multi MERCI Part I trials. *Stroke,* 38,1274–1280.

Forsman M., Fleischer J. E., et al. Superoxide dismutase and catalase failed to improve neurologic outcome after complete cerebral ischemia in the dog. *Acta Anaesthesiol. Scand.,* 1988; 32(2): 152–5.

Francis J. W., Ren J., et al. Postischemic infusion of Cu/Zn superoxide dismutase or SOD:Tet451 reduces cerebral infarction following focal ischemia/reperfusion in rats. *Exp. Neurol.,* 1997; 146(2):435–43.

Fukuda, S.; del Zoppo, G. J. Models of focal cerebral ischemia in the nonhuman primate. *ILAR J.,* 2003, 44, 96–104.

Ferrer I., Planas A. M. Signaling of cell death and cell survival following focal cerebral ischemia: life and death struggle in the penumbra. *J. Neuropathol. Exp. Neurol.*, 2003;62:329.

Feuerstein G. Z., Zaleska M. M., Krams M., et al. Missing steps in the STAIR case: a Translational Medicine perspective on the development of NXY-059 for treatment of acute ischemic stroke. *J. Cereb. Blood Flow Metab.*, 2008;28:217.

Furlan, A. J. et al. Closure or medical therapy for cryptogenic stroke with patent foramen ovale. *N. Engl. J. Med.*, 366, 991–999 (2012).

Furlan, A. et al. (1999) Intra-arterial prourokinase for acute ischemic stroke: the PROACT II study – a randomized controlled trial. Prolyse in Acute Cerebral Thromboembolism. *J. Amer. Med. Assoc.*, 282, 2003–2011.

Furlan, A. J. et al. (2006) Dose Escalation of Desmoteplase for Acute Ischemic Stroke (DEDAS): evidence of safety and efficacy 3 to 9 hours after stroke onset. *Stroke,* 37, 1227–1231.

Gibson, C. M. et al. (2006) Dose escalation trial of the efficacy, safety, and pharmacokinetics of a novel fibrinolytic agent, BB-10153, in patients with ST elevation MI: results of the TIMI 31 trial. *J. Thromb. Thrombolysis,* 22, 13–21.

Green A. R., Ashwood T. Free radical trapping as a therapeutic approach to neuroprotection in stroke: experimental and clinical studies with NXY-059 and free radical scavengers. *Curr. Drug Targets CNS Neurol. Disord.,* 2005;4:109.

Glickman, S. W.; Phillips, S.et al. Discriminative capacity of biomarkers for acute stroke in the emergency department. *J. Emerg. Med.,* 2011, 41, 333–339.

Gedikli O., Baykan M. Statins in stroke prevention. *Anadolu. Kardiyol. Derg.,* 2008; 8(3): 217–22.

Garcia J. H., Liu K. F., Yoshida Y., Lian J., Chen S., del Zoppo G. J. Influx of leukocytes and platelets in an evolving brain infarct (Wistar rat). *Am. J. Pathol.,* 1994; 144(1):188–99.

Goto H., Fujisawa H., S., et al. Neurotoxic effects of exogenous recombinant tissue-type plasminogen activator on the normal rat brain. *J. Neurotrauma*, 2007; 24(4):745–52.

Guyot L. L., Diaz F. G., et al. Real-time measurement of glutamate release from the ischemic penumbra of the rat cerebral cortex using a focal middle cerebral artery occlusion model. *Neurosci. Lett.,* 2001; 299(1–2):37–40.

Gotti B., Duverger D., et al. Ifenprodil and SL 82.0715 as cerebral anti-ischemic agents. I. Evidence for efficacy in models of focal cerebral ischemia. *J. Pharmacol. Exp. Ther.,* 1988; 247(3):1211–21.

Gribkoff V. K., Starrett J. E. et al. Targeting acute ischemic stroke with a calcium-sensitive opener of maxi-K potassium channels. *Nat. Med.*, 2001; 7(4):471–7.

Goldberg M.: Stroke Trials Registry, 2010. Available at: http://clinicaltrial. gov/ct2/show/ NCT00638781?term_DIAS&rank_4. http://clinicaltrial.gov/ ct2/show/NCT01349946? term_DEFUSE&rank_1; http://clinicaltrial.gov/ct2/show/NCT00638248?term_DEDAS& rank_1.

Hopkins L., Ecker R.: Cerebral endovascular neurosurgery. *Neurosurgery,* 62:1483-1501, 2008.

Hademenos G. J., Massoud T. F. Biophysical mechanisms of stroke. *Stroke,* 1997; 28(10): 2067–77.

Hemmen T. M., Raman R., et al. Intravenous thrombolysis plus hypothermia for acute treatment of ischemic stroke (ICTuS-L): final results. *Stroke,* 2010; 41(10):2265–70.

Hofmeijer J., Schepers J., et al. Delayed decompressive surgery increases apparent diffusion coefficient and improves peri-infarct perfusion in rats with space-occupying cerebral infarction. *Stroke,* 2004; 35(6):1476–81.

Horn J., Limburg M. Calcium antagonists for acute ischemic stroke. *Cochrane Database Syst. Rev.*, 2000; (2):CD001928.

Hacke W., Schwab S., et al. 'Malignant' middle cerebral artery territory infarction: clinical course and prognostic signs. *Archives of neurology*, 1996; 53(4):309–15.

Hacke, W. et al. (2008) Thrombolysis with alteplase 3 to 4.5 hours after acute ischemic stroke. *N. Engl. J. Med.,* 359, 1317–1329.

Hacke, W. et al. (2004) Association of outcome with early stroke treatment: pooled analysis of ATLANTIS, ECASS, and NINDS rtPA stroke trials. *Lancet,* 363, 768–774.

Haley, E. C., Jr. et al. (2005) A pilot dose-escalation safety study of tenecteplase in acute ischemic stroke. *Stroke,* 36, 607–612.

Hacke, W. et al. (1988) Intra-arterial thrombolytic therapy improves outcome in patients with acute vertebrobasilar occlusive disease. *Stroke,* 19, 1216–1222.

Henkes, H. et al. (2006) A device for fast mechanical clot retrieval from intracranial arteries (Phenox clot retriever). *Neurocrit. Care*, 5, 134–140.

Hussain, M. S. et al. (2010) Symptomatic delayed reocclusion after initial successful revascularization in acute ischemic stroke. *J. Stroke Cerebrovasc. Dis.,* 19, 36–39.

Haddad J. J. Redox regulation of pro-inflammatory cytokines and IkappaB-alpha/NF-kappaB nuclear translocation and activation. *Biochem. Biophys. Res. Commun.,* 2002; 296(4): 847–56.

Hasan, N.; McColgan, P.; Bentley, P.; Edwards, R. J.; Sharma, P. Towards the identification of blood biomarkers for acute stroke in humans: A comprehensive systematic review. *Br. J. Clin. Pharmacol.,* 2012, 74, 230–240.

Hayakawa, K.; Pham, L. D. et al. Astrocytic high-mobility group box 1 promotes endothelial progenitor cell-mediated neurovascular remodeling during stroke recovery. *Proc. Natl. Acad. Sci. USA,* 2012, 109, 7505–7510.

Hirano, K., Takashima, S.et al. Study of hemostatic biomarkers in acute ischemic stroke by clinical subtype. *J. Stroke Cerebrovasc. Dis.,* 2012, 21, 404–410.

Hara H., Friedlander R. M., Gagliardini V., et al. Inhibition of interleukin 1beta converting enzyme family proteases reduces ischemic and excitotoxic neuronal damage. *Proc. Natl. Acad. Sci. U S A,* 1997;94:2007.

Hayakawa, K.; Mishima, K.; et al.. Delayed treatment with minocycline ameliorates neurologic impairment through activated microglia expressing a high-mobility group box1-inhibiting mechanism. *Stroke,* 2008, 39, 951–958.

Healey, J. S. et al. Subclinical atrial fibrillation and the risk of stroke. *N. Engl. J. Med.,* 366, 120–129 (2012).

Hughes P. M., Allegrini P. R., Rudin M., et al. Monocyte chemoattractant protein-1 deficiency is protective in a murine stroke model. *J. Cereb. Blood Flow Metab.,* 2002; 22:308.

Imaizumi S., Woolworth V., Fishman R. A., Chan P. H. Liposome-entrapped superoxide dismutase reduces cerebral infarction in cerebral ischemia in rats. *Stroke,* 1990; 21(9):1312–7.

IMS Study Investigators, (2004) Combined intravenous and intra-arterial recanalization for acute ischemic stroke: the Interventional Management of Stroke Study. *Stroke,* 35, 904–911.

Internet Stroke Center WU: Stroke Trials Registry, 2010. Available at: http://www.strokecenter.org/trials/clinicalstudies/list

Janjua, N. et al. (2008) Impact of arterial reocclusion and distal fragmentation during thrombolysis among patients with acute ischemic stroke. *Am. J. Neuroradiol.*, 29, 253–258.

Jacobs S. E., Morley C. J., et al. Whole-body hypothermia for term and near-term newborns with hypoxic-ischemic encephalopathy: a randomized controlled trial. *Arch. Pediatr. Adolesc. Med.,* 2011; 165(8):692–700.

Janardhan V., Qureshi A. I. Mechanisms of ischemic brain injury. *Curr. Cardiol. Rep.*, 2004; 6(2): 117–23.

Jahan R. Solitaire flow-restoration device for treatment of acute ischemic stroke: safety and recanalization efficacy study in a swine vessel occlusion model. *AJNR.* 2010; 31(10):1938–43.

Jia J., Guan D., Zhu W., et al. Estrogen inhibits Fas-mediated apoptosis in experimental stroke. *Exp. Neurol.*, 2009;215:48.

Jean W. C., Spellman S. R., et al. Reperfusion injury after focal cerebral ischemia: the role of inflammation and the therapeutic horizon. *Neurosurgery,* 1998; 43(6):1382–96.

Jones T. H., Morawetz R. B., et al. Thresholds of focal cerebral ischemia in awake monkeys. *J. Neurosurg.,* 1981; 54(6):773–82.

Jonsson, H.; Johnsson, P. et al. S100B as a predictor of size and outcome of stroke after cardiac surgery. *Ann. Thorac. Surg.,* 2001, 71, 1433–1437.

Juurlink B. H., Sweeney M. I. Mechanisms that result in damage during and following cerebral ischemia. *Neurosci Biobehav Rev.,* 1997; 21(2):121–8.

Kim D. W., Eum W. S., et al. Transduced Tat-SOD fusion protein protects against ischemic brain injury. *Mol. Cells,* 2005; 19(1):88–96.

Kennea N. L., Mehmet H. Neural stem cells. *J. Pathol.,* 2002; 197(4):536–50.

Kuroda S., Siesjo B. K. Reperfusion damage following focal ischemia: pathophysiology and therapeutic windows. *Clin. Neurosci.,* 1997; 4(4):199–212.

Kelly, M. E. et al. (2008) Recanalization of an acute middle cerebral artery occlusion using a self-expanding, reconstrainable, intracranial microstent as a temporary endovascular bypass. *Stroke,* 39, 1770–1773.

Kerber, C. W. et al. (2007) Rapid intracranial clot removal with a new device: the alligator retriever. *Am. J. Neuroradiol.*, 28, 860–863.

Kaur, J. et al. (2004) The neurotoxicity of tissue plasminogen activator? *J. Cereb. Blood Flow Metab.*, 24, 945–963.

Levy, E. I. et al. (2009) First food and drug administration-approved prospective trial of primary intracranial stenting for acute stroke. SARIS (Stent-Assisted Recanalization in Acute Ischemic Stroke). *Stroke,* 40, 3552.

Lisboa, R. C. et al. (2002) Analysis of the safety and efficacy of intra-arterial thrombolytic therapy in ischemic stroke. *Stroke,* 33, 2866–2871.

Llevadot, J. et al. (2001) Bolus fibrinolytic therapy in acute myocardial infarction. *J. Amer. Med. Assoc.,* 286, 442–449.

Lapchak, P. A. et al. (2002) Microplasmin: a novel thrombolytic that improves behavioral outcome after embolic strokes in rabbits. *Stroke,* 33, 2279–2284.

Liebig, T. et al. (2008) Comparative in vitro study of five mechanical embolectomy systems: effectiveness of clot removal and risk of distal embolization. *Neuroradiology,* 50, 43–52.

Levy, E. I. et al. (2006) Stent-assisted intracranial recanalization for acute stroke: early results. *Neurosurgery,* 58, 458–463.

Lawrence, T.; Natoli, G. Transcriptional regulation of macrophage polarization: Enabling diversity with identity. *Nat. Rev. Immunol.,* 2011, 11, 750–761.

Lamy, C. et al. Clinical and imaging findings in cryptogenic stroke patients with and without patent foramen ovale: the PFO-ASA Study. *Stroke,* 33, 706–711 (2002).

Lees K. R., Zivin J. A., Ashwood T., et al. NXY-059 for acute ischemic stroke. *N. Engl. J. Med.,* 2006;354:588.

Leker R. R., Shohami E. Cerebral ischemia and trauma-different etiologies yet similar mechanisms: neuroprotective opportunities. *Brain Res. Brain Res. Rev.,* 2002; 39(1): 55–73.

Lewandowski C. A., Frankel M., et al. Combined intravenous and intra-arterial r-TPA versus intra-arterial therapy of acute ischemic stroke: Liebig T., Reinartz J., Hannes R., Miloslavski E., Henkes H. Comparative in vitro study of five mechanical embolectomy systems: effectiveness of clot removal and risk of distal embolization. *Neuroradiology,* 2008; 50(1):43–52.

Levy E. I., Siddiqui A. H., et al. First Food and Drug Administration-approved prospective trial of primary intracranial stenting for acute stroke: SARIS (stent-assisted recanalization in acute ischemic stroke). *Stroke,* 2009; 40(11):3552–6.

Lundbye J. B., Rai M., et al. Therapeutic hypothermia is associated with improved neurologic outcome and survival in cardiac arrest survivors of nonshockable rhythms. *Resuscitation,* 2011.

Li, L.; Lundkvist, A.; Andersson, D.; et al. Protective role of reactive astrocytes in brain ischemia. *J. Cereb. Blood Flow Metab.,* 2008, 28, 468–481.

Lo, E. H. A new penumbra: Transitioning from injury into repair after stroke. *Nat. Med.,* 2008, 14, 497–500.

Lalancette-Hebert, M.; Gowing, G.; et al. Selective ablation of proliferating microglial cells exacerbates ischemic injury in the brain. *J. Neurosci.,* 2007, 27, 2596–2605.

Lampl, Y.; Boaz, M.; Gilad, R.; et al. Minocycline treatment in acute stroke: An open-label, evaluator-blinded study. *Neurology,* 2007, 69, 1404–1410.

Lansberg, M. G.; Bluhmki, E.; Thijs, V. N. Efficacy and safety of tissue plasminogen activator 3 to 4.5 hours after acute ischemic stroke: A metaanalysis. *Stroke,* 2009, 40, 2438–2441.

Liebig T., Reinartz J., Hannes R., et al: Comparative in vitro study of five mechanical embolectomy systems: Effectiveness of clot removal and risk of distal embolization. *Neuroradiology,* 50:43-52, 2008.

Levy E., Siddiqui A., Crumlish A., et al: First food and drug administration-approved prospective trial of primary intracranial stenting for acute stroke. Saris (stent-assisted recanalization in acute ischemic stroke). *Stroke,* 40:3552-3556, 2009.

Lee, S. R.; Lo, E. H. Induction of caspase-mediated cell death by matrix metalloproteinases in cerebral endothelial cells after hypoxia-reoxygenation. *J. Cereb. Blood Flow Metab.,* 2004, 24, 720–727.

Lee, S. R.; Tsuji, K.; Lo, E. H. Role of matrix metalloproteinases in delayed neuronal damage after transient global cerebral ischemia. *J. Neurosci.*, 2004, 24, 671–678.

Lo, E. H.; Wang, X.; Cuzner, M. L. Extracellular proteolysis in brain injury and inflammation: Role for plasminogen activators and matrix metalloproteinases. *J. Neurosci. Res.*, 2002, 69, 1–9.

Liu T., McDonnell P. C., Young P. R., et al. Interleukin-1 beta mRNA expression in ischemic rat cortex. *Stroke,* 1993;24:1746.

Macleod M. R., O'Collins T., Horky L. L., et al. Systematic review and metaanalysis of the efficacy of FK506 in experimental stroke. *J. Cereb. Blood Flow Metab.,* 2005;25:713.

Mayeux, R. Biomarkers: Potential uses and limitations. *NeuroRx,* 2004, 1, 182–188.

Margaill I., Plotkine M., Lerouet D. Antioxidant strategies in the treatment of stroke. *Free Radic. Biol. Med.*, 2005; 39(4):429–43.

Marginean, I. C.; Stanca, D. M.; et al. Plasmatic markers in hemorrhagic stroke. *J. Med. Life,* 2011, 4, 148–150.

Metting, Z.; Wilczak, N.; Rodiger, L. A.; Schaaf, J. M.; van der Naalt, J. GFAP and S100B in the acute phase of mild traumatic brain injury. *Neurology,* 2012, 78, 1428–1433.

Montaner, J.; Mendioroz, M.; et al. Differentiating ischemic from hemorrhagic stroke using plasma biomarkers: The S100B/RAGE pathway. *J. Proteomics*, 2012, 75, 4758–4765.

Mbye, L. H.; Keles, E.; et al. VA64, a membrane-resealing agent, reduces histopathology and improves functional outcome after controlled cortical impact in mice. *J. Cereb. Blood Flow Metab.*, 2012, 32, 515–524.

Montaner, J.; Alvarez-Sabín, J. et al. Matrix metalloproteinase expression after human cardioembolic stroke: Temporal profile and relation to neurological impairment. *Stroke,* 2001, 32, 1759–1766.

Montaner, J.; Molina, C. A.; et al. Matrix metalloproteinase-9 pretreatment level predicts intracranial hemorrhagic complications after thrombolysis in human stroke. *Circulation,* 2003, 107, 598–603.

Morris M. C., Depollier J., Mery J., Heitz F., Divita G. A peptide carrier for the delivery of biologically active proteins into mammalian cells. *Nat Biotechnol.*, 2001; 19(12):1173–6.

Mosser, D. M.; Edwards, J. P. Exploring the full spectrum of macrophage activation. *Nat. Rev. Immunol.*, 2008, 8, 958–969.

Murray, P. J.; Wynn, T. A. Protective and pathogenic functions of macrophage subsets. *Nat. Rev. Immunol.*, 2011, 11, 723–737.

Montaner, J.; Mendioroz, M.; Ribó, M. et al. A panel of biomarkers including caspase-3 and D-dimer may differentiate acute stroke from stroke-mimicking conditions in the emergency department. *J. Intern. Med.,* 2011, 270, 166–174.

Muir K. W., Lees K. R. Clinical experience with excitatory amino acid antagonist drugs. *Stroke,* 1995;26:503.

Muir K. W. L. K. Intravenous magnesium sulphate in acute stroke: a randomised, double-blind, placebo-controlled pilot study. Cerebrovasc. Dis. 1994;4:255. Abstract. *Cerebrovasc. Dis.,* :255, 1994.

Mäurer M., Shambal S., Berg D., et al: Differentiation between intracerebral hemorrhage and ischemic stroke by transcranial color-coded duplex-sonography. *Stroke,* 29:2563, 1998.

Mellott, M. J. et al. (1995) Vampire bat salivary plasminogen activator evokes minimal bleeding relative to tissue-type plasminogen activator as assessed by a rabbit cuticle bleeding time model. *Thromb. Haemost.*, 73, 478–483.

Mayer, T. E. et al. (2002) Mechanical extraction of a basilar-artery embolus with the use of flow reversal and a microbasket. *N. Engl. J. Med.*, 347, 769–770.

Molina, C. A. and Saver, J. L. (2005) Extending reperfusion therapy for acute ischemic stroke: emerging pharmacological, mechanical, and imaging strategies. *Stroke,* 36, 2311–2320.

Muir K. W., Lees K. R., Ford I., et al: Magnesium for acute stroke (intravenous magnesium efficacy in stroke trial): Randomised controlled trial. *Lancet,* 363:439, 2004.

Nogueira, R. G. et al. (2008) Low-pressure balloon angioplasty with adjuvant pharmacological therapy in patients with acute ischemic stroke caused by intracranial arterial occlusions. *Neuroradiology,* 50, 331–340.

Nakano, S. et al. (2002) Direct percutaneous transluminal angioplasty for acute middle cerebral artery trunk occlusion: an alternative option to intra-arterial thrombolysis. *Stroke,* 33, 2872–2876.

Nogueira, R. G. and Smith, W. S. (2009) Safety and efficacy of endovascular thrombectomy in patients with abnormal hemostasis: pooled analysis of the MERCI and Multi MERCI trials. *Stroke,* 40, 516–522.

Nagai Y., Popiel H. A. Conformational changes and aggregation of expanded polyglutamine proteins as therapeutic targets of the polyglutamine diseases: exposed beta-sheet hypothesis.*Curr. Pharm. Des.,* 2008;14:3267.

Navarro-Sobrino, M.; Rosell, A.; et al. A large screening of angiogenesis biomarkers and their association with neurological outcome after ischemic stroke. *Atherosclerosis,* 2011, 216, 205–211.

Ning, M.; Sarracino, D. A.et al. Proteomic protease substrate profiling of tPA treatment in acute ischemic stroke patients: A step toward individualizing thrombolytic therapy at the bedside. *Transl. Stroke Res.,* 2010, 1, 268–275.

Natarajan S. K., Snyder K. V., et al. Safety and effectiveness of endovascular therapy after 8 hours of acute ischemic stroke onset and wakeup strokes. *Stroke,* 2009; 40(10):3269–74.

Nogueira, R. G. et al. (2008) Endovascular approaches to acute stroke. Part 1. Drugs, devices, and data. *Am. J. Neuroradiol.*, 30, 649–661.

Nogueira R. G., Schwamm L. H., Hirsch J. A. Endovascular approaches to acute stroke, part 1: Drugs, devices, and data. *AJNR,* 2009; 30(4):649–61.

Nogueira R. G., Yoo A. J., Buonanno F. S., Hirsch J. A. Endovascular approaches to acute stroke, part 2: a comprehensive review of studies and trials. *AJNR,* 2009; 30(5):859–75.

Noh S. J., Lee J. M. et al. SP-8203 shows neuroprotective effects and improves cognitive impairment in ischemic brain injury through NMDA receptor. *Pharmacol. Biochem. Behav.,* 2011, 100(1):73–80.

Offner H., Subramanian S., Parker S. M., et al. Experimental stroke induces massive, rapid activation of the peripheral immune system. *J. Cereb. Blood Flow Metab.,* 2006;26:654.

Oki, K. et al. Human-induced pluripotent stem cells form functional neurons and improve recovery after grafting in strokedamaged brain. *Stem Cells*, 30, 1120–1133 (2012).

Ogawa, A. et al. (2007) Randomized trial of intraarterial infusion of urokinase within 6 hours of middle cerebral artery stroke: the middle cerebral artery embolism local fibrinolytic intervention trial (MELT) Japan. *Stroke,* 38, 2633–2639.

Ohta K., Graf R., Rosner G., Heiss W. D. Calcium ion transients in peri-infarct depolarizations may deteriorate ion homeostasis and expand infarction in focal cerebral ischemia in cats. *Stroke,* 2001; 32(2):535–43.

Ostrowski R. P., Colohan A. R., Zhang J. H. Molecular mechanisms of early brain injury after subarachnoid hemorrhage. *Neurol. Res.*, 2006; 28(4):399–414.

O'Collins, V. E.; Macleod, M. R.; et al. 1026 experimental treatments in acute stroke. *Ann. Neurol.*, 2006, 59, 467–477.

Okada, S.; Nakamura, M.; et al. Conditional ablation of Stat3 or Socs3 discloses a dual role for reactive astrocytes after spinal cord injury. *Nat. Med.*, 2006, 12, 829–834.

Pancioli, A. M. et al. (2008) The combined approach to lysis utilizing eptifibatide and rtPA in acute ischemic stroke: the CLEAR stroke trial. *Stroke*, 39, 3268.

Pfefferkorn, T.; Rosenberg, G. A. Closure of the blood-brain barrier by matrix metalloproteinase inhibition reduces rtPA-mediated mortality in cerebral ischemia with delayed reperfusion. *Stroke,* 2003, 34, 2025–2030.

Palesch Y. Y., Hill M. D., Ryckborst K. J., et al: The alias pilot trial: A doseescalation and safety study of albumin therapy for acute ischemic stroke—II: Neurologic outcome and efficacy analysis. *Stroke*, 37:2107-2114, 2006.

Penumbra Pivotal Stroke Trial Investigators: The penumbra pivotal stroke trial: Safety and effectiveness of a new generation of mechanical devices for clot removal in intracranial large vessel occlusive disease. *Stroke,* 40:2761-2768, 2009.

Peric, B.; Zagar, I.; Novakovic, S.; Zgajnar, J.; Hocevar, M. Role of serum S100B and PET-CT in follow-up of patients with cutaneous melanoma. *BMC Cancer*, 2011, 11, 328.

Pettigrew, L. C.; Kasner, S. E.; et al. Arundic Acid (ONO-2506); Stroke Study Group. Safety and tolerability of arundic acid in acute ischemic stroke. *J. Neurol. Sci.,* 2006, 251, 50–56.

Polazzi, E.; Monti, B. Microglia and neuroprotection: From in vitro studies to therapeutic applications. *Prog. Neurobiol.,* 2010, 92, 293–315.

Popovich, P. G.; Longbrake, E. E. Can the immune system be harnessed to repair the CNS? *Nat. Rev. Neurosci*., 2008, 9, 481–493.

Qian, L.; Ding, L.; Cheng, L.; et al. Early biomarkers for post-stroke cognitive impairment. *J. Neurol.*, 2012, 259, 2111–2118.

Qureshi, A. I. et al. (2002) Aggressive mechanical clot disruption and low-dose intraarterial third-generation thrombolytic agent for ischemic stroke: a prospective study. *Neurosurgery*, 51, 1319–1327.

Ramos-Fernandez M., Bellolio M. F., Stead L. G.Matrix metalloproteinase-9 as a marker for acute ischemic stroke: A systematic review. *J. Stroke Cerebrovasc. Dis.,* 2011, 20, 47–54.

Reddy M. K., Wu L., et al. Superoxide Dismutase-Loaded PLGA Nanoparticles Protect Cultured Human Neurons Under Oxidative Stress. *Appl. Biochem. Biotechnol*., 2008; 151(2–3):565–77.

Reddy M. K., Labhasetwar V. Nanoparticle-mediated delivery of superoxide dismutase to the brain: an effective strategy to reduce ischemia-reperfusion injury. *FASEB J.* 2009; 23(5):1384–95.

Rha J. H., Saver J. L. The impact of recanalization on ischemic stroke outcome: a meta-analysis. *Stroke,* 2007; 38(3):967–73.

Roitberg B. Transplantation for stroke. *Neurol. Res.,* 2004; 26(3):256–64.

Rosamond, W. et al. (2008) Heart disease and stroke statistics: 2008 update – a report from the American Heart Association Statistics Committee and Stroke Statistics Subcommittee. *Circulation,* 117, 25–146.

rtPA Stroke Study Group, (1995) Tissue plasminogen activator for acute ischemic stroke: The National Institute of Neurological Disorders and Stroke. *N. Engl. J. Med.,* 333, 1581–1587.

Rosenberg G. A., Yang Y. Vasogenic edema due to tight junction disruption by matrix metalloproteinases in cerebral ischemia. *Neurosurg. Focus*, 2007; 22(5):E4.

Rosell, A.; Lo, E. H. Multiphasic roles for matrix metalloproteinases after stroke. *Curr. Opin. Pharmacol.,* 2008, 8, 82–89.

Rossi, D. J.; Brady, J. D.; Mohr, C. Astrocyte metabolism and signaling during brain ischemia. *Nat. Neurosci.,* 2007, 10, 1377–1386.

Saver J. L., Kidwell C., Eckstein M., Starkman S. Prehospital neuroprotective therapy for acute stroke: results of the Field Administration of Stroke Therapy-Magnesium (FAST-MAG) pilot trial. *Stroke*, 2004; 35(5):e106–8.

Schwab S., Steiner T., Aschoff A., et al. Early hemicraniectomy in patients with complete middle cerebral artery infarction. *Stroke,* 1998; 29(9):1888–93.

Schaller B., Graf R. Cerebral ischemia and reperfusion: the pathophysiologic concept as a basis for clinical therapy. *J. Cereb. Blood Flow Metab.,* 2004; 24(4):351–71.

Schurer L., Grogaard B., Gerdin B., Arfors K. E. Superoxide dismutase does not prevent delayed hypoperfusion after incomplete cerebral ischaemia in the rat. *Acta. Neurochir. (Wien),* 1990; 103(3–4):163–70.

Shintani Y., Terao Y., Ohta H. Molecular Mechanisms Underlying Hypothermia-Induced Neuroprotection. *Stroke Research and Treatment*, 2011; PMC2995905.

Siesjo B. K., Agardh C. D., Bengtsson F. Free radicals and brain damage. *Cerebrovasc. Brain Metab. Rev.*, 1989; 1(3):165–211.

Siesjo B. K. Cell damage in the brain: a speculative synthesis. *J. Cereb. Blood Flow Metab.,* 1981; 1(2):155–85.

Sinha J., Das N., Basu M. K. Liposomal antioxidants in combating ischemia-reperfusion injury in rat brain. *Biomed. Pharmacother*., 2001; 55(5):264–71.

Stroke, (1989) Recommendations on stroke prevention, diagnosis, and therapy: report of the WHOTask Force on Stroke and other Cerebrovascular Disorders. *Stroke,* 20, 1407–1431.

Switzer, J. A.; Hess, D. C.; et al. Matrix metalloproteinase-9 in an exploratory trial of intravenous minocycline for acute ischemic stroke. *Stroke,* 2011, 42, 2633–2635.

Sundstrom, J.; Vasan, R. S. Circulating biomarkers of extracellular matrix remodeling and risk of atherosclerotic events. *Curr. Opin. Lipidol*., 2006, 17, 45–53.

Sandercock, P. et al. The benefits and harms of intravenous thrombolysis with recombinant tissue plasminogen activator within 6 h of acute ischaemic stroke (the third international stroke trial (IST-3)): a randomised controlled trial. *Lancet,* 379, 2352–2363 (2012).

Sakata, H.; Niizuma, K.; Yoshioka, H.; et al. Minocycline-preconditioned neural stem cells enhance neuroprotection after ischemic stroke in rats. *J. Neurosci*., 2012, 32, 3462–3473.

Seidel G., Meairs S.: Ultrasound contrast agents in ischemic stroke. *Cerebrovasc. Dis*., 27:25-39, 2009 (suppl 2)

Smith W., Sung G., Starkman S., et al: Safety and efficacy of mechanical embolectomy in acute ischemic stroke results of the MERCI trial. *Stroke*, 36:1432-1438, 2005.

Smith W. S. Safety of mechanical thrombectomy and intravenous tissue plasminogen activator in acute ischemic stroke. Results of the multi Mechanical Embolus Removal in Cerebral Ischemia (MERCI) trial, part I. AJNR, 2006; 27(6):1177–82.

Smith, W. S. et al. (2008) Mechanical thrombectomy for acute ischemic stroke: final results of the Multi MERCI trial. *Stroke,* 39, 1205–1212.

Shuaib A., Lees K. R., Lyden P., et al. NXY-059 for the treatment of acute ischemic stroke. *N. Engl. J. Med.,* 2007;357:562.

Sims N. R., Muyderman H. Mitochondria, oxidative metabolism and cell death in stroke. *Biochim. Biophys. Acta.,* 2009 doi:10.1016/j.bbadis.2009.09.003.

Smith W. S., Sung G., Saver J., et al. Mechanical thrombectomy for acute ischemic stroke: final results of the Multi MERCI trial. *Stroke,* 2008; 39(4):1205–12.

Soriano S. G., Amaravadi L. S., Wang Y. F., et al. Mice deficient infract alkine are less susceptible to cerebral ischemia-reperfusion injury. *J. Neuroimmunol.,* 2002;125:59.

Struffert T., Kohrmann M., et al. The penumbra pivotal stroke trial: safety and effectiveness of a new generation of mechanical devices for clot removal in intracranial large vessel occlusive disease. *Stroke,* 2009; 40(8):2761–8.

Struffert T., Köhrmann M., et al. Stroke System as an "add-on" for the treatment of large vessel occlusive disease following thrombolysis: first results. *European radiology,* 2009; 19(9):2286–93.

Strobel, K.; Skalsky, J.; Kalff, V. et al. Tumour assessment in advanced melanoma: Value of FDG-PET/CT in patients with elevated serum S-100B. *Eur. J. Nucl. Med. Mol. Imaging,* 2007, 34, 1366–1375.

Su E. J., Fredriksson L., et al. Activation of PDGF-CC by tissue plasminogen activator impairs blood-brain barrier integrity during ischemic stroke. *Nat. Med.,* 2008; 14(7): 731–7.

Sugrue P. A., Hage Z. A., Surdell D. L., et al: Basilar artery occlusion following c1 lateral mass fracture managed by mechanical and pharmacological thrombolysis. *Neurocrit. Care,* 11:255-260, 2009.

Thijs V., Peeters A., Vosko M., et al: Randomized, placebo-controlled, dose-ranging clinical trial of intravenous microplasmin in patients with acute ischemic stroke. *Stroke,* 40:3789-3795, 2009.

The NINDS Stroke Study Investigators, (2005) Recombinant tissue plasminogen activator for minor strokes: the National Institute of Neurological Disorders and Stroke rt-PA Stroke Study experience. *Ann. Emerg. Med.,* 46, 243–252.

Takahashi, K. and Yamanaka, S. Induction of pluripotent stem cells from mouse embryonic and adult fibroblast cultures by defined factors. *Cell,* 126, 663–676 (2006).

Than, M.; Cullen, L.; Aldous, et al. 2-Hour accelerated diagnostic protocol to assess patients with chest pain symptoms using contemporary troponins as the only biomarker: The ADAPT trial. *J. Am. Coll. Cardiol.,* 2012, 59, 2091–2098.

Tayebjee, M. H.; Lim, H. S.; et al. Matrix metalloproteinase-9 and tissue inhibitor of metalloproteinase-1 and -2 in type 2 diabetes: Effect of 1 year's cardiovascular risk reduction therapy. *Diabetes Care,* 2004, 27, 2049–2051.

Tsai, T. H.; Chen, Y. L.; et al. Link between lipoprotein-associated phospholipase A2 gene expression of peripheral-blood mononuclear cells and prognostic outcome after acute ischemic stroke. *J. Atheroscler. Thromb.,* 2012, 19, 523–531.

Tsubokawa T., Jadhav V., Solaroglu I., et al. Lecithinized superoxide dismutase improves outcomes and attenuates focal cerebral ischemic injury via antiapoptotic mechanisms in rats. *Stroke,* 2007; 38(3):1057–62.

Takano, T.; Oberheim, N.; Cotrina, M. L.; Nedergaard, M. Astrocytes and ischemic injury. *Stroke,* 2009, 40, S8–S12.

Tateishi, N.; Mori, T.; Kagamiishi, Y.; et al.. Astrocytic activation and delayed infarct expansion after permanent focal ischemia in rats. Part II: Suppression of astrocytic activation by a novel agent (R)-(−)-2-propyloctanoic acid (ONO-2506) leads to mitigation of delayed infarct expansion and early improvement of neurologic deficits. *J. Cereb. Blood Flow Metab*., 2002, 22, 723–734.

Taylor C. P. Mechanism of action of new anti-epileptic drugs. New Trends in Epilepsy Management: The Role of Gabapentin. 1994;13-40 ea. Chadwick D.

The Interventional Management of Stroke (IMS) II Study. *Stroke,* 2007; 38(7):2127–35.

The penumbra pivotal stroke trial: safety and effectiveness of a new generation of mechanical devices for clot removal in intracranial large vessel occlusive disease *Stroke,* 2009; 40(8):2761–8.

The Ancrod Stroke Study Investigators, (1994) Ancrod for the treatment of acute ischemic brain infarction. *Stroke*, 25, 1755–1759.

Turner R., Vink R. Inhibition of neurogenic inflammation as a novel treatment for ischemic stroke. *Timely Top Med. Cardiovasc. Dis.,* 2007; 11:E24.

Ueda, T. et al. (1997) Endovascular treatment for acute thrombotic occlusion of the middle cerebral artery: local intra-arterial thrombolysis combined with percutaneous transluminal angioplasty. *Neuroradiology,* 39, 99–104.

Vangilder, R. L.; Huber, J. D.; Rosen, C. L.; Barr, T. L. The transcriptome of cerebral ischemia. *Brain Res. Bull*., 2012, 88, 313–319.

Voskuhl, R. R., Peterson, R. S.; Song, B.; et al. Reactive astrocytes form scar-like perivascular barriers to leukocytes during adaptive immune inflammation of the CNS. *J. Neurosci.*, 2009, 29, 11511–11522.

Valko M., Leibfritz D., et al. Free radicals and antioxidants in normal physiological functions and human disease. *Int. J. Biochem. Cell Biol.,* 2007; 39(1):44–84.

Veronese F. M., Caliceti P., Schiavon O., Sergi M. Polyethylene glycol-superoxide dismutase, a conjugate in search of exploitation. *Adv. Drug Deliv. Rev.,* 2002; 54(4):587–606.

Wagner K. R., Jauch E. C. Extending the window for acute stroke treatment: thrombolytics plus CNS protective therapies. *Exp. Neurol*., 2004; 188(2):195–9.

Weant, K. A.; Baker, S. N. New windows, same old house: An update on acute stroke management. *Adv. Emerg. Nurs. J.,* 2012, 34, 112–121.

Wester P. O. A. K., Eriksson S., Hagg E., et al. Infusion of magnesium in patients with acute brain infarction.Acta Neurol Scand. 1985:143. Abstract. *Acta. Neurol. Scand*., 143. :143, 1985.

Wiesmann, M.; Steinmeier, E.; Magerkurth, O.; Linn, J.; Gottmann, D.; Missler, U. Outcome prediction in traumatic brain injury: Comparison of neurological status, CT findings, and blood levels of S100B and GFAP. *Acta. Neurol. Scand.,* 2010, 121, 178–185.

Wiltrout C., Lang B., Yan Y., Dempsey R. J., Vemuganti R. Repairing brain after stroke: a review on post-ischemic neurogenesis. *Neurochem. Int.,* 2007; 50(7–8):1028–41.

Wolf, P. A., Abbott, R. D. and Kannel, W. B. Atrial fibrillation as an independent risk factor for stroke: the Framingham Study. *Stroke*, 22, 983–988 (1991).

Wolpert, S. M. et al. (1993) Neuroradiologic evaluation of patients with acute stroke treated with recombinant tissue plasminogen activator: the rtPA Acute Stroke Study Group. *Am. J. Neuroradiol.*, 14, 3–13.

Wu T. W., Li W. W., Li H. Netrin-1 attenuates ischemic stroke-induced apoptosis. *Neuroscience,* 2008;156:475.

Wakhloo A., Gounis M.: Retrievable closed cell intracranial stent for foreign body and clot removal. *Neurosurgery,* 62:ONS390-ONS393, 2008 (5 suppl 2).

Xu, L.; Fagan, S. C.; Waller, J. L.; et al. Low dose intravenous minocycline is neuroprotective after middle cerebral artery occlusion-reperfusion in rats. *BMC Neurol.*, 2004, 4, 7.

Yang Y., Candelario-Jalil E., Thompson J. F., et al. Increased intranuclear matrix metalloproteinase activity in neurons interferes with oxidative DNA repair in focal cerebral ischemia. *J. Neurochem.*, 2009.

Yenari, M. A.; Kauppinen, T. M.; Swanson, R. A. Microglial activation in stroke: Therapeutic targets. *Neurotherapeutics*, 2010, 7, 378–391.

Yenari, M. A.; Xu, L.; Tang, X. N.; Qiao, Y.; Giffard, R. G. Microglia potentiate damage to blood-brain barrier constituents: Improvement by minocycline in vivo and in vitro. *Stroke,* 2006, 37, 1087–1093.

Yrjanheikki J., Keinanen R., Pellikka M., et al. Tetracyclines inhibit microglial activation and are neuroprotective in global brain ischemia. *Proc. Natl. Acad. Sci. U S A,* 1998;95: 15769.

Yrjanheikki J., Tikka T., Keinanen R., et al. A tetracycline derivative, minocycline, reduces inflammation and protects against focal cerebral ischemia with a wide therapeutic window. *Proc. Natl. Acad. Sci. U S A,* 1999;96:13496.

Yepes M., Sandkvist M., et al. Tissue-type plasminogen activator induces opening of the blood-brain barrier via the LDL receptor-related protein. *J. Clin. Invest.,* 2003; 112(10): 1533–40.

Yasui K., Baba A. Therapeutic potential of superoxide dismutase (SOD) for resolution of inflammation. *Inflammation Res.,* 2006; 55(9):359–63.

Zaidat O. O., Wolfe T., Hussain S. I., et al: Interventional acute ischemic stroke therapy with intracranial self-expanding stent. *Stroke*, 39:2392, 2008.

Zhang Z., Zhang R. L., et al. A new rat model of thrombotic focal cerebral ischemia. *J. Cereb. Blood Flow Metab.,* 1997; 17(2):123–35.

Zaidat O. O., Suarez J. I., et al. Response to intraarterial and combined intravenous and intra-arterial thrombolytic therapy in patients with distal internal carotid artery occlusion. *Stroke,* 2002; 33(7):1821–6.

Zamanian, J. L.; Xu, L.; Foo, L. C.; et al. Genomic analysis of reactive astrogliosis. *J. Neurosci.,* 2012, 32, 6391–6410.

Zaidat, O. O. et al. (2008) Interventional acute ischemic stroke therapy with intracranial self-expanding stent. *Stroke,* 39, 2392–2395.

Zeumer, H. et al. (1983) Interventional neuroradiology: local intra-arterial fibrinolysis in acute vertebrobasilar thromboembolic disease. *Am. J. Neuroradiol.*, 4, 401–404.

Zhao, B. Q.; Wang, S.; Kim, H. Y.; et al. Role of matrix metalloproteinases in delayed cortical responses after stroke. *Nat. Med.,* 2006, 12, 441–445.

Zonta, M.; Angulo, M. C.; Gobbo,S.; et al. Neuron-to-astrocyte signaling is central to the dynamic control of brain microcirculation. *Nat. Neurosci.,* 2003, 6, 43–50.

In: Recent Advances in Stroke Therapeutics
Editor: Manzoor Ahmad Mir
ISBN: 978-1-63117-754-5

Chapter V

Stem Cells and Treatment of Strokes

Abstract

Stroke is a leading cause of death and disability worldwide. Stem cell therapy is an emerging therapeutic modality with evidence of significant benefits in preclinical stroke models. A number of phase I and II clinical trials have now been completed, with several more currently under way. Translation to the bedside, however, remains a long way off, and there are many questions that remain unanswered. This chapter will summarize the current evidence and ongoing clinical trials worldwide, and explore the challenges to making this a realistic treatment option for the future. Despite advances in acute care and secondary preventive strategies, stroke remains a major burden on health-care resources worldwide. Thrombolysis with tissue plasminogen activator is now a well-established treatment for acute ischemic stroke and is associated with significant improvements in outcomes. However, its use is limited to a narrow time window of only 4.5 hours from symptom onset, and in the UK only 5% of stroke patients currently receive this treatment. Stem cell therapy is an emerging therapeutic modality in the treatment of stroke. Its basis stems from the observation that certain parts of the adult brain are capable of regeneration (a relatively recent discovery). Neurogenesis in the adult brain has been demonstrated in the dentate nucleus of the hippocampus and the subventricular zone. In a study of patients with ischemic stroke, neurogenesis was demonstrated in the ischemic penumbra, where cells were found to preferentially localize to the vicinity of blood vessels. These findings are suggestive of poststroke compensatory neurogenesis, which may contribute to recovery after the insult. While the regenerative capacity of certain parts of the brain has been demonstrated, it is clear that this endogenous repair process is unable to overcome the devastating damage to brain tissue that occurs after acute, severe stroke. Cell-based therapies have the potential to open up new avenues of treatment in this arena. Targets for stem cell therapy include neuroprotective approaches aimed at protecting at-risk tissue during the acute phase of stroke, as well as neuroreparative approaches which may involve direct replacement of damaged brain tissue, or alternatively promotion of the brain's endogenous repair processes.

Introduction

Stem cells (SCs) are characterized by self-renewability, i.e., the ability to divide themselves rapidly and continuously and to create new SCs and progenitors more differentiated than the mother cells. SCs show high plasticity, i.e., the ability to transform into cells from various different tissues. The plasticity can be explained by trans-differentiation (direct or indirect) and fusion. Trans-differentiation is the acquisition of the identity of a different phenotype through the expression of the gene pattern of other tissue. By fusion with a cell of another tissue, a SC can express a gene from that cell and acquire a phenotypic element of another tissue (Zhonw W 2008, Fortier LA 2005). In the human body, adult stem cells (ASCs) maintain the tissue homeostasis. ASCs usually differentiate in a restricted range (multi-potent) of progenitors and terminal cells to replace old and damaged cells.SCs derived from early human embryos (Embryonic stem cells (ESCs)), on the other hand, are pluri-potent and can generate all committed cell types (Perra MF 2000, Pessina A 2006). Fetal stem cells (FSCs) derive from the placenta, membranes, amniotic fluid or fetal tissues.

Today living in the 21st century, we still do not have proper treatments for many neurological diseases like Parkinson's disease, Alzheimer's disease, etc. Some light of hope for the treatment of these incurable diseases is - the stem cells. Stem cells are a special kind of cell that has the ability to divide indefinitely and have the potential to give rise to specialized cells (that is, any cell of the body). All stem cells regardless of their source have three general properties

- They are capable of dividing and renewing themselves for long periods
- They are unspecialized
- They can give rise to specialized cell types

Stem cells are capable of dividing and renewing themselves for long periods. Unlike muscle cells, blood cells, or nerve cells—which do not normally replicate themselves—stem cells may replicate many times, or proliferate. A starting population of stem cells that proliferates for many months in the laboratory can yield millions of cells. If the resulting cells continue to be unspecialized, like the parent stem cells, the cells are said to be capable of long-term self-renewal.

Broadly speaking, clinical approaches to stem cell therapy can be divided into “endogenous” and “exogenous” approaches:

1) The endogenous approach aims to stimulate mobilization of stem cells already present within the individual. Examples of this approach include the use of granulocyte-colony stimulating factor (G-CSF) used to mobilize hematopoietic stem cells into the peripheral blood. G-CSF use has been shown to have both neuroprotective as well as neuroregenerative properties, (Shabitz WR 2003, Shyu WC 2004) and additionally appears to have direct effects beyond simply mobilization of stem cells.
2) The exogenous approach involves transplantation of the patient with stem cells delivered locally (e.g, direct intracerebral implantation) or systemically (e.g., intravenous or intra-arterial) and may involve in vitro culture of cells for the

expansion of cell numbers prior to administration. There is a large body of preclinical data and now mounting data from clinical trials that have utilized exogenous approaches to stem cell therapy for stroke. In this chapter, we will discuss these, and the challenges posed in translating this therapy to the bedside, in more detail. Of note, the vast majority of work has focused on ischemic rather than hemorrhagic stroke, and therefore we refer to data from ischemic stroke studies, unless stated otherwise.

Stem Cell Therapy in Stroke Patients: The Challenges

Significant advances have been made in the field of stem cell therapy for stroke, and the potential benefits of such treatments are vast. However, several important questions remain unanswered, and translation to the bedside remains distant. The important areas of uncertainty are discussed below.

Table 1. Showing the Potency of Stem Cells

Stem Cell Type	Description	Examples
Totipotent	Each cell can develop into a new individual	Cells from early (Morula) (1-3 days) embryos
Pluripotent	Cells can vary form any (over 200) cell types	Some cells of blastocyst (5 to 14 days)
Miltipotent	Cells differentiated, but can form a number of other tissues	Fetal tissue, cord blood, and adult stem sells
Oligopotent	Cells differentiated, but can give rise to few different cells	Lymphoid and myeloid stem cells
Unipotent	Cells can give rise to their own type only	Mucles stem cells

Which Stem Cells Should Be Used?

Stem cells can be defined as clonogenic cells that have the capacity to self-renew and differentiate into multiple cell lineages (Weissman II 1998). The two major types of stem cells, as classified by source, are embryonic stem cells (ESCs) and adult stem cells (Figure 2). Human ESCs are pluripotent and are isolated from 5-day-old human blastocysts. However, several factors limit the widespread use of ESCs. These include ethical concerns regarding the use of unwanted embryos and concerns regarding tumorigenicity, specifically the risk of teratoma formation in vivo (Thomson JA 1998). In contrast to ESCs, adult stem cells are multipotent stem cells that can be obtained from adults as well as children, including from umbilical cord blood. They are present within various organs, including the brain and bone marrow, and have the advantage of being suitable for autologous as well as allogeneic use. Of note, one disadvantage of these cells is that they have less differentiation potential than ESCs.

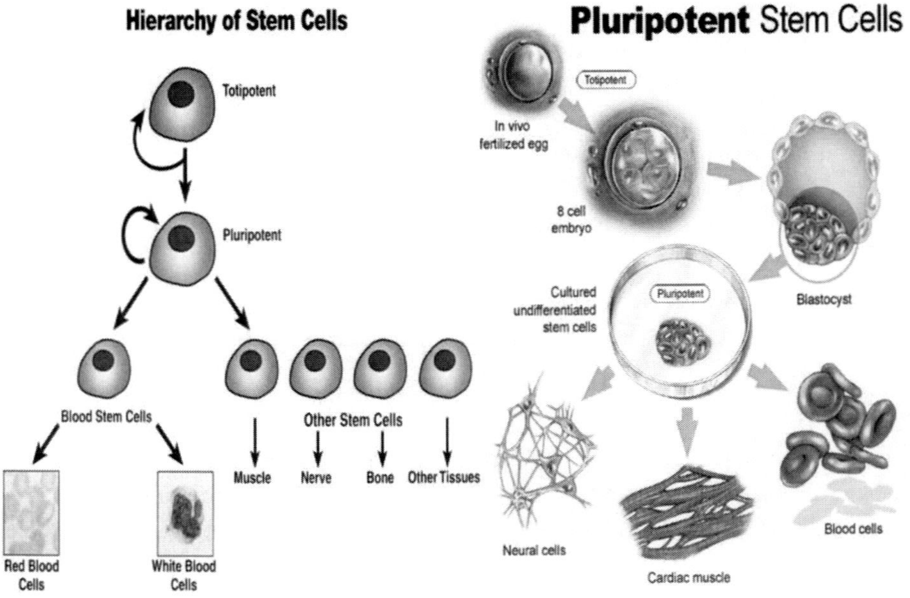

Figure 1. Stem cells can give rise to any cell type in the body. All stem cells, regardless of their source have three general properties: they are capable of dividing and renewing themselves for long periods; they are unspecialized; and they can give rise to specialized cell types.

A number of different types of stem cells, obtained from different sources, have been shown to improve clinical and radiological outcomes in preclinical models of stroke. The choice of cell type for clinical trial use should consider not only efficacy, but also ease of obtaining the cells, issues regarding cell culture for expansion, the need for immunosuppression and questions regarding dosage. A number of autologous and allogeneic cells have been tested in the preclinical arena. Issues specific to autologous cells include questions regarding extraction of consistent, adequate numbers of cells, as well as potency of the cells obtained (e.g., potency may fall with the age of the donor). Allogeneic cells must have the capacity for expansion to provide adequate numbers for widespread use, while ethical issues regarding the source will also need to be considered when using ESCs or fetal tissue, as previously mentioned. Cell-culturing techniques used for autologous or allogeneic cells will need to be consistent and adhere to strict safety criteria (good manufacturing practice). Long-term biological safety of any cell-based therapy is a further area of great importance. There is therefore a host of factors to consider when deciding which cell type is best to use. The different types of cells tested in preclinical studies are discussed in more detail below.

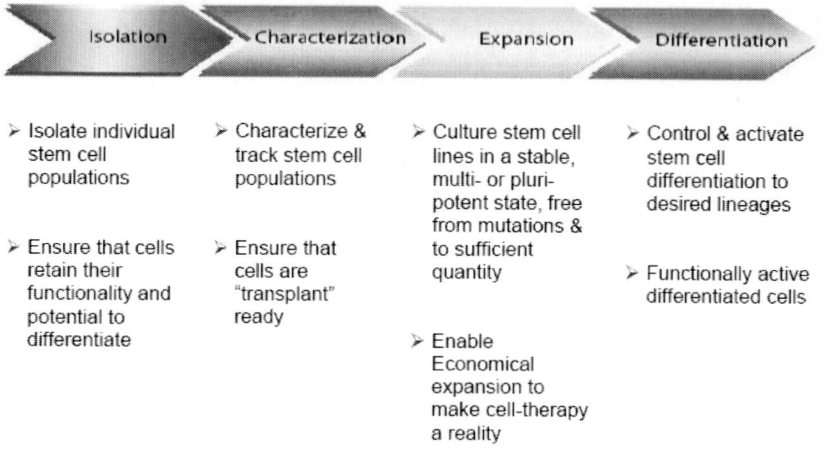

(A)

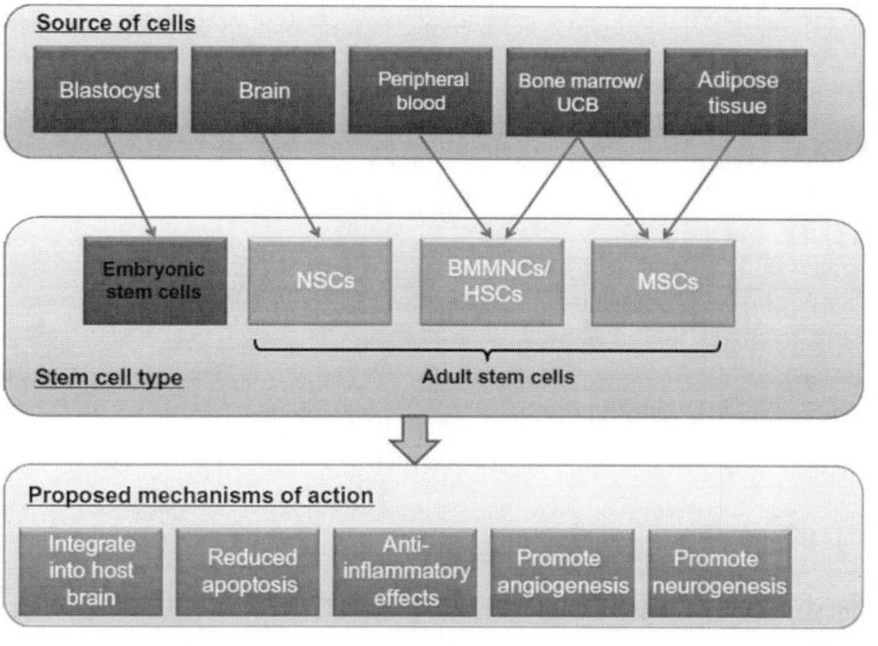

(B)

Abbreviations: UCB, umbilical cord blood; NSC, neuronal stem cell; BMMNC, bone marrow mononuclear cell; HSC, hematopoietic stem cell; MSC, mesenchymal stem cell.

Figure 2. A) Stages in using Stem cells for Therapeutic Use. B) Stem cell types used in stroke trials, and the proposed mechanisms of action.

Neural Stem/Progenitor Cells

Neural stem cells (NSCs) have the capacity to differentiate into neurons, astrocytes, and oligodendrocytes. There are a wide variety of sources of exogenous neural stem cells, with much work being done on transplantation of embryonic and fetal-derived NSCs in experimental stroke models (Chu K 2003, and 2004Jeong SW 2003, Kelly S 2004, Hicks AU 2009) However, the use of such embryonic or fetal tissue is limited by ethicolegal implications, in addition to important biological questions regarding the long-term risk of teratoma formation by ESCs. The emergence of induced pluripotency, whereby skin fibroblasts from patients can be transformed into ESC-like cells, may overcome the ethical issues of using fetal or embryonic tissue in future studies, while also providing a source of autologous cells, thereby removing any questions regarding immune rejection (Takashi K 2006 and 2007, Yu J 2007).

Neural stem cells derived from the adult central nervous system are a possible alternative source of cells for transplantation. Studies have documented the isolation of NSCs from the adult rodent brain (Wachs FP 2003) as well as (more recently) the adult human brain (Nunes MC 2003). One study demonstrated that adult NSCs derived from the subventricular zone of young adult rats could survive and migrate towards the lesion in rats with an ischemic stroke following intracisternal administration (Zheng ZG 2003). Electron microscopy examination also suggested that the transplanted cells showed signs of neuronal differentiation.

Although possible in principle, brain biopsies for isolation of adult human NSCs and autologous transplantation poststroke is technically difficult, and no clinical trials utilizing adult NSCs have been undertaken. A number of human immortalized cell lines have been shown to improve functional outcomes after experimental stroke in rodent models. These cell lines have the advantage of providing an abundant source of cells for transplantation, available ready-prepared, at the time of a stroke. Biological safety of such cell lines, however, remains a concern in the long term.

The immortalized cell line NTera-2 (NT2) was derived from a human teratocarcinoma (Andrews PW 1984). After several weeks' exposure to retinoic acid and mitotic inhibitors, these cells differentiate into postmitotic neuron-like cells, named NT2N cells (also known as hNT neurones).23 Terminal differentiation of these cells only occurs following transplantation into an adult brain.24 The transplantation of NT2N cells into the ipsilateral striatum of ischemic rat brains improved functional recovery, with some parameters of behavioral improvement persisting for up to 6 months post-transplantation (Klepner SR 1995, Borlongan CV 1995).

No evidence of tumorigenicity was found following post-mortem examination of the rats. The CTX0E03 cell line developed by ReNeuron (Guildford, UK) is a fetally derived multipotent neural stem cell line that is conditionally immortalized with c-myc-ER, such that proliferation only occurs in the presence of the drug 4-hydroxy-tamoxifen (Stromer P 2008). It has been shown to effect a dose-dependent improvement in sensorimotor function in rodent models of middle cerebral artery ischemic stroke when delivered intracerebrally (Taguchi A 2004).

Hematopoietic Stem/Progenitor Cells

Hematopoietic stem cells (HSCs) can be obtained from bone marrow, peripheral blood, or umbilical cord blood. The advantage of such cells is that they are suitable for both autologous as well as allogeneic use, and furthermore are not associated with the ethical issues surrounding ESC or fetally derived stem cells. It is contentious whether these cells can differentiate into neuronal cells. However, preclinical studies of CD34+ cells have shown significant benefits in rodent models of stroke, with evidence of functional improvement as well as reduced infarct volume. Potential disadvantages of these cells include issues with consistency of numbers and potency of cells obtained from the bone marrow, as well as the need for ex vivo expansion of cells, when using umbilical cord blood as the source.

In one study, CD34+ cell transplantation delivered intravenously resulted in increased perilesional angiogenesis and subsequent neurogenesis in mice at 48 hours poststroke (Taguchi A 2004). A further study investigating direct intracerebral implantation of CD34+ cells 1 week after induced stroke was also able to show evidence of neurogenesis and angiogenesis, with differentiation of transplanted cells into cells expressing markers for neurons, glial cells, and vascular endothelial cells (Shyu WC 2006).

Mesenchymal Stem Cells

Mesenchymal stem cells (MSCs), also known as bone marrow stromal cells, can be obtained from bone marrow as well as such other sources as adipose tissue. As with HSCs, they are suitable for autologous as well as allogeneic use. One disadvantage of this cell type is the requirement for several weeks of cell culture to generate sufficient numbers, thereby making the use of autologous MSCs in the acute phase of stroke an unviable option.

These cells have shown significant functional benefits in rodent models of stroke in the acute as well as chronic setting (up to 1 months poststroke) and when delivered by a variety of routes (intravenous, intra-arterial and intracerebral) (Chen J 2001, Shen LH 2007, Li Y 2001). The mechanism of improvement remains unclear, though promotion of endogenous neurogenesis, reduction of apoptosis, and induction of angiogenesis have been demonstrated in different studies (Chen J 2003).

Bone Marrow Mononuclear Cells (BMMNCs)

Mononuclear cells obtained from bone marrow contain populations of both mesenchymal and hematopoietic stem cells. They have been shown to reduce neurological deficits as well as infarct size in animal models of stroke (Brenneman 2010, Giraldi-Guimareas A 2009). These cells are easy to obtain from bone marrow, and are suitable for autologous and allogeneic use. Transplantation with HSCs (CD34+ cells) or MSCs provides purer, more concentrated cell populations, though BMMNCs have the advantage of being easier to prepare and separate from bone marrow, making them theoretically more practical, particularly in the acute setting. As with HSCs, there are issues with obtaining consistent numbers of cells from bone marrow aspiration and questions regarding the potency of cells, particularly in older patients (Li TS 2009). Potential mechanisms of action include paracrine effects secreting trophic factors (such as vascular endothelial growth factor (VEGF) and stromal cell–derived factor-1), as well as possible immunomodulatory benefits (Sharma S 2010).

Mechanism of Action of Stem Cell Therapy

The possible mechanisms of stem cell therapy include the formation of neuronal cavity, reduced apoptosis, promotion of angiogenesis and reduced inflammation. Elucidation of potential mechanisms of action is vital to the further development of stem cell therapy techniques and ultimately translation to the bedside. There are a number of proposed mechanisms that have been investigated in preclinical stroke models (Figure 1). There is very little evidence that adult stem cells integrate into the ischemic brain and form functional neurons with adequate synaptic connections. Most studies have shown very limited numbers of engrafted cells, with functional benefits in excess of what would be expected based on the degree of engraftment. Following an ischemic stroke, neurons and glia die by a mixture of necrosis and apoptosis. Cell transplantation may elicit a neuroprotective response by rescuing the apoptotic cells, particularly in penumbral tissue. This is likely to be mediated by the secretion and upregulation of certain trophins, such as basic fibroblast growth factor, brain-derived neurotrophic factor, VEGF, glial cell-line-derived factor, and nerve growth factor. Several studies have suggested that a reduction in apoptosis in the ischemic boundary area occurs following cellular therapy that is associated with improved neurological recovery in experimental models (Kurozumi K 2005, Llado J 2004). Immunomodulatory effects of transplanted cells may have a role in neuroprotection. Preclinical studies have shown evidence of upregulation of anti-inflammatory cytokines and attenuation of expression of proinflammatory cytokines in both ischemic and hemorrhagic stroke (Lee ST 2008, Jiang Q 2005). If an anti-inflammatory effect is to play an important role, delivery of the cells will need to be in the early stages of the stroke. Following a stroke, regenerative strategies should be aimed at not only restoration of neural elements, but also supporting structures such as blood vessels. Angiogenesis have been demonstrated after cell transplantation with various stem cells, including NSCs, CD34+ cells and MSCs. Direct incorporation of the transplanted cells into new blood vessels has also been demonstrated. However, more likely mechanisms of action include the release of VEGF and also the increase in endogenous levels of other factors (such as brain-derived neurotrophic factor and fibroblast growth factor) that play a role in neovascularization (Jiang Q 2005, Cheng X 2011).

Promotion of Neurogenesis and Other Endogenous Repair Processes by Stem Cell Therapy

Endogenous neurogenesis is increased per se after a stroke, likely reflecting an intrinsic host-repair mechanism (Arvidissson A 2002). Administration of cord blood cells and mesenchymal cells have been reported to enhance endogenous neurogenesis, (Nakatomi H 2002) although whether this is likely to be functionally significant is still unclear. It is possible that transplantation of various stem cells may amplify endogenous plasticity responses, again mediated by the secretion of trophic factors. One study suggested that intracarotid administration of MSCs facilitated host neuronal and synaptic plasticity, with increased synaptophysin expression in the ischemic penumbra (Shen LH 2006). Furthermore, axonal sprouting from the nonischemic to the contralateral hemisphere was observed following the intravenous administration of human cord blood cells (Xia J 2005).

Other stem/progenitor cells are also increased following cerebral ischemia. Under physiological conditions, a relatively small pool of CD34+ stem/progenitor cells circulates in the peripheral blood. An Ischemic stroke is known to increase levels of CD34+ cells (mobilized from the bone marrow) in the peripheral blood (Paczkowaska E 2005). In addition, there is evidence that increased CD34+ mobilisation into the peripheral blood in patients with acute ischemic stroke correlates with neurological recovery, with high counts associated with better recovery (Dunac A 2007). Treatment with G-CSF, for example, which mobilizes CD34+ cells into the peripheral circulation, may potentially enhance this endogenous repair mechanism.

Benefits of Stem Cell Therapy to Patients

A crucial question for upcoming clinical trials is which patients will benefit from stem cell therapy. The pathological type and anatomical location of the stroke are important issues, which are discussed in more detail below. In addition, demographic differences, in particular differences in age and gender, are also likely to affect how patients respond to treatment.54 The vast majority of preclinical work has been conducted on young, previously healthy, male animals. Elderly patients, who represent the largest subset of stroke victims, may not derive the same benefit as that seen in such animal studies. As stated previously, the majority of preclinical work has focused on ischemic rather than hemorrhagic strokes. In view of this, the ongoing and completed clinical trials have almost exclusively concentrated on ischemic stroke patients. Of the published clinical trials to date, only one has included any patients with hemorrhagic strokes (Kondziolka D 2005).

Within the ischemic stroke subgroup, the majority of preclinical evidence for benefit has been obtained from animal models with predominantly striatal infarcts. A smaller number of trials have investigated cortical models of stroke, with mixed results (Hicks AU 2008). Cortical strokes are associated with larger, more damaging infarcts, and it may be that these are too large to affect any repair. A direct comparison between subcortical and cortical infarcts in addition to various doses of cells would be useful in order to optimize patient selection. For example, one preclinical study that compared anatomical location found the benefit of stem cell therapy to be more pronounced in striatal infarcts, rather than larger cortical lesions (Smith EJ 2012). Further issues to consider when designing clinical trials are stability of patients and associated comorbidities. Patients with larger strokes are commonly medically unwell due to multiple reasons (e.g., aspiration pneumonia, cardiac arrhythmias), which could preclude them from entry into acute trials despite being eligible. Furthermore, multiple comorbidities are also likely to affect the response of the patient to stem cell therapy.

Optimal Timing for Treatment

Preclinical studies have shown benefits of stem cell therapy in both acute and chronic models of stroke. Decisions regarding the ideal timing need to take into account the likely mechanism of action. A neuroprotective mechanism would require acute delivery, although graft survival may be affected by the damaging effects of ischemia and reperfusion, mediated via excitotoxic neurotransmitters, free radicals, and other inflammatory mediators (Mitsiosis N 2006). If the aim is to enhance endogenous repair mechanisms and inhibit neuronal apoptosis, then acute or subacute delivery would be desirable, as these processes occur predominantly in the first few weeks postischemia (Hayashi T 2003). A neuroreparative approach aiming for direct replacement of damaged tissue with new neuronal circuitry (using intracerebral transplantation), would benefit from a later timescale, once neuroinflammation has subsided. Such a strategy would be looking at treatment delivered weeks to months after the stroke, in keeping with ongoing host plasticity during that time.

Future studies will need to address questions regarding timing, with direct comparisons between acute and chronic delivery. One animal study demonstrated significant neurological improvements with intravenous injection of BMMNCs at 24 and 72 hours, poststroke but showed no improvement in animals treated at 7 days poststroke (Yang B 2011). Other studies comparing acute to chronic delivery of cells have shown conflicting results, though there were important differences between these trials in terms of the cells used, animal model, and exact timing of transplantation. (Grabowski M 1994, Darsalia V 2011) Such comparative data is sparse in the preclinical arena and sorely lacking in the clinical arena, and at present the optimal timing of treatment is yet to be determined.

Delivery Route of Stem Cells

Studies in the preclinical and clinical settings have used a variety of different routes of stem cell delivery, illustrating the point that the best delivery method remains unclear. Benefits have been seen using direct intracerebral implantation as well as systemic delivery using the intravenous and intra-arterial routes. Intracerebral implantation allows direct delivery of cells to the affected site, but is invasive and may present issues of disrupting the underlying brain tissue. Use of a general anesthetic for intracerebral delivery, particularly in the acute stroke patient, is problematic, though alternatively a local anesthetic can be used. The intravenous route is the safest, easiest route of delivery, though there are issues regarding accumulation of cells in nontarget organs, with only a small proportion reaching the brain (Fisher UM 2009). The size of the cells used is important in this regard. The intra-arterial route allows more direct delivery of cells, allowing better first-pass delivery while being less invasive than direct surgical implantation.

Decisions regarding the route of delivery will need to take into account issues regarding the practicality and safety, as well as cell type/dosage and proposed mechanism of action. The best route of delivery is yet to be determined, and there is a paucity of preclinical data comparing the different available delivery methods. One study of ischemic stroke in rats compared intravenous to intra-arterial delivery of neural progenitor cells. Their data showed a superior cell delivery to the ischemic hemisphere, with the intra-arterial route (Lappalainen RS 2008). However, as mentioned previously, all three modes of delivery have clearly shown benefits in different preclinical studies, which raise the question: is it necessary for cells to enter the brain to have their beneficial effect? More well-designed trials are needed to directly compare different routes of delivery using standardized criteria, in order to help answer these vital questions.

How Can Transplanted Cells Be Tracked?

Tracking of cells is paramount to improving our understanding of cell migration and mechanisms of action. Currently there is no ideal method of doing this, with the techniques available being suboptimal for a number of reasons.

One commonly employed tracking method in preclinical studies is cell labeling with superparamagnetic iron oxide particles, which allows the anatomical location of transplanted cells to be determined using magnetic resonance imaging (MRI) (Bulte JW 2002). Other examples of imaging modalities used to track labeled cells include positron emission tomography (PET), bioluminescence imaging (BLI), and single-photon-emission computed tomography (SPECT) (Love Z 2007). One drawback of many cell-labeling techniques is the difficulty tracing the labeled cells when they divide, either due to failure of uptake of the label or the presence of a weaker signal in the new cells. In addition, if the cell dies and is phagocytosed by macrophages, any signal received will be misleading (MrColgan P 2011). BLI overcomes this issue, as it picks up luminescence signals emitted from living cells. However, one of the concerns with BLI is poor spatial resolution, an important drawback of this modality (Bliss T 2010).

To date, only one clinical trial of stem cell therapy in stroke patients has investigated the role of tracking the transplanted cells. A study of BMMNCs labelled with technetium-99m (99mTc) looked at cell homing and uptake using whole-body scintigraphy and SPECT scans (Barbossa LM 2010). They confirmed the presence of cells in the brain at 2 hours, as well as distributed to the liver, lungs, spleen, kidneys, and bladder. Furthermore, preferential accumulation of radioactivity was seen in the ipsilateral affected hemisphere (compared to the contralateral hemisphere) in all patients at 2 hours postinfusion. In addition to tracking cells, imaging modalities are also required to evaluate the functional outcome of transplanted cells. Diffusion-weighted MR studies can be used to assess for neovascularization, PET scanning to assess metabolic changes, diffusion-tensor imaging to assess fiber-tract integrity, and functional MRI to assess neuroplasticity. It is likely, therefore, that a combination of imaging modalities will eventually be required to give a better overall assessment of the fate of transplanted cells, in order to further the understanding of their mechanisms of action.

Stem Cell Therapy in Stroke Patients: Clinical Trials

Clinical trials of stem cell therapy in stroke patients are still in their infancy. There have been a number of recent phase I/II trials, primarily investigating the role in ischemic stroke patients. However, these trials have not clearly defined the best cell type, route of delivery, or timing of therapy, and more coordinated research is needed to better answer these uncertainties.

The majority of preclinical work has focused on treatment in the acute or subacute phases of stroke. In contrast, all the early clinical trials have concentrated on chronic stroke patients. There is certainly preclinical evidence pointing to benefit in the chronic subgroup. In addition, patients are more stable and chronic delivery occurs well after the acute inflammatory response has subsided. There are now an emerging number of acute human trials that have also been completed. Reasons for acute delivery of cells have been discussed previously. It is important to note that the pathophysiological processes and proposed mechanisms of action in the acute phase are quite different to the chronic phase of stroke, and it is not possible to extrapolate data gleaned from one setting to the other. Future studies will need to address questions regarding the ideal timing of transplantation.

The currently available clinical trial data utilizing human stem cells will be discussed further, as well as a discussion on ongoing trials, of which there are now several scattered across different centers worldwide.

Chronic Stroke Trials

NT2N Cells

NT2N were the first human cells to be tested in stroke clinical trials. A phase I trial examined the safety of direct stereotactic transplantation of cells into patients with basal ganglia stroke that had occurred 6 months to 6 years previously (Kondziolka D 200). Twelve patients with stable motor deficits were treated, along with an immunosuppressive regimen of cyclosporine-A due to the allogeneic nature of the treatment. Two doses of cells were used: 2 × 106 and 6 × 106 cells. There was a trend towards improved functional outcomes in the four patients who received the higher dose of cells. Autopsy on one patient, who died of myocardial infarction 27 months post-transplantation, showed apparent survival of NT2N cells in the brain. Furthermore, PET scans at 6 months post-transplantation showed increased metabolic activity at the site of infarct in six patients (Nelson PT 2002). This initial safety trial led to a phase II study assessing the effect of NT2N cell transplantation in 18 patients with a basal ganglia stroke between 1 and 6 years previously. Stereotactic cellular transplantation plus two months of rehabilitation (n = 14) was compared to control patients who received rehabilitation alone (n = 4). Six of the 14 patients who received a transplant appeared to show improvement on a standardized stroke scale, but this was not statistically significant against control patients. Of note, this trial included ischemic (n = 9) and hemorrhagic strokes (n = 9).

Mesenchymal Stem Cells

The extensive preclinical work on MSCs described previously led to a phase I/II clinical trial using autologous culture-expanded MSCs in patients with ischemic middle cerebral artery (MCA)- territory stroke.75 Thirty patients with established stroke (1 month postinfarct) were randomized to receive MSCs by the intravenous route (n = 5) or no MSCs (n = 15). Cells were extracted by bone marrow aspiration and culture-expanded prior to infusion. There was no cell-related toxicity related to the MSC administration, and the authors suggested that functional improvement may have been better in the transplanted group compared with the control group, although this was not statistically significant. There were no significant differences between the two groups in relation to changes in infarct volume at 1-year follow-up. Following on from this study, the same group conducted a trial looking at the long-term (5-year) effects of MSC transplantation in patients with severe MCA-territory stroke (Lee JS 2010). Sixteen patients (versus 36 controls) were treated with intravenous delivered, autologous, culture-expanded MSCs. There was no difference in adverse events between the two groups. Functional outcome appeared to be better in the treated group, with a significantly increased proportion of patients with a modified Rankin score of 0–3, compared to the controls.

A further trial of autologous MSCs administered in ischemic stroke patients, within 6 months of their event, was recently reported (Honmou O 2011). Cells were delivered intravenously 36–133 days poststroke in an open-label study of 12 patients. MSCs were serum-expanded prior to infusion. The treatment was shown to be safe and feasible, with no significant adverse events. Furthermore, mean infarct volume as assessed by MRI was reduced by .20% at 1 week postinfusion. Of note, the culturing conditions and media were different between the two MSC trials described above.

Bone Marrow Mononuclear Cells

Two trials utilizing BMMNCs have been reported in chronic stroke patients. One open-label study treated six male patients with the MCA-territory ischemic stroke within 90 days of the event.78 Autologous BMMNCs were isolated after bone marrow aspiration. The cells were then delivered intra-arterially, with a proportion of these labeled with 99mTc. There were no treatment-related adverse events up to 6 months follow-up. Evidence was seen of cell migration in the brain at 2 hours postinfusion in all six patients, though at 24 hours this number had dropped to two patients (Barbosa LM 2010). All patients showed improvements in their National Institutes of Health Stroke Scale scores by 6 months. In a separate study, autologous bone marrow stem cells obtained by bone marrow aspiration were transplanted stereotactically in five patients with established stroke (Saurez C 2009). The procedure was well tolerated, with no adverse events up to 1 year follow-up.

Ongoing Chronic Trials

There are at least ten other ongoing or completed trials in chronic (4 weeks post event) stroke patients that are yet to report. Details of these unreported trials are listed in Table 5.2. A number of different cell types at different time points and via different methods of delivery are being tested. These include allogeneic cells, such as the CTX0E03 neural stem cell line, which has been discussed previously.

Such commercially developed cell lines, if shown to be beneficial, are an exciting prospect owing to the ability to develop them for "off the shelf" use, available ready-prepared at the time of a stroke. The results of these various trials are awaited with interest, though it is clear to see that meaningful comparisons between the different trials will be difficult to make, and how far these trials will go towards answering the outstanding questions in this field is difficult to say.

Table 2. Summary of ongoing or completed (but unreported) chronic stroke trials

Cell type	Study design	Expected no of patients	Timing of delivery post stroke	Route of delivery	Clinical trial identifier	Trial status
Chronic trials (4 weeks post event)						
CTX0E03 neural stem cells	PI, NR-OL	12	6 months–5 years	IC	NCT01151124	Recruiting
MSCs	PII, R-OL	30	,6 weeks	IV	NCT00875654	Recruiting
CD34+	PII, R-OL	30	6–60 months	IC	NCT00950521	Complete
CD34+	PI, NR-OL	6	6–60 months	IC	NCT01438593	Not yet recruiting
CD34+	PI, R-OL	40	,1 year	IA	NCT01518231	Recruiting
MSCs, EPCs	PI/II, R-DB	90	5 weeks	IV	NCT01468064	Recruiting
MSCs	PII, R-OL	50	1 week–2 months	IV	NCT01461720	Recruiting
MSCs	PI/II, NR-OL	35	.6 months	IV	NCT01297413	Recruiting
SB623	PI/II, NR-OL	18	6–36 months	Unclear	NCT01287936	Recruiting
OECs	PI, R-SB	6	6 months–5 years	IC	NCT01327768	Recruiting

Note: CTX0E03 and SB623 are commercially developed stem cell lines.

Abbreviations: BMMNC, bone marrow mononuclear cells; MSCs, mesenchymal stem cells; OECs, olfactory ensheathing cells; EPCs, endothelial progenitor cells; NR, nonrandomized; OL, open-label; PI and II, phase I and II trials; R, randomized; SB, single-blind; DB, double-blind; IV, intravenous; IA, intra-arterial; IC, intracerebral.

Acute Stroke Trials

Bone Marrow Mononuclear Cells

There are currently three published trials of stem cell therapy in acute stroke patients. All three trials utilized BMMNCs and were able to demonstrate safety and feasibility in the treated subjects. One study treated ischemic stroke (MCA territory) patients at 24–72 hours post event with intravenously delivered cells (Friedrich M 2012). Ten patients were treated in an open-label study, with no evidence of study-related serious adverse events up to 6 months follow-up. All patients had shifted down by at least 1 point on the modified Rankin Scale (mRS) at 6 months compared to at day 7. The second study (also open-label) treated 20 patients with MCA-territory ischemic stroke at 3–7 days post event, with the cells delivered intra-arterially (Friedrich M 2010). There were no procedure-related adverse events reported up to 6 months follow-up. A good outcome (defined as an mRS of #2) was seen in eight of the 20 patients at 90 days. The third, most recently published trial treated ten patients with BMMNCs delivered intra-arterially at 5–9 days after stroke (Monichie F 2012). This was a single-blind, controlled study (ten consecutive controls; nonrandomized). Two of the treated patients had isolated partial seizures at 3 months. There were no significant differences in neurological outcome between the two groups at final 180-day follow-up. None of these trials were powered to demonstrate efficacy.

Ongoing Acute/Subacute Trials

A further six acute/subacute trials (4 weeks poststroke) are ongoing or yet to report (Table 5.3). As with the chronic stroke trials, these are utilizing a variety of different cell types, including BMMNCs, CD34+ cells, and MSCs, as well as commercially developed stem cell lines. We have investigated the use of intra-arterially delivered CD34+ cells in patients with severe MCA-territory ischemic stroke, recruited within 7 days of the event (ClinicalTrials.gov identifier NCT00535197).

To date, no trial has reported on the effects of immunoselected CD34+ cells for acute or chronic ischemic stroke. Such cells have been shown to improve functional outcome and infarct size in preclinical models. Furthermore, a recently published trial of BMMNC treatment of acute ischemic stroke showed a trend towards a positive correlation between number of CD34+ cells injected and functional outcome at 1 month (Monichie F 2012). We have demonstrated safety and feasibility in our patient cohort, as well as improvements in clinical scores and functional status at 6-month follow-up (unpublished data). Of the other ongoing studies, one is investigating the use of MSCs in hemorrhagic as well as ischemic strokes.

This will be of interest, as the use of stem cells for hemorrhagic stroke has not been well investigated in the clinical arena. It must be borne in mind however, that the underlying pathophysiological processes at play and therefore the mechanisms of recovery are quite different between these subtypes of stroke. The completed results of these various trials are eagerly awaited.

Table 3. Summary of ongoing or completed (but unreported) acute/subacute stroke trials

Cell type	Study design	Expected no of patients	Timing of delivery poststroke	Route of delivery	Clinical trialidentifier	Trial status
Acute and subacute trials (,4 weeks postevent)						
BMMNC	PII, R-OL	120	7–30 days	IV	NCT01501773	Complete
MSCs	PII, NR-OL	120	7–14 days (infarct)or 10–21 days (ICH)	IV, then intrathecal 7 days later	NCT01389453	Recruiting
CD34+	PI/II, NR-OL	10	7 days	IA	NCT00535197	Recruiting
MSCs	PI/II, R-DB	78	,10 days	IV	NCT01091701	Not yet recruiting
MultiStem	PII, R-DB	140	1–2 days	IV	NCT01436487	Recruiting
ALD-401	PI/II, R-DB	100	13–19 days	IA	NCT01273337	Recruiting

Note: MultiStem and ALD-401 are commercially developed stem cell lines.

Abbreviations: BMMNC, bone marrow mononuclear cells; MSCs, mesenchymal stem cells; OECs, olfactory ensheathing cells; EPCs, endothelial progenitor cells; NR, nonrandomized; OL, open-label; PI and II, phase I and II trials; R, randomized; SB, single-blind; DB, double-blind; IV, intravenous; IA, intra-arterial; IC, intracerebral; ICH, intracerebral hemorrhage.

Table 4. Stroke Therapy Academic Industry Roundtable (STAIR) II recommendations

Considerations for designing phase IIb stroke trials
• Route of administration
• Dose range
• Duration of treatment
• Time from stroke onset to initiation of treatment (a key variable)
• Pharmacokinetic profile
• Side effects and their frequency (with attention to side-effect management)
• Interactions with other commonly used medications
• Drug distribution to the proposed site of action
• Refinement and identification of the target population (e.g, drugs without preclinical evidence of activity in white-matter ischemia should not be studied in patients with subcortical stroke or even large cortical events with attendant subcortical injury)
• Obtain evidential measurement of therapeutic activity by evaluation of clinical and/or surrogate markers (hints of potential effectiveness)

Adapted from Stroke Therapy Academic Industry Roundtable II (STAIR-II). Recommendations for clinical trial evaluation of acute stroke therapies. *Stroke*. 2001;32:1598–1606.83.

Note: Important factors relevant to stem cell therapy *underlined.*

Table 5. Stem Cell Therapies as an Emerging Paradigm in Stroke (STEPS) recommendations

Considerations for animal and human testing of cellular therapy
Mechanism of action
• Trophic factors
• Cell replacement
• Local environment support
• Other
Pathological substrate
• Ischemic versus hemorrhagic
• Peri-infarct versus intra-infarct
Location of pathology
• Cortical versus subcortical
• Brain stem
Timing after stroke
• Acute
• Subacute, chronic

Adapted from Stem Cell Therapies as an Emerging Paradigm in Stroke participants. Stem Cell Therapies as an Emerging Paradigm in Stroke (STEPS): bridging basic and clinical science for cellular and neurogenic factor therapy in treating stroke. *Stroke*. 2009;40:510–515.85.

The Future

Routine use of stem cells at the bedside for stroke patients is an exciting prospect, though realistically remains a long way off. The future may well see the availability of "off-the shelf" stem cell products available for immediate use. Perhaps patients will receive individually tailored stem cell products, engineered to secrete specific trophic factors, to suit their specific subtype and duration of stroke. There is clearly a long way to go in both preclinical and clinical research, and long-term biosafety measures will be an essential consideration in this regard.

A number of clinical trials have now begun to demonstrate the safety and feasibility of different approaches to stem cell therapy. However, there are a large number of unanswered questions that remain. The great variation in the stem cell trials completed to date means that it is difficult to make any meaningful comparisons between them. Future clinical trials will need to start trying to address the important outstanding questions. It is imperative that trials are therefore designed with this in mind. Careful planning and collaborative work need to take place in order to maximize the likelihood of getting a useful answer from these studies. This includes such considerations as incorporation of a dose-escalation design and comparisons between different methods of delivery as well as different time points for delivery. The Stroke Therapy Academic Industry Roundtable (STAIR) II meeting elucidated the important considerations when designing future phase IIb studies. Many of these recommendations are particularly relevant to the field of stem cell research (see Figure 2; important factors highlighted). They emphasized that "lack of establishing the optimal dose, duration of therapy, and time window may have contributed to the failure of neuroprotection trials." Therefore, refinement and identification of the target population is essential. In addition, narrowing selection criteria in phase IIb studies to target patients more likely to respond based on clinical and imaging characteristics may optimize the chances of detecting a biologically relevant drug effect (STAIR IV recommendations). Subsequent to these public cations, the Stem Cell Therapies as an Emerging Paradigm in Stroke (STEPS) meeting sought to develop a framework specifically to help guide design of future preclinical and clinical studies in the field of cell-based therapies (STEPS 2009). These recommendations from experts from the preclinical and clinical arenas should be carefully borne in mind before commencing any future trials.

In conclusion, there have been significant advances made in the field of stem cell research over the last two decades, with evidence of significant benefits in both acute and chronic animal models of stroke. Translation to clinical practice, however, remains a long way off. A number of trials are under way, though future work will need to concentrate on overcoming the still-significant challenges standing in the way of this becoming a realistic treatment option for the future.

Sources of Transplant Cells

Stem cells must possess two characteristics: they must be able to replicate and they must have the capacity for differentiation into multiple cell lines (Preston SL 2003). Stem cells vary in their degree of potential for differentiation. Totipotent cells can form the embryo, as well as any cell line. Pluripotent cells cannot form an embryo, but can differentiate into cells of multiple different tissue cell lines. Multipotent cells can only produce a limited set of cell lines, appropriate for a given tissue environment. Unipotent cells can only generate one cell type. Thus, fetal tissue can possibly yield pluripotent stem cells and certainly generate organ-specific multipotent stem cells. Of course, the use of human fetal tissue is controversial for ethical reasons and limited (in the USA) by recent legislative restrictions. Other potential sources for stem cells exist. Multipotent stem cells have been identified within adult tissue, including brain, although not in sufficient numbers to be reasonably extracted for clinical use (Gu W 2000). In some organs, notably the bone marrow, multipotent cells have shown a capacity to "change their minds" and transdifferentiate into lineages of other organs, including neural cells (Sanchez Ramos J 2000, Woodbery D 2000). There is evidence that human umbilical cord blood cells (HUBCs) may also manifest transdifferentiation (Sanchez Ramos JR 2001). Finally, tumor cell lines occasionally yield lines of immortal, organ-specific, multipotent stem cells. An example of a tumor cell line that may prove useful in neurotransplantation is the Ntera 2/cl.D12 (NTs) human embryonic carcinomaderived cell line (Kleppner SR 1995). These cells replicate and differentiate into human neuronal cells (Trojanowaski JQ 1993). Thus, NTs have the characteristics of multipotent neural stem cells. When transplanted, these neuronal cells survive, extend processes, express neurotransmitters, form functional synapses, and integrate with the host. The final cells appear virtually indistinguishable from terminally differentiated, postmitotic neurons. The cells are capable of differentiation to express different neuronal markers characteristic of mature neurons. Their neuronal phenotype makes them a promising candidate for replacement in central nervous system disorders, as a virtually unlimited supply of pure, postmitotic, terminally differentiated human neuronal cells.

Multipotent Cell Transplants in Animal Models of Stroke

In 1998, Borlongan et al. showed that transplants of LBS-neurons could reverse the deficits caused by a stroke (Borlongan CV 1998). They used a rat model of permanent focal ischemia. At 1 month postischemia surgery, they selected all rats that showed significant behavioral deficits and randomized this group to receive transplantation either of fetal rodent striatal cells (n = 8) or human embryonic carcinoma-derived (hNT) neurons (n = 14). They had an existing set of 22 control rats that received transplants of either cerebellar cell or cell medium. They tested all animals at 1, 2, 3, and 6 months after surgery, having noted previously that ischemic animals continue to display significant deficits for >3 months postischemia. They used the passive avoidance test (the same test used to identify rats with significant deficits poststroke) and the elevated body swing test (EBST), a measure of motor asymmetry. The rats who received either striatal fetal cells or hNT neurons significantly outperformed the controls; rats receiving hNT had a significantly earlier recovery of behavioral deficits compared to those who received the striatal fetal cells. Similarly, rats who received hNT neurons recovered motor symmetry significantly faster than those receiving striatal fetal cells, while both of these groups significantly outperformed the controls.

Immunohistochemical staining done on treatment rats showed that there was survival of the grafted cells after 6 months.

Cell Transplants in Human Stroke

The transplantation of hNT neurons into the brains of humans with stroke has now undergone Phase I and Phase II trials, with promising results. The first clinical study of transplantation of the immortalized line of hNT cells into human stroke victims was conducted at the University of Pittsburgh. The goal was to demonstrate the safety and feasibility of the neuronal cell implantation procedure. The study was an openlabel trial with observer-blinded neurologic evaluation of patients with stroke who received stereotactic implants of human neuronal cells. Patients with basal ganglia infarcts and stable motor deficits were enrolled. They had to have had strokes between 6 months and 6 years prior to transplantation. The mean time since onset of the stroke was actually 27 months (range 7 to 55). Cells were delivered stereotactically via three 20-_l injections along a single trajectory through the infarct. The first four patients received 2 million cells via single-pass injections into the area of infarction. The next eight patients were randomized to receive either 2 or 6 million cells (three separate stereotactic trajectories with three injections each around the stroke). Because of concerns for cell rejection, the patients were given intravenous methylprednisolone during the procedure, followed by cyclosporine-A administration beginning 1 week before surgery and for 8 weeks following. Patients were evaluated for safety and efficacy at ten intervals over the 52 weeks following surgery. Disability was assessed using the National Institutes of Health Stroke Scale (NIHSS), European Stroke Scale (ESS), and Barthel Index (BI). Positron emission tomography using fluorodeoxyglucose (FDG-PET) and magnetic resonance imaging (MRI) scans were obtained at baseline; MRI was repeated at weeks 4 and 24, while PET was repeated at weeks 24 and 52. The goals of demonstrating safety were met, with no adverse events related to implantation. One patient developed renal insufficiency attributed to the cyclosporine-A. One patient, whose infarct involved temporal lobe cortical tissue, had a generalized seizure 6months after the surgery and was treated successfully with anticonvulsant medication. On patient had a subsequent stroke, remote from the site of neuronal transplantation, 6 months after the surgery. No malignancies, deaths, or cell-related adverse events occurred in the follow-up period. Although the study was not designed as an efficacy study, the functional outcomes suggested clinical benefit. The ESS, which had been stable between the preoperative evaluation and the day of surgery, improved in 6 of the 12 patients, remained unchanged in 3, and deteriorated in 3, compared with baseline scores. The mean improvement in ESS from baseline to week 24 was 2.9 points, achieving significance (p = 0_046). Motor improvement accounted for much of the clinical improvement in the ESS in the patients enrolled in this first study. The NIHSS seemed to improve overall in the group, without achieving significance: eight patients had improved, one was unchanged, and three deteriorated at the 24-week follow-up. The BI did not change significantly. Serial MRI scans showed no changes in the brain after the surgery when compared with baseline. The serial PET scans, however, manifested differences between the baseline and follow-up studies done 6 months later. There was an increase in $\geq$15% in the relative uptake of FDG within the transplant site, in 6 of 11 patients. This increased metabolic activity suggests the return of viable neurons to the areas of infarction. While an inflammatory response could produce such findings, there was no sign of inflammation on serial MRI. The suggestion of cell survival in the serial PET studies was corroborated by some pathological data. One of the patients, a 71-year-old man, died of a presumed myocardial infarction 27 months following the transplantation surgery. He was one of the patients who demonstrated no motor recovery. Histochemical stains of his brain demonstrated a population of neurons at the graft site. Many of these were NF protein immunoreactive, suggesting that they were nNT neurons. This was confirmed with a special single chromosome 21-specific probe (specific for hNT neurons) that detected multiple signals in nuclei within the area of the graft. Therefore, in the Phase I study, transplantation of the hNT neurons into areas of stroke was shown to be both safe and feasible. The transplant cells survived, and there was even a suggestion of clinical benefit. A Phase II dose–response trial was undertaken at two centers (University of Pittsburgh and Stanford University). Patients were randomized. The first seven of these received 5 million cells along five trajectories with five injections each (i.e., one million cells per trajectory), while another seven patients received 10 million cells, along five trajectories and with five injections each. There were four control patients. All patients received cyclosporine for 6 months as well as focused stroke rehabilitation. The primary outcome was the motor ESS at 6 months. NIHSS, ESS, and MRI were done on routine follow-up. The safety results of the Phase II trial were similar to those of Phase I, with no major medical complications of the procedure and no lasting effects due to implantation or cyclosporine administration. One patient experienced a syncopal episode, 1 month following surgery. One patient experienced a seizure 1 day after surgery. One patient, who was on aspirin and clopidogrel combination therapy, underwent surgical drainage of a chronic subdural hematoma, 1 month following transplant. Two of the four control patients experienced improvements in their motorESS scores after 6 months of physical therapy. The range of change on this scale was −0.5 to +3.5 points. Of the transplant group, 8 of the 14 improved after 6 months, and the range was −5.5 to +14.5. Overall, the transplant group had a statistically insignificant improvement in motor ESS over the control group ($p = 0\text{-}148$). However, the relatively large degree of improvement of some of the transplant patients was notable. Unexpected improvements were also noted in some of the secondary outcome measurements. For example, there seemed to be a trend toward improvement in the treatment group with respect to hand and wrist movement. Interestingly, there were significant improvements in certain neuropsychological measurements, such as visuospatial construction and retention, and nonverbal memory, in the treatment group compared with the controls. These results were recently published (Kondziolka D 2005, Stilley CS 2004).

From these first two trials, it is inferred that stereotactic cell implantation of immortalized multipotent neural stem cells, derived from a tumor cell line, is relatively safe and devoid of delayed cell-related adverse effects; the transplanted cells survive in vivo; and some patients that received cell transplants showed motor and cognitive improvements. Future trials using this cell line will have to address optimal patient selection, timing of surgery, number of cells needed, optimal implant location, and the need for immunosuppression.

Possible Mechanisms

It remains unclear exactly how hNT neuron transplants exert their effects in animal stroke models and their possible effects in humans with stroke. There is suggestive evidence that the transplanted cells do survive. It remains to be proven whether they also integrate into the existing neural network that surrounds them, although the surprising improvement in cognition that was observed in some of the transplant patients, if a There must also be other mechanisms involved. The improvements noted in the bone marrow stromal cell (Bang Oy 2005) pilot trial and in the HUBC animal models (Chen A 2001) occurred too soon to be attributable to neuronal integration. Perhaps, the transplanted cells induced a host response, such as the secretion of neurotrophic factors, which independently promoted recovery. BMSCs are known to secrete interleukins (IL)-6, IL-7, IL-8, IL-12, IL-14, IL-15, along with macrophage stimulating factor, Flt-3 ligand, and stem cell factor (Eaves CJ 1991). These cytokines have been identified as promoters of growth and survival of mouse hippocampal neuron progenitor cells (Mehler MF 1993). BMSCs also release neurotransmitters which can supplement for lost neurons after ischemia. It is therefore possible that these or other trophic factors could perhaps stimulate synaptic sprouting in damaged brain tissue.

Conclusion

Stroke is a major cause of disability, and a repair strategy needs to be developed. Cell therapies have the potential for providing a means of repairing brain tissue that has been permanently injured by stroke. There are several sources of neuronal progenitor cells that are under investigation. In animal models, it has been successfully shown that fetal cell transplants are able to survive and convey functional recovery. BMSCs and HUBCs seem to be able to transdifferentiate into neuronal cells and survive in the brains of animals with stroke. On the other hand, further research is required to determine the functional significance of this mode of transplantation. Implanted tumor-derived neuronal progenitor cells (hNT neurons) survive and convey functional improvement in animals. There is promising preliminary evidence that the same holds true for humans. Once a source of neuronal progenitor cells can be found that can consistently differentiate into viable neuronal cells and then survive within stroke-injured brain tissue, further research will then be able to refine the process. Future research would then focus on determining the ideal timing of transplantation, selection of the best size and location of the cellular implant, and possibly even optimizing the cellular environment by controlling local trophic factor concentrations. The goal is to replace lost neurons in a self-sustainable tissue milieu, and reintegrate the replacement cells into existing neural networks, in order to ultimately restore functions that have been lost.

References

Arvidsson A, Collin T, Kirik D, Kokaia Z, Lindvall O. Neuronal replacement from endogenous precursors in the adult brain after stroke. *Nat Med*. 2002;8:963–970.

Andrews PW, Damjanov I, Simon D, et al. Pluripotent embryonal carcinoma clones derived from the human teratocarcinoma cell line Tera-2. Differentiation in vivo and in vitro. *Lab Invest*. 1984;50: 147–162.

Bang OY, Lee JS, Lee PH, Lee G. Autologous mesenchymal stem cell transplantation in stroke patients. *Ann Neurol*. 2005;57:874–882.

Bliss T, Andres RH, Steinberg GK. Optimizing the success of cell transplantation therapy for stroke. *Neurobiol Dis*. 2010;37:275–283.

Bulte JW, Duncan ID, Frank JA. In vivo magnetic resonance tracking of magnetically labeled cells after transplantation. *J Cereb Blood Flow Metab*. 2002;22:899–907.

Barbosa da Fonseca LM, Gutfilen B, Rosado de Castro PH, et al. Migration and homing of bone-marrow mononuclear cells in chronic ischemic stroke after intra-arterial injection. *Exp Neurol*. 2010;221: 122–128.

Borlongan CV, Tajima Y, Trojanowski JQ, Lee VM, Sanberg PR. Transplantation of cryopreserved human embryonal carcinoma-derived neurons (NT2N cells) promotes functional recovery in ischemic rats. *Exp Neurol*. 1998;149:310–321.

Borlongan CV, Tajima Y, Trojanowski JQ, Lee VM, Sanberg PR. Cerebral ischemia and CNS transplantation: differential effects of grafted fetal rat striatal cells and human neurons derived from a clonal cell line. *Neuroreport*. 1998;9:3703–3709.

Brenneman M, Sharma S, Harting M, et al. Autologous bone marrow mononuclear cells enhance recovery after acute ischemic stroke in young and middle-aged rats. *J Cereb Blood Flow Metab*. 2010;30:140–149.

Battistella V, Freitas G, Dias V, et al. Safety of autologous bone marrow mononuclear cell transplantation in patients with nonacute ischemic stroke. *Regen Med*. 2011;6:45–52.

Bjorklund A, Steveni U. Growth of central catecholamine neurones into smooth muscle grafts in the rat mesencephalon. *Brain Res* 1971;31(1):1–20.

Borlongan CV, Tajima Y, Trojanowski JQ, Lee VM, Sanberg PR. Transplantation of cryopreserved human embryonal carcinoma-derived neurons (NT2N cells) promotes functional recovery in ischemic rats. *Exp Neurol* 1998;149(2):310–321.

Bang OY, Lee JS, Lee PH, Lee G. Autologous mesenchymal stem cell transplantation in stroke patients. *Ann Neurol* 2005;57:874–882. *Safety and Efficacy of Transplanting Neural Stem Cells* 9.

Chen J, Sanberg PR, Li Y, et al. Intravenous administration of human umbilical cord blood reduces behavioral deficits after stroke in rats. *Stroke* 2001;32(11):2682–2688.

Curtis MA, Kam M, Nannmark U, et al. Human neuroblasts migrate to the olfactory bulb via a lateral ventricular extension. Science. 2007; 315:1243–1249.

Chu K, Kim M, Jeong SW, Kim SU, Yoon BW. Human neural stem cells can migrate, differentiate, and integrate after intravenous transplantation in adult rats with transient forebrain ischemia. *Neurosci Lett*. 2003;343:129–133.

Chu K, Kim M, Park KI, et al. Human neural stem cells improve sensorimotor deficits in the adult rat brain with experimental focal ischemia. *Brain Res*. 2004;1016:145–153.

Chen J, Li Y, Wang L, et al. Therapeutic benefit of intravenous administration of bone marrow stromal cells after cerebral ischemia in rats. *Stroke*. 2001;32:1005–1011.

Chen J, Li Y, Katakowski M, et al. Intravenous bone marrow stromal cell therapy reduces apoptosis and promotes endogenous cell proliferation after stroke in female rat. *J Neurosci Res*. 2003;73:778–786.

Chen J, Zhang ZG, Li Y, et al. Intravenous administration of human bone marrow stromal cells induces angiogenesis in the ischemic boundary zone after stroke in rats. *Circ Res.* 2003;92:692–699.

Cheng X, Wang Z, Yang J, et al. Acidic fibroblast growth factor delivered intranasally induces neurogenesis and angiogenesis in rats after ischemic stroke. *Neurol Res.* 2011;33:675–680.

Dunac A, Frelin C, Popolo-Blondeau M, et al. Neurological and functional recovery in human stroke are associated with peripheral blood CD34+ cell mobilization. *J Neurol.* 2007;254:327–332.

Darsalia V, Allison SJ, Cusulin C, et al. Cell number and timing of transplantation determine survival of human neural stem cell grafts in stroke-damaged rat brain. *J Cereb Blood Flow Metab.* 2011;31: 235–242.

Eriksson PS, Perfilieva E, Bjork-Eriksson T, et al. Neurogenesis in the adult human hippocampus. *Nat Med.* 1998;4:1313–1317.

Eaves CJ, Cashman JD, et al. Mechanisms that regulate the cell cycle status of very primitive hematopoietic cells in long-term human marrow cultures: analysis of positive and negative regulators produced by stromal cells within the adherent layer. *Blood* 1991;78:110–117.

Fischer UM, Harting MT, Jimenez F, et al. Pulmonary passage is a major obstacle for intravenous stem cell delivery: the pulmonary first-pass effect. *Stem Cells Dev.* 2009;18:683–692.

Friedrich M. Intra-arterial infusion of autologous bone-marrow mononuclear cells in patients with moderate to severe middle-cerebral-artery acute ischemic stroke. *Cell Transplant.* 2012;21 Suppl 1:13–21.

Fisher M, Albers GW, Donnan G, et al. Enhancing the development and approval of acute stroke therapies: Stroke Therapy Academic Industry Roundtable. *Stroke.* 2005;36:1808–1813.

Freed CR, Greene P, Breeze RE, et al. Transplantation of embryonic dopamine neurons for severe Parkinson's disease. *N Engl J Med* 2001;344(10):710–719.

Grabowski M, Johansson BB, Brundin P. Survival of fetal neocortical grafts implanted in brain infarcts of adult rats: the influence of postlesion time and age of donor tissue. *Exp Neurol.* 1994;127:126–136.

Gu W, Brannstrom T, Wester P. Cortical neurogenesis in adult rats after reversible photothrombotic stroke. *J Cereb Blood Flow Metab* 2000;20: 1166–1173.

Giraldi-Guimaraes A, Rezende-Lima M, Bruno FP, Mendez-Otero R. Treatment with bone marrow mononuclear cells induces functional recovery and decreases neurodegeneration after sensorimotor cortical ischemia in rats. *Brain Res.* 2009;1266:108–120.

Hayashi T, Noshita N, Sugawara T, Chan PH. Temporal profile of angiogenesis and expression of related genes in the brain after ischemia. *J Cereb Blood Flow Metab.* 2003;23:166–180.

Honmou O, Houkin K, Matsunaga T, et al. Intravenous administration of auto serum-expanded autologous mesenchymal stem cells in stroke. *Brain.* 2011;134(Pt 6):1790–1807.

Jin K, Wang X, Xie L, et al. Evidence for stroke-induced neurogenesis in the human brain. *Proc Natl Acad Sci U S A.* 2006;103: 13198–13202.

Jeong SW, Chu K, Jung KH, Kim SU, Kim M, Roh JK. Human neural stem cell transplantation promotes functional recovery in rats with experimental intracerebral hemorrhage. *Stroke*. 2003;34:2258–2263.

Hicks AU, Lappalainen RS, Narkilahti S, et al. Transplantation of human embryonic stem cell-derived neural precursor cells and enriched environment after cortical stroke in rats: cell survival and functional recovery. *Eur J Neurosci*. 2009;29:562–574.

Intercollegiate Stroke Working Party. National Sentinel Stroke Clinical Audit 2010: Public Report for England, Wales and Northern Ireland. London: Royal College of Physicians 2011.

Hicks AU, MacLellan CL, Chernenko GA, Corbett D. Long-term assessment of enriched housing and subventricular zone derived cell transplantation after focal ischemia in rats. *Brain Res*. 2008;1231: 103–112.

Jiang Q, Zhang ZG, Ding GL, et al. Investigation of neural progenitor cell induced angiogenesis after embolic stroke in rat using MRI. *Neuroimage*. 2005;28:698–707.

Kleppner SR, Robinson KA, Trojanowski JQ, Lee VM. Transplanted human neurons derived from a teratocarcinoma cell line (NTera-2) mature, integrate, and survive for over 1 year in the nude mouse brain. *Comp Neurol* 1995;357(4): 618–632.

Kelly S, Bliss TM, Shah AK, et al. Transplanted human fetal neural stem cells survive, migrate, and differentiate in ischemic rat cerebral cortex. *Proc Natl Acad Sci U S A*. 2004;101:11839–11844.

Kondziolka D, Steinberg GK, Wechsler L, et al. Neurotransplantation for patients with subcortical motor stroke: a phase 2 randomized trial. *J Neurosurg*. 2005;103:38–45.

Kondziolka D, Wechsler L, Goldstein S, et al. Transplantation of cultured human neuronal cells for patients with stroke. *Neurology*. 2000;55:565–569.

Kondziolka D, Steinberg GK, Wechsler LR, et al. Neurotransplantation for patients with subcortical motor stroke: a phase 2 randomized trial. *J Neurosurg* 2005;103(1):38–45.

Kurozumi K, Nakamura K, Tamiya T, et al. Mesenchymal stem cells that produce neurotrophic factors reduce ischemic damage in the rat middle cerebral artery occlusion model. *Mol Ther*. 2005;11: 96–104.

Kleppner SR, Robinson KA, Trojanowski JQ, Lee VM. Transplanted human neurons derived from a teratocarcinoma cell line (NTera-2) mature, integrate, and survive for over 1 year in the nude mouse brain. *J Comp Neurol*. 1995;357:618–632.

Li Y, Chen J, Wang L, Lu M, Chopp M. Treatment of stroke in rat with intracarotid administration of marrow stromal cells. *Neurology*. 2001;56:1666–1672.

Li TS, Kubo M, Ueda K, et al. Identification of risk factors related to poor angiogenic potency of bone marrow cells from different patients. *Circulation*. 2009;120(Suppl 11):S255–S261.

Li Y, Chopp M, Chen J, et al. Intrastriatal transplantation of bone marrow nonhematopoietic cells improves functional recovery after stroke in adult mice. *J Cereb Blood Flow Metab*. 2000;20:1311–1319.

Llado J, Haenggeli C, Maragakis NJ, Snyder EY, Rothstein JD. Neural stem cells protect against glutamate-induced excitotoxicity and promote survival of injured motor neurons through the secretion of neurotrophic factors. *Mol Cell Neurosci*. 2004;27:322–331.

Lee ST, Chu K, Jung KH, et al. Anti-inflammatory mechanism of intravascular neural stem cell transplantation in haemorrhagic stroke. *Brain*. 2008;131:616–629.

Liu F, Yuan R, Benashski SE, McCullough LD. Changes in experimental stroke outcome across the life span. *J Cereb Blood Flow Metab*. 2009;29:792–802.

Lappalainen RS, Narkilahti S, Huhtala T, et al. The SPECT imaging shows the accumulation of neural progenitor cells into internal organs after systemic administration in middle cerebral artery occlusion rats. *Neurosci Lett*. 2008;440:246–250.

Love Z, Wang F, Dennis J, et al. Imaging of mesenchymal stem cell transplant by bioluminescence and PET. *J Nucl Med*. 2007;48: 2011–2020.

Lee JS, Hong JM, Moon GJ, et al. A long-term follow-up study of intravenous autologous mesenchymal stem cell transplantation in patients with ischemic stroke. *Stem Cells*. 2010;28:1099–1106.

McColgan P, Sharma P, Bentley P. Stem cell tracking in human trials: a meta-regression. *Stem Cell Rev*. 2011;7:1031–1040.

Meltzer CC, Kondziolka D, Villemagne VL, et al. Serial (18F) fluorodeoxyglucose positron emission tomography after human neuronal implantation for stroke. *Neurosurgery*. 2001;49:586–591; discussion 591–592.

Moniche F, Gonzalez A, Gonzalez-Marcos JR, et al. Intra-arterial bone marrow mononuclear cells in ischemic stroke: a pilot clinical trial. *Stroke*. 2012;43:2242–2244.

Mehler MF, Rozental R, Dougherty M, Spray DC, Kessler JA. Cytokine regulation of neuronal differentiation of hippocampal progenitor cells. *Nature* 1993;362:62–65.

Nelson PT, Kondziolka D, Wechsler L, et al. Clonal human (hNT) neuron grafts for stroke therapy: neuropathology in a patient 27 months after implantation. *Am J Pathol*. 2002;160:1201–1206.

Mitsios N, Gaffney J, Kumar P, Krupinski J, Kumar S, Slevin M. Pathophysiology of acute ischaemic stroke: an analysis of common signalling mechanisms and identification of new molecular targets. *Pathobiology*. 2006;73:159–175.

Nakatomi H, Kuriu T, Okabe S, et al. Regeneration of hippocampal pyramidal neurons after ischemic brain injury by recruitment of endogenous neural progenitors. Cell. 2002;110:429–441.

Olanow CW, Goetz C, Kordower JH, et al. A double-blind controlled trial of bilateral fetal nigral transplantation in Parkinson's disease. *Ann Neurol* 2003;54(3):403–414.

Pleasure SJ, Lee VM. NTera 2 cells: a human cell line which displays characteristics expected of a human committed neuronal progenitor cell. *J Neursci Res* 1993;35(6):585–602.

Preston SL, Alison M, et al. The new stem cell biology: something for everyone. *Mol Pathol* 2003;56(2):86–96.

Paczkowska E, Larysz B, Rzeuski R, et al. Human hematopoietic stem/progenitor-enriched CD34(+) cells are mobilized into peripheral blood during stress related to ischemic stroke or acute myocardial infarction. *Eur J Haematol*. 2005;75:461–467.

Roitberg B, Urbaniak K, Emborg M. Cell transplantation for Parkinson's disease. *Neurol Res* 2004;26(4):355–362.

Stilley CS, Ryan CM, et al. Changes in cognitive function after neuronal cell transplantation for basal ganglia stroke. *Neurology* 2004;35:585–602.

Sanchez-Ramos JR, Song S, Kamath SG. Expression of neural markers in human umbilical cord blood. *Exp Neurol* 2001;171:109–115.

Sanchez-Ramos J, Song S, Cardozo-Pelaex F. Adult bone marrow stromal cells differentiate into neural cells in vitro. *Exp Neurol* 2000;164:247–256.

Stilley CS, Ryan CM, et al. Changes in cognitive function after neuronal cell transplantation for basal ganglia stroke. *Neurology* 2004;35:585–602.

Sanchez-Ramos JR, Song S, Kamath SG. Expression of neural markers in human umbilical cord blood. *Exp Neurol* 2001;171:109–115.

Sanchez-Ramos J, Song S, Cardozo-Pelaex F. Adult bone marrow stromal cells differentiate into neural cells in vitro. *Exp Neurol* 2000;164:247–256.

Stem Cell Therapies as an Emerging Paradigm in Stroke participants. Stem Cell Therapies as an Emerging Paradigm in Stroke (STEPS): bridging basic and clinical science for cellular and neurogenic factor therapy in treating stroke. *Stroke*. 2009;40:510–515.

Savitz SI, Misra V, Kasam M, et al. Intravenous autologous bone marrow mononuclear cells for ischemic stroke. *Ann Neurol*. 2011;70:59–69.

Stroke Therapy Academic Industry Roundtable II (STAIR-II). Recommendations for clinical trial evaluation of acute stroke therapies. *Stroke*. 2001;32:1598–1606.

Shen LH, Li Y, Chen J, et al. Intracarotid transplantation of bone marrow stromal cells increases axon-myelin remodeling after stroke. *Neuroscience*. 2006;137:393–399.

Smith EJ, Stroemer RP, Gorenkova N, et al. Implantation site and lesion topology determine efficacy of a human neural stem cell line in a rat model of chronic stroke. *Stem Cells*. 2012;30:785–796.

Suárez-Monteagudo C, Hernández-Ramírez P, Alvarez-González L, et al. Autologous bone marrow stem cell neurotransplantation in stroke patients. An open study. *Restor Neurol Neurosci*. 2009;27:151–161.

Saporta S, Borlongan CV, Sanberg PR. Neural transplantation of human neuroteratocarcinoma (hNT) neurons into ischemic rats. A quantitative dose-response analysis of cell survival and behavioral recovery. *Neuroscience*. 1999;91:519–525.

Stroemer P, Hope A, Patel S, Pollock K, Sinden J. Development of a human neural stem cell line for use in recovery from disability after stroke. *Front Biosci*. 2008;13:2290–2292.

Stroemer P, Patel S, Hope A, et al. The neural stem cell line CTX0E03 promotes behavioral recovery and endogenous neurogenesis after experimental stroke in a dose-dependent fashion. *Neurorehabil Neural Repair*. 2009;23:895–909.

Shyu WC, Lin SZ, Chiang MF, Su CY, Li H. Intracerebral peripheral blood stem cell (CD34+) implantation induces neuroplasticity by enhancing beta1 integrin-mediated angiogenesis in chronic stroke rats. *J Neurosci*. 2006;26:3444–3453.

Shen LH, Li Y, Chen J, et al. Therapeutic benefit of bone marrow stromal cells administered 1 month after stroke. *J Cereb Blood Flow Metab*. 2007;27:6–13.

Sharma S, Yang B, Strong R, et al. Bone marrow mononuclear cells protect neurons and modulate microglia in cell culture models of ischemic stroke. *J Neurosci Res*. 2010;88:2869–2876.

Shyu WC, Lin SZ, Yang HI, et al. Functional recovery of stroke rats induced by granulocyte colony-stimulating factor–stimulated stem cells. *Circulation*. 2004;110:1847–1854.

Schäbitz WR, Kollmar R, Schwaninger M, et al. Neuroprotective effect of granulocyte colony stimulating factor after focal cerebral ischemia. *Stroke*. 2003;34:745–751.

Thomson JA, Itskovitz-Eldor J, Shapiro SS, et al. Embryonic stem cell lines derived from human blastocysts. *Science*. 1998;282: 1145–1147.

Taguchi A, Soma T, Tanaka H, et al. Administration of CD34+ cells after stroke enhances neurogenesis via angiogenesis in a mouse model. *J Clin Invest*. 2004;114:330–338.

Takahashi K, Yamanaka S. Induction of pluripotent stem cells from mouse embryonic and adult fibroblast cultures by defined factors. *Cell*. 2006;126:663–676.

Takahashi K, Tanabe K, Ohruki M, et al. Induction of pluripotent stem cells from adult human fibroblasts by defined factors. *Cell*. 2007; 131:861–872.

Tissue plasminogen activator for acute ischemic stroke. The National Institute of Neurological Disorders and Stroke rt-PA Stroke Study Group. *N Engl J Med* 1995;333(24):1581–1587.

Trojanowski JQ, Mantione JR, Lee JH, et al. Neurons derived from a human teratocarcinoma cell line establish molecular and structural polarity following transplantation into the rodent brain. *Exp Neurol* 1993;122(2):283–294.

Trojanowski JQ, Mantione JR, Lee JH, et al. Neurons derived from a human teratocarcinoma cell line establish molecular and structural polarity following transplantation into the rodent brain. *Exp Neurol* 1993;122(2):283–294.

Vendrame M, Gemma C, de Mesquita D, et al. Anti-inflammatory effects of human cord blood cells in a rat model of stroke. *Stem Cells Dev*. 2005;14:595–604.

Weissman IL, Anderson DJ, Gage F. Stem and progenitor cells:origins, phenotypes, lineage commitments, and transdifferentiations. *Annu Rev Cell Dev Biol*. 2001;17:387–403.

Wachs FP, Couillard-Despres S, Engelhardt M, et al. High efficacy of clonal growth and expansion of adult neural stem cells. *Lab Invest*. 2003;83:949–962.

Woodbury D, Schwarz EJ, Prockop DJ, Black IB. Adult rat and human bone marrow stromal cells differentiate into neurons. *J Neursci Res* 2000;61:364–370.

Xiao J, Nan Z, Motooka Y, Low WC. Transplantation of a novel cell line population of umbilical cord blood stem cells ameliorates neurological deficits associated with ischemic brain injury. *Stem Cells Dev*. 2005;14:722–733.

Yu J, Vodyanik MA, Smuge-Otto K, et al. Induced pluripotent stem cell lines derived from human somatic cells. *Science*. 2007;318: 1917–1920

Zhang ZG, Jiang Q, Zhang R, et al. Magnetic resonance imaging and neurosphere therapy of stroke in rat. *Ann Neurol*. 2003;53: 259–263.

Summary

Strokes are a leading cause of brain injury that strike approximately 800,000 people per year in the US alone, killing about 150,000 meaning one death in every four minutes. According to World Health Organization, 15 million people suffer strokes worldwide each year and out of these, 5 million die and another 5 million are permanently disabled. Despite advances in stroke research during last decade, current strokes remain a vexing public health problem.

The current therapeutic strategies for strokes have been largely unsuccessful. One possible explanation is that research and pharmacological management have focused on very early events in brain ischemia. New research has shown that brain ischemia and trauma elicit strong inflammatory reactions driven by both external and brain cells. The recognition of inflammation as a fundamental response to brain ischemia provides novel opportunities for new anti-inflammatory therapies. Cerebral ischemia results in a number of hemodynamic, biochemical, and neurophysiologic alterations. A series of complex acute, subacute and chronic events occur after the incidence of stroke and reperfusion. Ischemic injury involves energy failure, loss of cell ion homeostasis, acidosis, increased intracellular calcium excitotoxicity, free radical-mediated toxicity, and pathological permeability of the blood-brain barrier (BBB). Free radicals, specifically reactive oxygen species (ROS) that are generated soon after ischemia, as well as in later stages of ischemic reperfusion (e.g., by inflammatory cells), are the fundamental mediators of reperfusion injury. Two important pathophysiological mechanisms involved during ischemic stroke are oxidative stress and inflammation. Brain tissue is not well equipped with antioxidant defenses, so reactive oxygen species and other free radicals/oxidants, released by inflammatory cells, threaten tissue viability in the vicinity of the ischemic core. This book will discuss the molecular aspects of oxidative stress and inflammation in ischemic strokes and some potential therapeutic strategies that target neuroinflammation and the innate immune system. Although for many years the CNS was considered an immune-privileged organ, it is now well accepted that the immune and the nervous systems are engaged in bi-directional crosstalk. Moreover, mounting data suggests that in the brain, as in peripheral organs, inflammatory cells participate in tissue remodeling after injury. Microglial cells are the resident macrophages of the brain and play a critical role as resident immunocompetent and phagocytic cells in the CNS. Currently, little is known about endogenous counterregulatory immune mechanisms. However, recent studies showing that regulatory T cells are major cerebroprotective immunomodulators after a stroke suggest that targeting the endogenous adaptive immune response may offer novel promising neuroprotectant therapies.

Even with the onset of the 21st century, there is still no effective therapy for strokes beyond a limited group of patients who are treated with thrombolytics, which have significant adverse effects. This situation prevails despite intense research efforts and numerous clinical trials that have attempted to develop drugs to reduce morbidity and mortality from strokes. So far, drug development efforts have targeted modulators of ion channels ($Ca^{2+}$and Na^{+}), scavengers of oxygen radicals, and antagonists of excitotoxic neurotransmitters (primarily glutamate and glycine receptors).

However, clinical trials with modulators of these targets have failed so far because of their lack of efficacy, adverse effects, or other developmental difficulties. Debates on the reasons for this grim reality have sprung up in recent meetings, with finger-pointing about major possible causes of failure including incorrect animal models, misidentified mechanisms of action, poor clinical designs, inadequate timing of treatment, and other variables. An acute ischemic stroke is treatable, and our ability to treat patients with an ischemic stroke continues to improve. With the recent publications on stroke diagnostics and treatment, important changes in stroke patient management will surely occur, and most of the latest publications will be reflected in this book. The most important advances have been the widening of the time window for both intravenous thrombolysis as well as endovascular arterial recanalization treatments. This change in the expansion of the time window has major implications because it could dramatically increase the number of potential patients for treatment. Further expansion of the time window is possible with the likelihood that imaging will provide the necessary information for identifying suitable, individual patients. The basic imaging approaches to acute ischemic stroke patients have evolved slightly in last few years.

Despite tremendous progress in understanding the pathophysiology of a stroke, translation of this knowledge into effective therapies has largely failed, with the exception of thrombolysis, which only benefits a small proportion of patients. Systemic and local immune responses have important roles in causing stroke and are implicated in the primary and secondary progression of ischaemic lesions, as well as in repair, recovery, and overall outcome after a stroke. However, potential therapeutic targets in the immune system and inflammatory responses have not been well characterised. The development of novel and effective therapeutic strategies for strokes will require further investigation of these pathways in terms of their temporal profile (before, during, and after stroke) and risk-to-benefit therapeutic ratio of modulating them.

We postulate that a better understanding of the interactions between the immune system and the CNS will foster the development of innovative therapeutic strategies for stroke patients. Therefore, the latest updates discussed in this book on the cellular and humoral aspects of immune and inflammatory reactions in strokes will increase our understanding about the roles that infections and immune reactions play in the brain milieu, which may have an impact on the treatment of neuroinjuries and ancillary brain diseases.

Index

A

B

C

D

E

F

G

H

T

U

V